Bernd Spiessl

Internal Fixation of the Mandible

A Manual of AO/ASIF Principles

With a Contribution by Berton Rahn

Translator Terry C. Telger

With 397 Figures in 645 Separate Illustrations

Springer-Verlag Berlin Heidelberg New York
London Paris Tokyo

Authors

Bernd Spiessl, M. D., D. D. S.
Professor Emeritus of Maxillofacial Surgery,
University of Basel. Formerly Chief of Clinic
for Plastic and Reconstructive Surgery,
Department of Surgery, University of Basel.
CH-4031 Basel (Kantonsspital)
Formerly Chief of Maxillofacial Surgery,
Department of Surgery, Kantonsspital Aarau

Berton A. Rahn, M. D., D. D. S.
Assistant Director of
Laboratory of Experimental Surgery
Swiss Research Institute
CH-7270 Davos

Translator
Terry C. Telger
6112 Waco Way, Ft. Worth, TX 76133, USA

Title of the German Edition
Osteosynthese des Unterkiefers
ISBN 3-540-17511-3 Springer-Verlag Berlin
Heidelberg New York London Paris Tokyo

ISBN 3-540-16282-8 Springer-Verlag Berlin Heidelberg New York
ISBN 0-387-16282-8 Springer-Verlag New York Berlin Heidelberg

Library of Congress Cataloging-in-Publication Data
Spiessl, Bernd. [Osteosynthese des Unterkiefers. English] Internal fixation of the mandible : a manual of AO/ASIF principles / Bernd Spiessl ; translator, Terry C. Telger. p. cm.
Translation of: Osteosynthese des Unterkiefers. Bibliography: p. Includes index.
ISBN 0-387-16282-8
1. Mandible – Fractures – Treatment. 2. Internal fixation in fractures. I. Title. RD526.S6513
1989 617'.156 – dc19 88-21839 CIP

Typesetting, printing and bookbinding: Appl, Wemding
2124/3145-543210 – Printed on acid-free paper

Dedicated to my colleagues

Preface

The rigid internal fixation of mandibular fractures has become a widely accepted practice among European surgeons. The caution or even outright rejection voiced at a congress of the German Society of Maxillofacial Surgeons held in the late 1970s is no longer prevalent. Through a process of critical review and implementation, rigid internal fixation has become an established treatment modality at numerous centers, especially in Switzerland, the Federal Republic of Germany, and the Netherlands.

By comparison, the method has received very little attention in North America and the Anglo-Saxon countries. By and large, surgeons in these countries continue to treat mandibular fractures by intermaxillary fixation, possibly supplemented by the use of interosseous wires. Many recent editions of surgical texts confirm this.

Lately, however, there appears to be a surge of interest in methods of functionally stable internal fixation, especially in the United States of America, and AO/ASIF instruction courses are increasingly in demand. This book is intended to aid course participants in their lessons and practical exercises and also to guide the clinical practitioner in the application of AO/ASIF principles.

Basel, September 1988 B. SPIESSL

Acknowledgments

I have received help from many sources. The colleagues of the past 20 years who have contributed to the case material upon which this manual is based are too numerous to credit by name.

I thank my secretary, Mrs. Helga Reichel, for her flawless typing of the manuscript. As in earlier publications, she helped to make this book possible through her technical expertise, accuracy, and perseverance.

Dr. Stephan Hauk was of great assistance in selecting the case presentations and preparing preliminary sketches of X-ray findings. Special thanks are due to Dr. Alan Schwimmer, D.D.S., Beth Israel Medical Center, New York, NY, USA, who proofread the English translation.

I am also grateful to Mr. Julius Pupp, illustrator at Springer-Verlag, for his excellent work in depicting radiographic findings and surgical techniques. Although the field was new to him, he approached it with great interest and offered valuable suggestions on how to present the material most effectively.

I express my sincere thanks to Springer-Verlag for the final editing of the text and illustrations and for their customary excellence in the organization, design, and production of this volume.

Basel, September 1988 B. SPIESSL

Table of Contents

Part II: Internal Fixation of Fresh Fractures

Part III: Reconstructive Surgery

List of Abbreviations

ASIF	AO Study Group for Internal Fixation
AO	Arbeitsgemeinschaft für Osteosynthesefragen
DCP	Dynamic compression plate
EDCP	Eccentric dynamic compression plate
IMF	Intermaxillary fixation
OPG	Orthopantomograph
Reco plate	Reconstruction plate
	Symbol for lag screw

Introduction

Internal fixation continues to be a subject of controversy among maxillofacial surgeons. While the opponents of operative fixation have become less vehement in recent years, there continues to be diversity of opinion on fundamental issues. This is due largely to the fact that intermaxillary fixation is a simple and classic concept and is not associated with complications that might be ascribed to the direct actions of the therapist.

Rigid internal fixation, on the other hand, is more demanding technically and in the type of instrumentation that is required. In careless or inexperienced hands, the method will invariably lead to complications for which the surgeon can be held accountable. The increasing popularity of internal fixation, then, relates less to its convenience for the therapist than to its potential benefit for the patient: the ability to move the jaw, without pain, immediately after treatment. Other significant advantages are the ability to eat normally, better access for intensive care in victims of multiple trauma a reduced risk of infection, and fewer late sequelae.

The key *therapeutic principle* in this type of fixation is *stability*. Stability is the product of a perfect anatomic reduction and interfragmental compression. Achieving it requires the selection of an optimum treatment method, experience in bone surgery, and a sound grasp of biomechanics. Neglecting these requirements in favor of a "do it yourself" approach will inevitably lead to failures that are erroneously ascribed to the method itself.

The standard for judging the quality of any treatment modality is its reproducibility. To be acceptable, a method should have a success rate of at least 90%. It was this quest for quality that led, in 1958, to the founding of the AO Study Group for Internal Fixation (AO/ASIF). The function of the group is to investigate questions that are of topical interest in modern bone surgery.

Numerous treatment centers in Switzerland and the AO International, headquartered in Bern, are responsible for the acquisition and exchange of experience with the "AO method." Periodic AO/ASIF conferences are held to present and discuss the results of hospital-wide and multicenter studies. Basic research is conducted at the Laboratory for Experimental Surgery in Davos and at the M.E. Müller Institute for Biomechanics in Bern.

The *goal* of internal fixation is *early mobilization* of the affected part. Thus, the technical and biologic criteria for selecting the treatment method are absolute stability and primary bone healing. Both require a departure from traditional concepts of bone surgery. The plausibility of the concepts presented in this text is based not only on clinical experience and scientific research, but also on a new type of *instrumentation*. The AO/ASIF has formed a large *technical committee* whose task is to ensure that a high standard of quality is maintained in the instruments and implants that are manufactured for use by surgeons who practise AO/ASIF techniques. Every instrument must satisfy technical, biologic, and metallurgical requirements that are appropriate for its intended use. Particular subcommittees are designated to deal with specific questions of instrument development. The Subcommittee for Maxillofacial Surgery has overseen the development of complete sets of instruments and implants including the standard instrument set, the mandibular set, and the special set for sagittal split osteotomies.

Right from the founding of the AO/ASIF, it was clear that specialized courses of instruction would be needed to guide surgeons in the proper handling and use of the instrument system. The first of these courses was held in Davos, Switzerland, in 1960. To date more than 40 such courses have been held there and have been attended by participants from 60 countries.

The AO/ASIF does not espouse eccentric viewpoints but strives to be wholly pragmatic in its orientation. Thousands of operative cases are systematically documented, and the data are stored in a computer at the Documentation Center in Bern. Data on mandibular fractures also may be stored and evaluated at the Center free of charge. At present the files include more than 800 internal fixations of the mandible that have been performed in Basel (see statistical analyses by Eschmann 1974; von Euw 1982; Bornand 1984; Philps 1987). This type of documentation permits a quality control process that goes beyond just instrumentation to therapeutic results. The experience derived from these cases forms an important basis for the principles of functionally stable internal fixation that are presented in this text.

These principles are detailed in Part 1, which addresses the essential aspects of stability, biomechanics, and operating technique.

Part 2 is a guide to the practical application of the principles. Organized by fracture type, and with the focus on individual case reports, this part of the text should be a valuable aid to patient selection and treatment planning. Details on the surgical anatomy of approaches will be of equal value to the practitioner.

Part 3 demonstrates the expanding range of indications for functionally stable internal fixations of the mandible. Three major areas are discussed: the operative treatment of nonunions, the primary bridging of defects created by mandibular resections, and fragment fixation and condylar replacement in orthopedic procedures.

Part I

Basic Principles

1 Goals of the AO/ASIF Technique

Analogous to the goals stated in the original *Manual of Internal Fixation* (Müller et al. 1969), modern bone surgery of the mandible aims at a *rapid recovery of form and function*. Four basic conditions must be met in order to accomplish this goal:

1) anatomic reduction of the bone fragments;
2) functionally stable fixation of the fragments;
3) preserving the blood supply to the fragments by atraumatic operating technique;
4) early, active, pain-free mobilization.

The knowledge and experience needed to satisfy these requirements cannot be improvised, nor can they be acquired without appropriate theoretical and practical training.

The *first* requirement, an accurate *anatomic reduction*, implies that the *occlusal* and *basal* reduction are of equal importance. For successful internal fixation, it is necessary to secure the occlusal reduction preoperatively by means of Ernst ligatures (see p. 61) or a partial or full splint. The choice depends on which device will permit the surest handling of the fragments during the internal fixation, and facilitate the reduction while preventing displacement.

The *second* requirement, *stability*, is a major determinant of the quality of the fixation. It requires a sound understanding of the concept of stability and a disciplined approach to the planning and conduct of the internal fixation.

The *third* requirement is equally important, since *blood flow* and stability are the elemental factors that dictate the course of healing. Preserving the *blood supply* to the bone fragments and soft tissues by using an atraumatic surgical technique is an essential preventive measure against poor healing and infection. The same imperative applies to internal fixations of the facial skeleton.There is no reliable evidence to support the notion that improved blood flow to the head and neck region will necessarily protect against disturbances of wound healing. However, it is certain that the fracture-producing trauma disrupts the local blood flow to the mandible, the degree of the disturbance varying with the extent of the injury. Thus, the need to limit the denudation of bone is no less a basic rule for open reduction and fixation of the mandible than it is for internal fixations of the extremities. This is a major reason why we consider the principle of exclusive, intraoral internal fixation to be unacceptable. It is inconsistent with the search for the most atraumatic means of handling the soft tissues (see p. 30ff.).

The *fourth* requirement aims at avoiding fracture disease through *early mobilization*. "Fracture disease" refers to the changes in bone and soft tissue that occur as a result of postfracture neurovascular disturbances. Although late sequelae of this type are not characteristic of mandibular injuries, the principle of early mobilization carries major therapeutic benefits. The capacity for immediate, pain-free, oral opening is so critically important for posttraumatic regeneration that it greatly outweighs the advantages of conservative therapy.

The reduced morbidity that comes with early mobilization offers the most striking benefits for trauma patients in shock, patients with multiple injuries, and tumor patients. It is manifested by:

1) avoidance of tracheotomy, which would otherwise be necessary in patients undergoing certain tumor operations and in patients with severe maxillofacial injuries
2) avoidance of pulmonary complications due to impaired oropharyngeal clearance;
3) normal food intake, which shortens the catabolic phase;
4) the ability to speak and interact socially.

Through research, teaching and clinical experience, and with emphasis on the basic requirements stated above, the AO/ASIF has succeeded in developing universally valid principles of operative fracture treatment. Our task now is to apply these principles to the surgery of the mandibular motor apparatus.

2 The Stability Principle

Early mobilization relies on the intrinsically rigid fixation of the bone fragments. There is another fact that compels one to recognize the importance of stability: Experience demonstrates that postfracture osteitis, osteomyelitis, and nonunion correlate rather well with instability. The alternatives, then, are either to follow the stability principle consistently, or disregard it in favor of traditional conservative methods such as wire sutures, minimal internal fixation, or traditional pin fixation.

2.1 Instability and Its Consequences

A proper balance of function and stability is essential to a successful internal fixation. The correctness of this statement is underscored by the complications that consistently develop when gross instability is present. One example is the result of three unstable fixation methods that were applied in the same patient (Fig. 1 a). In this case the mandibular fracture was managed initially by interosseous wiring and intermaxillary fixation. When osteitis developed six weeks later (Fig. 1 b), pin fixation was added. Six months later the patient was hospitalized with osteomyelitis and a sequestrum in the fracture line.

Another case illustrates the results of an unstable plate fixation of a

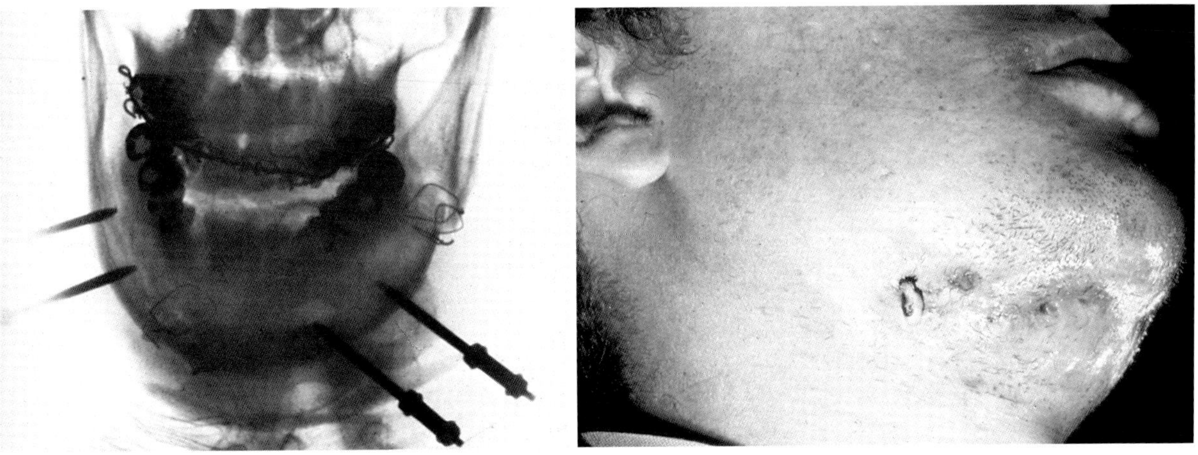

a b

Fig. 1. **a** Applied therapeutic principles: 1) intermaxillary fixation, 2) interosseous wiring, 3) external skeletal fixation. **b** Fistula associated with fracture-line osteomyelitis mandibular angle fracture that occurred following extraction of a third molar in the line of fracture (Fig. 2 a). Instability in this case was caused by a loose screw that had been driven into the alveolus of the extracted tooth. The lack of bony substance in that area caused the screw to strip its hole when tightened.

The loose screw then initiated a sequence of events in which other screws became loose. Early infection ensued, and the fracture went on to nonunion (Fig. 2 b). The fixation was revised using a tension band and stabilization plate (Fig. 2 c), and the nonunion healed without sequelae (Fig. 2 d).

Finally, the link between instability and infection is demonstrated by a third case in which the wrong plate was selected for the fixation of a comminuted fracture. Because the plate was too short and contained too few holes, the first screw in the right half of the plate had to be driven into the area of comminution (Fig. 3 a), which was unable to hold the screw securely. A contoured reconstruction plate should have been used, enabling the placement of at least three screws in each main fragment. This is the minimum number of screws needed to ensure adequate strength. As initially treated, only one screw in the right half of the plate was anchored securely in bone, and excessive tensile loading caused it to loosen.The result was osteomyelitis with sequestration (Fig. 3 b). The infection resolved with several weeks' of intermaxillary fixation, culminating in a nonunion (Fig. 3 c). This was managed by revision with internal fixation and bone grafting. Under the protection of the stable reconstruction plate (Fig. 3 d), the bone graft healed and the nonunion consolidated without intermaxillary fixation (Fig. 3 e).

The following lessons on the *primary importance of avoiding instability* may be drawn from the examples above:

1) If the bone fragments are unstable, any type of metallic foreign body will promote resorption and infection.
2) When the fragments are adequately immobilized by stable internal fixation, a bone graft will heal despite previous infection, and the fracture will become consolidated.

It is known from research and clinical experience that instability can be prevented, but first it is necessary to understand the concept of stability. To make the role of stability in operative fracture treatment as clear as possible, we add the word "absolute." "*Absolute stability*" is a clinical concept. It would be more correct to say "relative stability," which exists in the present dynamic system when pressure variations remain within specified limits in response to the action of an external force on the plate-bone system, and a state of equilibrium is restored when the force is removed. However, because a system is often called "relatively stable" in clinical parlance when in fact it is unstable (e.g., an interosseous wire suture), we prefer the term "absolute stability" when referring to a condition in which true stability has been achieved. It is clear, of course, that there is no such thing as an "absolute" stability covering all the parameters in a dynamic system for an indefinite period of time. That is why the term "biostable" is occasionally used, in acknowledgment of the fact that the quality of the stability has a critical bearing on the biology of fracture union.

Nevertheless, "absolute" is a much more appropriate concept for clinical practice. It conveys the sense of "extreme" or "maximum." In terms of

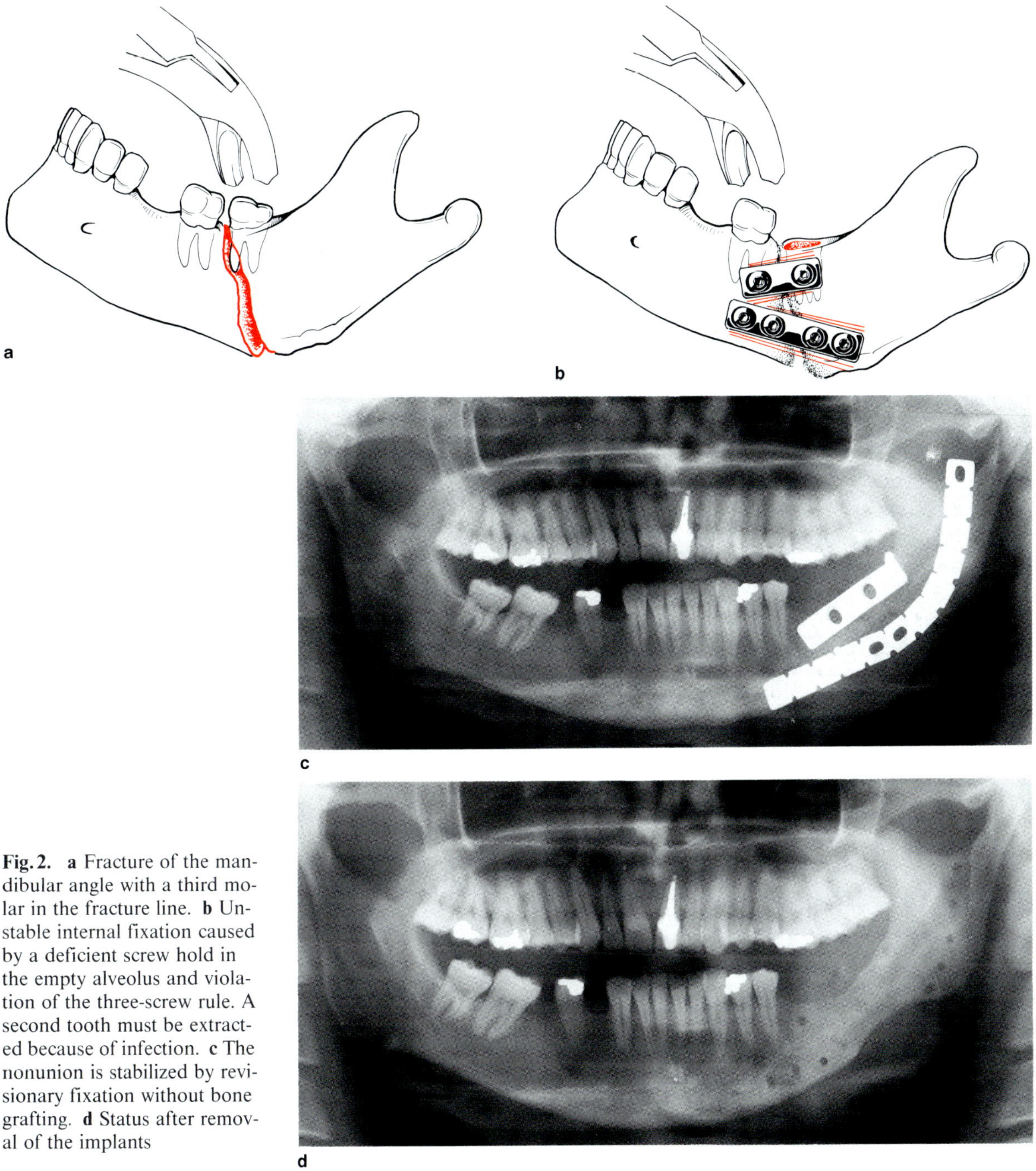

Fig. 2. **a** Fracture of the mandibular angle with a third molar in the fracture line. **b** Unstable internal fixation caused by a deficient screw hold in the empty alveolus and violation of the three-screw rule. A second tooth must be extracted because of infection. **c** The nonunion is stabilized by revisionary fixation without bone grafting. **d** Status after removal of the implants

Fig. 3. **a** Unstable internal fixation caused by a deficient screw hold in an area of comminution. **b** Multiple sequestra in association with a preangular fracture (see p. 196). The proximal plate length is insufficient in relation to the lever arm of the distal fragment. **c** Operation disclosed a nonunion with fibrous entrapment of the nerve. **d** Reconstruction of the mandible by autologous bone grafting around the nerve, supported with a reconstruction plate. **e** Status after implant removal

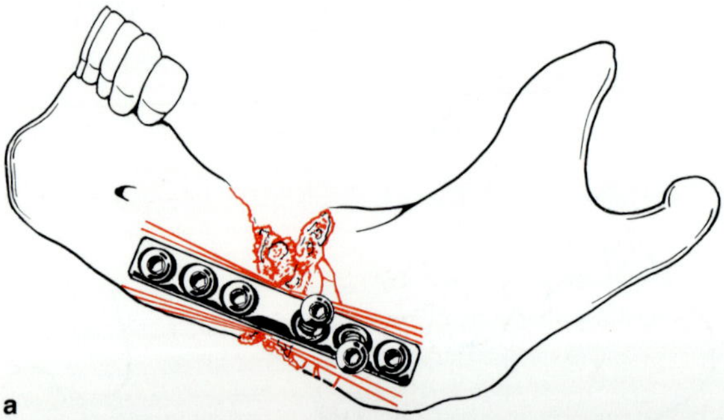

a

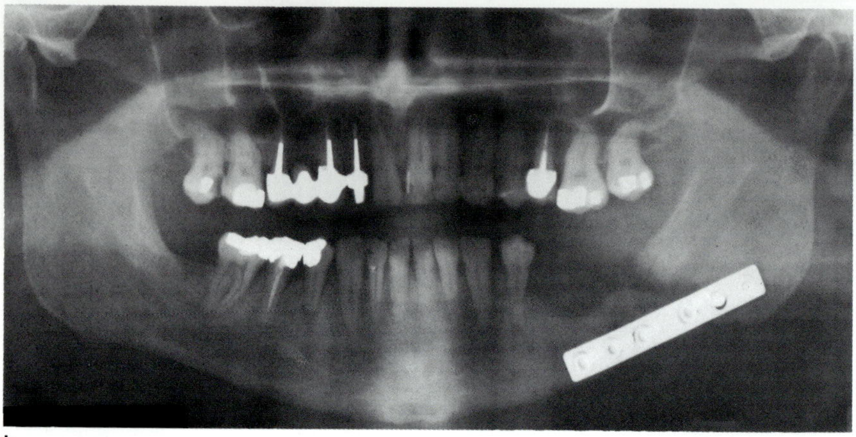

b

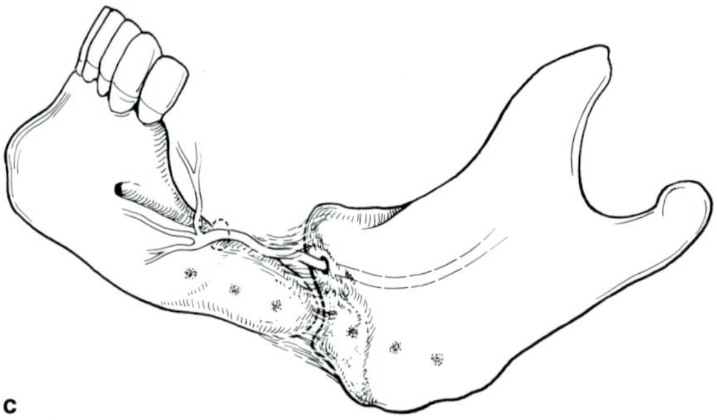

c

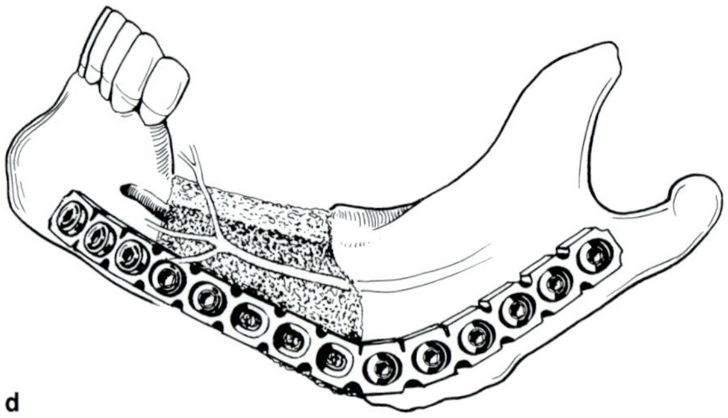

d

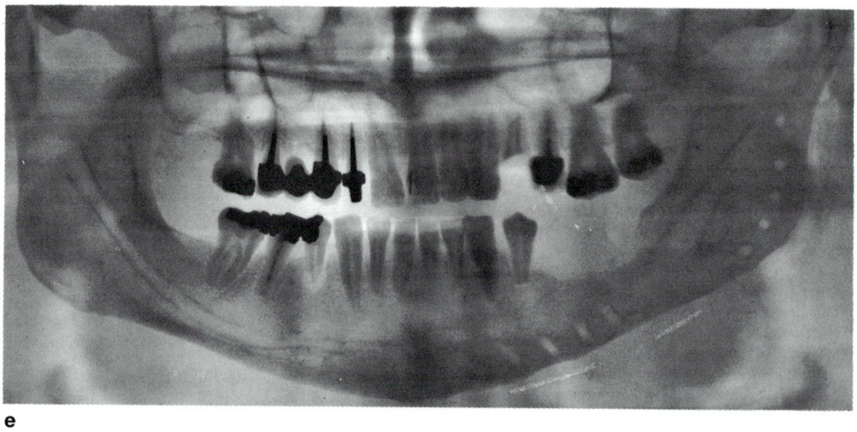

e

technique, it implies rigorousness and consistency. The opposite of this is compromise. The tendency toward compromise is great when problems arise intraoperatively that either cannot be solved or can be managed only with specialized experience.

This differs from the "a priori" compromise in which, from the outset, a minimal solution is chosen for a problem of methodology. This may relate to a difficult surgical approach, a technically complex and time-consuming freehand dental splinting procedure for a complicated fracture, or the application of a Reco plate to a segmental fracture. The a priori compromise is exemplified by minimal internal fixation, characterized by use of the intraoral approach, the Ivy splint, and mini plates.

Internal fixation *without compromise*, based on the principle of *absolute stability*, continues to be our guiding policy for the operative treatment of fractures.

2.2 Experimental Investigations of Stability and Instability

What is meant, then, by absolute stability? We define it as the absence of relative motion between the implant and bone and also between the bone ends. This is illustrated by the classic animal experiment performed by Perren et al. (1975). A compression plate was attached to the intact tibia of a live sheep. One end of the plate was fixed to the bone with two screws placed so that a compressive force was generated between them; the other end was left free (Fig. 4 a). When intermittent weight is placed on the tibia, a measurable relative motion takes place between the free end of the plate and the surface of the bone (shift of the arrowheads in Fig. 4 b). *Relative motion is the reversible displacement of a more rigid implant in relation to the less rigid bone due to elastic deformation of the bone in response to an alternating load.*

This relative motion can be prevented by anchoring the free end of the plate with a single screw that is inserted under tension. This technique is known as "prestressing" or "preloading" the screw (Fig. 5 a). The level of the primary stress can be measured by fitting the plate with strain gauges. In this way it can be demonstrated that the elimination of relative motion is dependent on *one* condition: *The primary compressive stress exerted by the single screw must be greater than the functional load on the extremity.* This primary stress diminishes when the bone comes under an axial load acting in the same direction, but it retains a positive value. That is, the pressure of the screw in the bone does not pass through the zero-load point, which would indicate cycling between tension and compression (Fig. 5 b).

This type of measurement provides a visible and objective means of confirming "absolute stability." The absence of movement between the plate, the bone, and the single screw enables new bone to form along the surface of the screw, with no intervening fibrous tissue (Fig. 6).

However, if the single screw is inserted without prestressing (Fig. 7 a), intermittent loading produces a continual cycling between tension and compression. The strain gauge registers this as a deflection past the zero point on the scale (Fig. 7 b). This indicates that the screw is not stable, and that relative motion is taking place between the bone and implant. The ini-

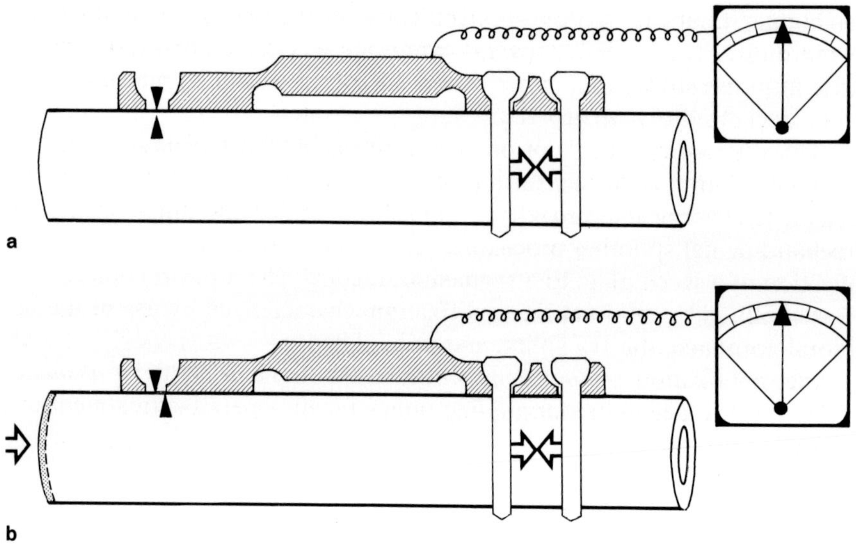

Fig. 4. **a** A strain-gauge-instrumented dynamic compression plate is fixed to the proximal tibia of a live sheep with two screws prestressed relative to each other. **b** Intermittent loading during gait causes shortening of the relatively elastic bone. *Relative motion* is measured between the free end of the plate and the bone

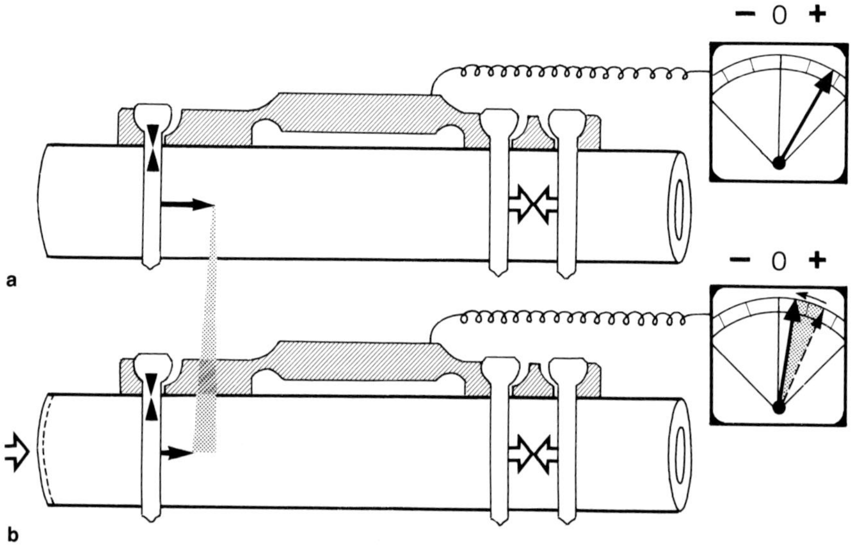

Fig. 5. **a** The free end of the plate is fixed to the bone with a screw inserted under tension. The tensile force measured on the plate with the strain gauges corresponds to the pressure of the screw in the bone (= "primary stress" or "prestress"). **b** Under the same conditions as in Fig. 5a, relative motion is no longer measurable under axial loading (see *arrows* in the area of the prestressed screw). The pressure of the screw diminishes under the load, but the indicator does not reach the zero point on the scale, so deleterious "load cycling" does not occur

tial micromovements incite resorption of the adjacent bone and connective tissue formation (Fig. 8 a), a process known as "*motion-induced osteolysis*." The resorbed bone is replaced by fibrous and granulation tissue, which leads to further loosening of the screw. In the best instance an irritation callus may form (Fig. 8 b), depending on the extent of the micromovements and the integrity of the blood supply.

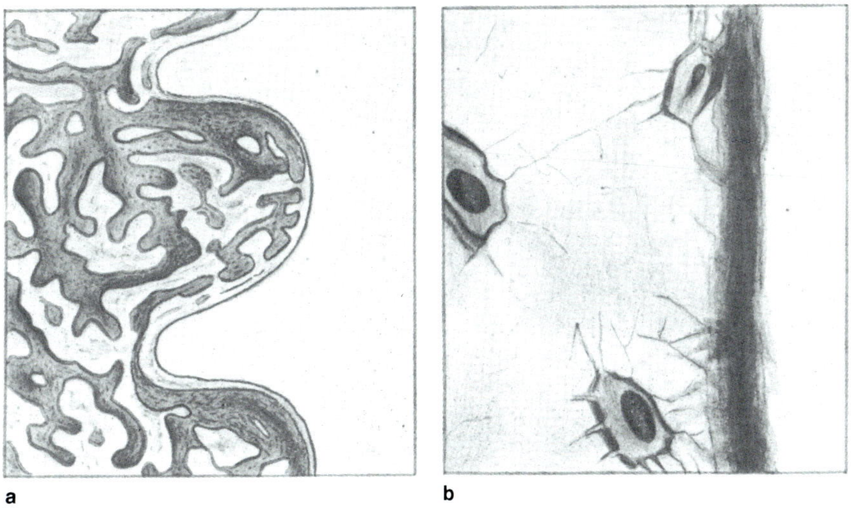

Fig. 6. **a** Interfacial area of an ASIF cortex screw inserted into bone. New bone has grown in apposition to the screw threads. Only a thin bony lamella separates the hematopoietic tissue from the metal. There is no evidence of resorption or marrow fibrosis. The screw was in place for two months. **b** We observe living osteocytes in lacunae in close proximity to the metal. Their canaliculi extend to the screw surface. There is not evidence of resorption. The screw was in place for nine months. (From Müller et al. 1977)

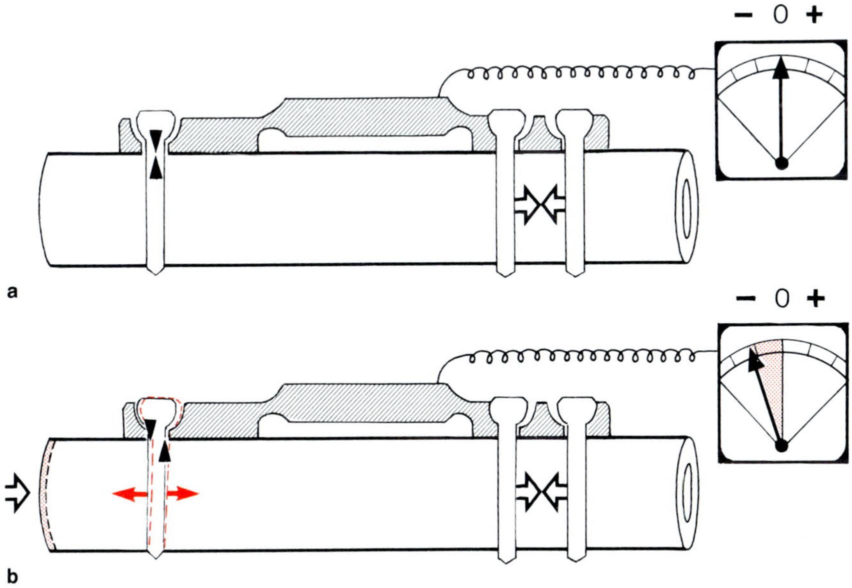

Fig. 7. **a** The plate end has been anchored to the bone with a *non-prestressed* screw. **b** Intermittent axial loading under these conditions produces relative motion between the plate and bone. The indicator dips below the zero point on the scale (= load cycling)

On the whole, the experiment clearly demonstrates the differences between stability and instability. This brings us to an elemental law of the biomechanics of internal fixation:

Relative motion will not occur at the metal-bone interface as long as the preload is greater than the functional load.[1] *If this condition is met, a state of absolute stability exists.*

The effects of instability are easily seen on roentgenograms (Fig. 9 a). On the *right* side of the figure, bone resorption is evident grossly and histologically (Fig. 9 b) about the screw that was inserted without prestressing. The screws on the *left* side were prestressed with respect to each other. There is no evidence of bone resorption around the screws, and microscopic examination shows no intervening fibrous tissue (Fig. 9 c). This is con-

[1] The preload represents a static force, the functional load a dynamic force.

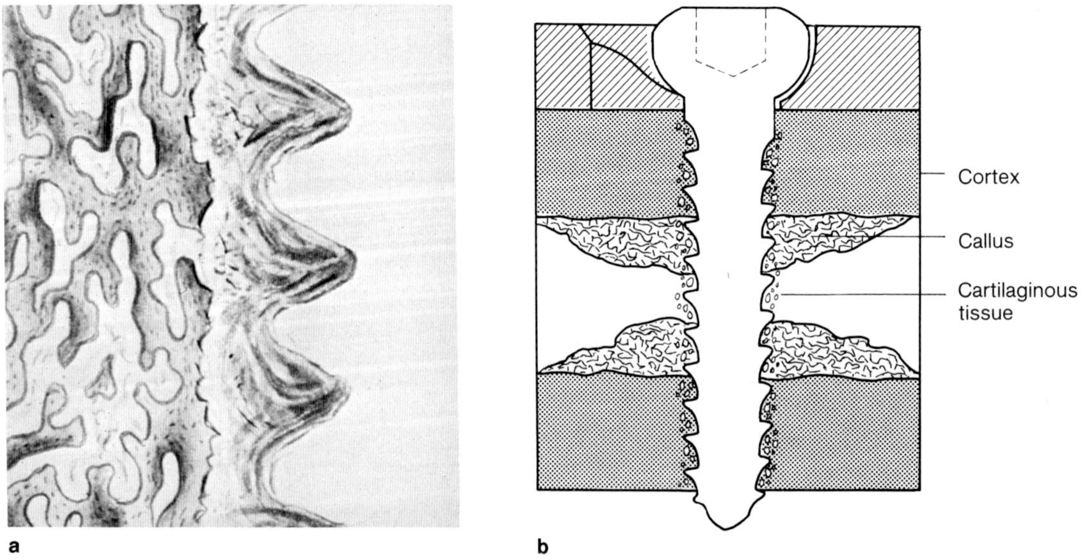

Fig. 8. **a** Interfacial area of a conventional self-tapping bone screw driven into an untapped pilot hole. Three months after screw insertion, the damaged bone has been replaced by a fibrous layer that does not afford a secure hold. (From Müller et al. 1969). **b** Tissue formation at the metal-bone interface in the presence of instability: granulation tissue, callus (depends on degree of instability), and cartilaginous tissue

sistent with the clinical observation that resorption on X-rays signifies an unstable internal fixation, since osteolysis also occurs at the fracture interface.

Summary: Bone resorption and reactive fibrous tissue growth are characteristic biologic processes that accompany instability. There is an associated danger of infection and nonunion, the risk of infection varying in proportion to the quantity or size of the material implanted.

On the other hand, intervening tissue does not form when the fragments are absolutely stable, and direct bony union of the fracture can occur. In this case the implant material per se does not pose a danger of infection.

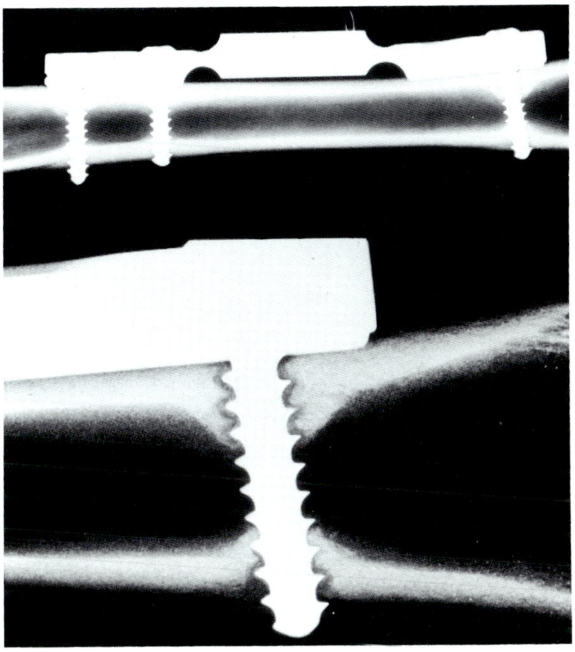

a

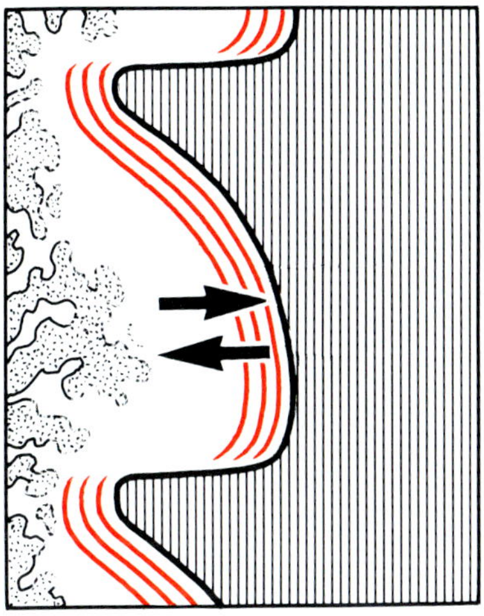

b

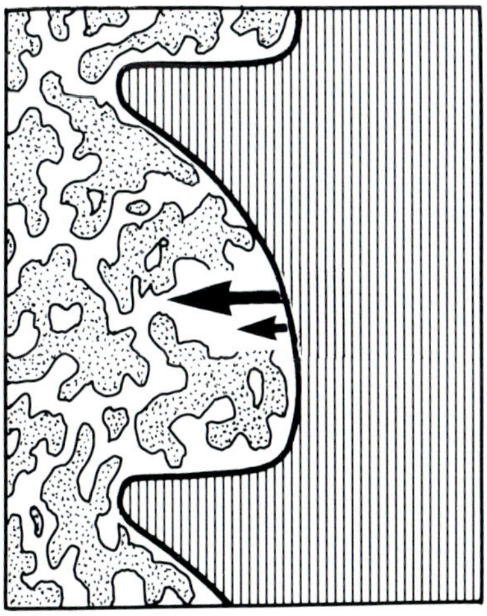

c

Fig. 9. **a** Radiographic appearance of osseous changes associated with experimentally produced stability and instability. The two screws in the left side of the plate were prestressed relative to each other at insertion; the screw on the right was inserted without prestressing. The interfacial zones on the left show no evidence of bony changes. On the right we find bone resorption all along the screw as well as callus formation; both are radiographic criteria of instability (from Müller et al. 1977). **b** Histologic appearance of a resorption zone (granulation tissue) along the surface of the unstable screw. The equal-size *arrows* pointing in opposite directions indicate that the static force of the screw is *not* greater than the functional forces under alternating loads. The resultant load cycling leads to secondary loosening of the implant. **c** In the prestressed screw, histologic examination shows direct contact between the implant and bone with no intervening tissue. The larger *arrow* indicates that the static force of this screw is greater than the functional forces under alternating loads (= no load cycling)

2.3 Significance of the Stability Principle

Absolute stability, then, is an ideal therapeutic principle. This principle has specific *biologic* and *clinical* significance in bone surgery. Its biologic aspect is that primary bone formation can occur only under conditions of mechanical rest. Its clinical one lies in the capacity for immediate, pain-free movement of bone that has been fixed using a functionally stable method.

2.3.1 Indirect (Secondary) and Direct (Primary) Bone Healing

Indirect (*secondary*) bone healing is the familiar result of *conventional* immobilization by intermaxillary fixation. Given an adequate vascular supply, consolidation of the fracture occurs gradually through the progressive replacement of cartilage and fibrous tissue by bone. The blood supply must be sufficient to meet the increased metabolic demand of the newly formed cells and enable their survival.

Any motion at the fracture site affects healing by destroying newly formed cells and capillaries. This is especially true in fractures with a long lever arm, such as fractures of the mandibular angle. Nature provides for this in that the periosteum and endosteum, together with the intracortical Haversian system, are induced by the trauma to form fibroblastic and cartilaginous tissue that fills the gap between the fracture fragments.The ultimate thickness of this tissue, called the callus, is proportional to the degree of motion at the fracture site. As the callus becomes thicker, it shortens the transverse lever arm and thus reduces motion of the fragments (Fig. 10). Meanwhile the callus, which initially is confined to the gap between the fragments, is converted to fibrocartilage, which in turn ossifies and increasingly stabilizes the fracture (Fig. 11). From that point on the newly formed bone, stimulated by functional loading, is gradually converted to lamellar bone that follows the pattern of the Haversian system.

The reduction or elimination of motion at the fracture site is a major goal of fracture treatment. The more successfully this can be accomplished, the less tendency there will be for callus formation and bone resorption to occur.

Intermaxillary fixation fails to produce immobility (mechanical rest), because methods employing elastic bands or loop wiring cannot eliminate interfragmental micromotion caused by the muscular pulls associated with the swallowing and yawn reflexes. Relative immobilization is also produced by interosseous wires and miniplates used without rigid intermaxillary fixation.These devices provide complication-free healing only in the absence of infection and with excessive callus formation.

The situation is quite different when *absolute stability* is achieved. It is our experience that *primary* bone healing is an attainable goal in fracture treatment when the stability principle is systematically followed. Krompecher discovered this biologic principle in 1937 in experiments on the skulls of embryonic rats. He found that defects in the cranial vault free from mechanical forces heal primarily, without intermediate fibrous tissue, by direct *vascular* bone formation. He postulated that the same reparative process could occur in fracture healing if the fragments were adequately

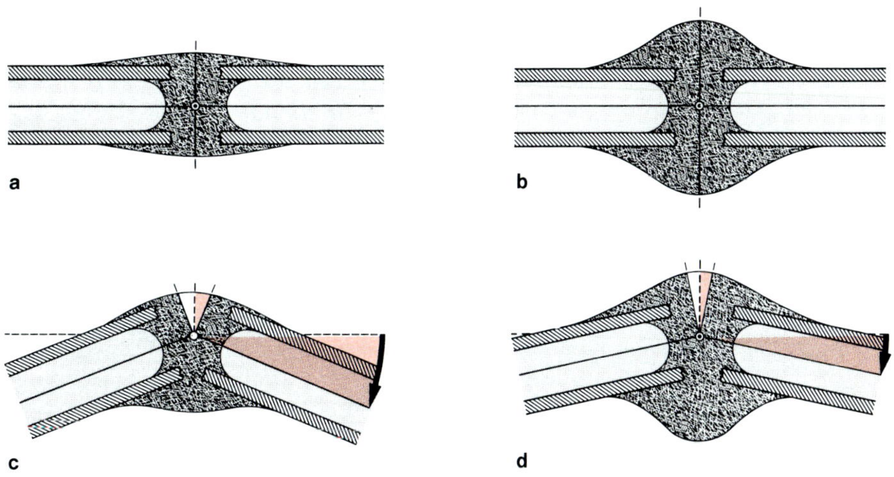

Fig. 10 a–d. As the thickness of the callus increases **(a)**, so does transverse surface area (vertical dimension), and therefore the lever arm of the stabilizing callus tissue becomes longer **(b)**. Under a constant functional load, the radius of fracture mobility is restricted *less* with a small callus (less stiffness) **(c)** than with a larger callus **(d).** (From Brinker et al. 1984)

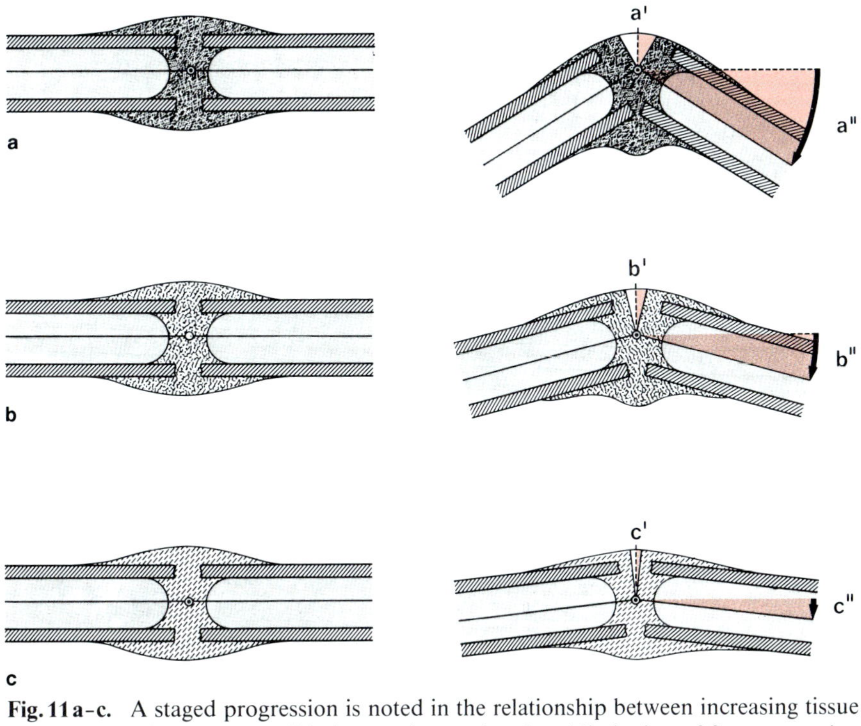

Fig. 11 a–c. A staged progression is noted in the relationship between increasing tissue thickness and fracture consolidation on the one hand and limitation of fracture motion on the other. Thus, for the three substrates of granulation tissue **(a)**, fibrocartilage **(b)**, and bone **(c)**, the *radius of the callus increases* **(a′, b′, c′)** while *fracture motion decreases* **(a″, b″, c″)** under a constant functional load. (From Brinker et al. 1984)

immobilized. In 1963 Schenk and Willenegger demonstrated the practical importance of this theory in the osteotomized radius of a dog.

When a compression plate is applied over a fracture or osteotomy in the prestressed condition, there will be a minute gap directly beneath the plate and a considerably wider gap opposite the plate. At both sites we observe a characteristic histomorphologic pattern of bone healing, known respectively as *contact healing* and *gap healing.*

The fracture ends in intimate contact with each other (those directly beneath to the plate) unite primarily by a proliferation of Haversian canals which grow across the fracture site (Fig. 12 a). The wider gap opposite the plate is permeated by blood vessels (Fig. 12 b). These are accompanied by osteoblasts, which form lamellar bone that initially is oriented at right angles to the long axis of the extremity. From about the fourth week on, a function-induced remodeling process begins in which the transversely oriented lamellae are replaced by axially oriented osteons.

These observations prompted numerous investigations conducted in various animal species under analogous conditions (e. g., Rahn et al. 1975; Gunst et al. 1982; Schenk 1986). Clinical experience, too, has fully confirmed the validity of the biologic principle of primary vascular bone healing (see also Figs. 20 and 21).

From a clinical standpoint, primary bone healing is not the true therapeutic goal. This may sound paradoxical, yet in terms of curative effect it is immaterial whether bony consolidation is accomplished indirectly through the differentiation of fibrous tissue or by the direct regeneration of osteons. This rule does not apply, however, in certain orthopedic procedures. For example, it is known that the recurrence rate after sagittal splitting of the mandibular ramus is highest when the osteotomy heals secondarily, i. e., when the fragments are separated by intermediate cartilage and fibrous tissue, whose lack of rigidity allows the fragments to migrate under loading even after a period of months. It matters little whether a wire suture or wire loop is used to approximate the fragments. A substantially lower recurrence rate is seen when the fragments heal primarily (see p. 333).

The major therapeutic value of stability in traumatology and tumor surgery lies in the rapid recovery of function. This implies a capacity for immediate active, pain-free closure of the mandible in habitual occlusion. There is absolutely no need for postoperative intermaxillary fixation, which is an essential part of conservative therapy and an indispensible adjunct to all other internal fixation methods that do not yield absolute stability.

The omission of intermaxillary fixation makes it much easier for the trauma patient to tolerate fracture treatment, for the orthopedic patient to tolerate corrective operations, and for the tumor patient to tolerate a mandibular resection. A shorter hospital stay and an earlier return to work are additional sociomedical benefits (see Graphs 1 and 2).

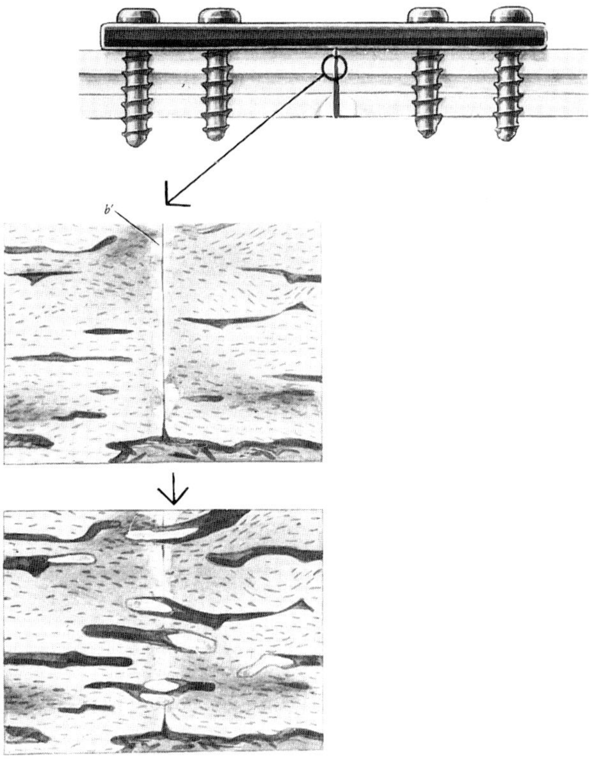

a

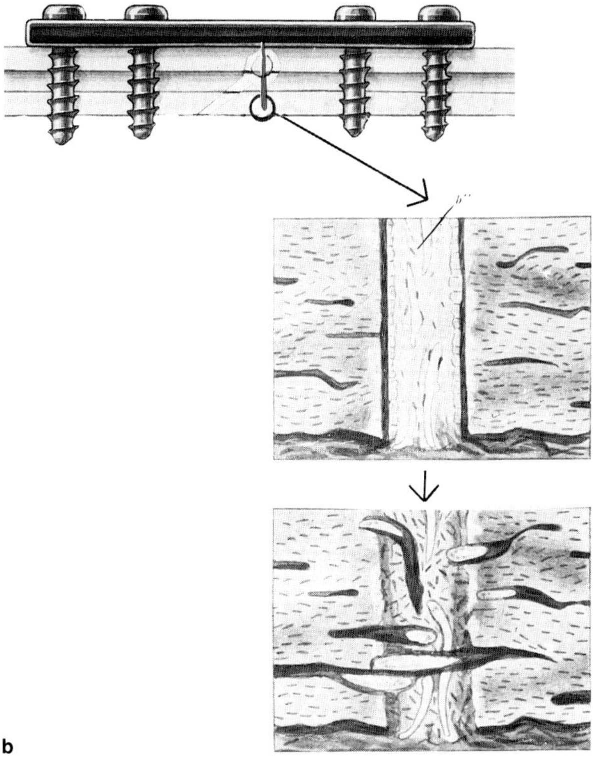

b

Fig. 12 a, b. Vascular bone formation. **a** *Contact healing* occurs by the primary formation of axially oriented lamellar bone. **b** In *gap healing*, transversely oriented bony lamellae are replaced secondarily by axially oriented osteons

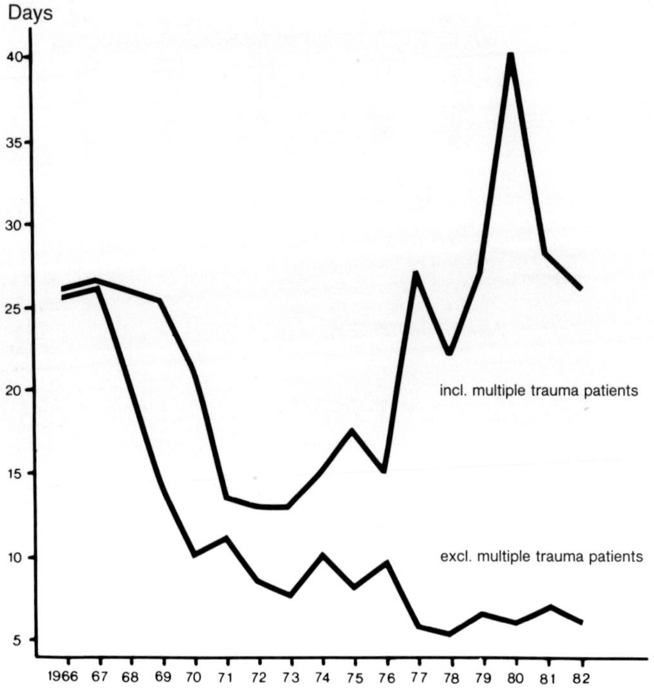

Graph 1. Length of hospital stay after internal fixation of the mandible

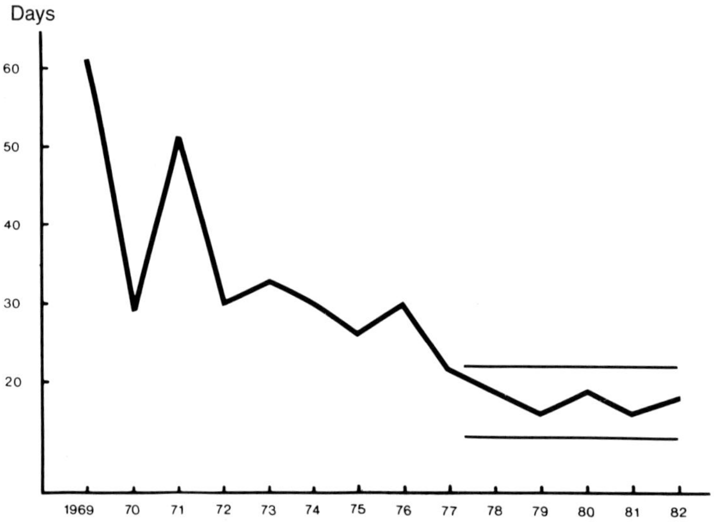

Graph 2. Time away from work after internal fixation of the mandible (70% of cases treated early)

3 Biomechanics

3.1 Anatomic Aspects of Biomechanics

Certain biomechanical principles must be understood in order to apply the stability principle successfully to the various types of mandibular fracture that can occur. Here "biomechanics" refers to the science of mechanics as it is applied to the mandibular motor apparatus.

3.1.1 Form and Structure of the Mandible

The mandible is the only freely movable bone of the face, being supported at two points. Each half of the mandible takes the shape of a vaulted beam that is convex in the direction where functional stresses are greatest. The beams function as lever arms, and very large stresses can develop within the bone even under relatively small compressive loads.

In experiments with a model of the mandibular motor apparatus, Junier (1980) found that stresses of 34–420 kg/mm^2 can develop within the mandible. Torsion and shear forces acting alternately in the lingual and buccal directions place additional demands on the architecture of the bone. The mandible is structured in a way that gives the bone a very high resistance to compressive, tensile, and shear loads. This combination also makes it highly resistant to bending loads. The mandible derives its strength from two major trajectory systems (Fig. 13). Numerous investigations begun by Walkhoff (1900), Levin (1913) and Benninghoff (1927) and continued by

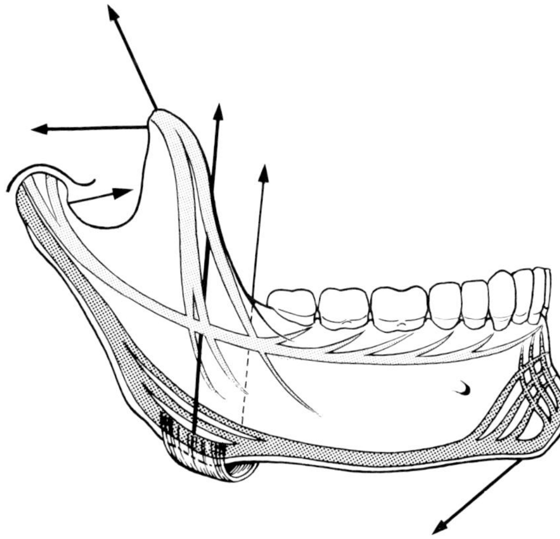

Fig. 13. Trajectory system of the mandible

Küppers (1971) confirm the observation of Pauwels (1948) that the internal trabeculae of bone tend to assume a trajectorial alignment that converts the various types of imposed stress into pure tension and compression. The mandible features a lightweight type of construction in which the chief *tension trajectory* is in its alveolar portion and the chief *pressure trajectory* is in its basal portion. The *compact bone* also adapts to functional loads in its cross-sectional geometry and distribution, especially in the basal region and along the oblique line. The very high transverse stress in the horseshoe-shaped part of the mandible (the body) determines the almost vertical course of the ascending rami, which is also necessitated by the articular fossae at the base of the skull. The mental protuberance forms a prominent buttress of compact bone to protect against the formidible transverse stresses that develop. In summary, the mandible features a minimum-maximum type of construction that is appropriate for its static and dynamic functions.

3.1.2 Muscular Apparatus of the Mandible

The mandible is suspended bilaterally by a system of muscles, tendons, and ligaments that enable it to move like a two-arm lever around an imaginary transverse axis. This axis is approximately in the area of the mandibular foramen, so that the inferior alveolar nerve enters the mandibular canal at the least mobile and most protected site. This point marks one end of the "line of zero force," along which forces are largely neutralized by virtue of the unequal stress distribution in the bone. Normally the zero-force line coincides with the mandibular canal (Fig. 14).

Most functional loads, then, are distributed along the base and alveolar part of the mandible. How are they generated? The angle of the mandible, the midpiece of the two-arm lever, is held firmly within the masseter-pterygoid sling. This system moves the mandible and also holds it the position it must maintain during its excursions. This sling principle, together with the most powerful muscle of mastication, the temporal muscle, which has its own apophysis (muscular process), not only permits elevation of the mandible to approximate the teeth but also provides for an occlusive force of between 50 and 80 kg (see Rahn et al. 1975) - pressures that would be

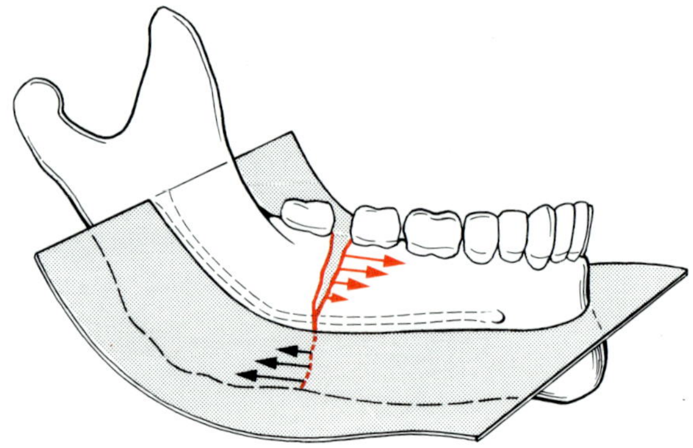

Fig. 14. The "line of zero force" roughly coincides with the mandibular canal and demarcates the basal arch from the alveolar process. A fracture is subjected to tensile forces above the line and to compressive forces below the line

needed for the mastication of tough meat, for example. While this trimuscular complex is concerned with the actual *working movement* of the jaw or mastication, the muscles that open the mouth, and a number of accessory muscles, provide for the side-to-side or anterior-posterior movements of the mandible that may be executed as a prelude to mastication. In their capacity as antagonists, these muscles impose bending and tensile stresses upon the jaw.

3.1.3 Implications for the Biomechanics of Internal Fixation

We may summarize the anatomic aspects of mandibular biomechanics as follows: The two chief trajectories of the mandible and the buttresses of compact bone are clearly an adaptation to the pattern of functional stresses that are imposed upon the jaw. Most of these stresses result from the action of muscular forces. In cases where mandibular continuity is disrupted and intermaxillary fixation is not part of the treatment plan, the neutralization of these forces is necessary in order to achieve a funtionally stable reduction.

The most reliable way to neutralize the forces is by restoring the tension and pressure trajectories of the mandible. A variety of methods and techniques may be used to implement this principle, depending on the location and type of the fracture. The tension trajectory along the alveolar border can be reconstructed with a *splint* placed in a dentulous area of the mandible or with a *small plate* applied behind the molars in the area of the oblique line. Each of these devices functions as a *tension band* to minimize bending stresses (see p. 51 ff.).

The pressure trajectory along the base of the mandible can be restored with a *stabilization plate* (neutralization plate). In this case the primary function of the device is to neutralize torsion and shear forces. The plate and tension band combination has proved highly effective for restoring the continuity of the tension and pressure trajectories in the mandible (Fig. 15).

The special anatomy of the mandible requires the use of other methods as well. For example, mechanical reconstruction of the tension trajectory can be replaced by static compression with a prestressed plate if circum-

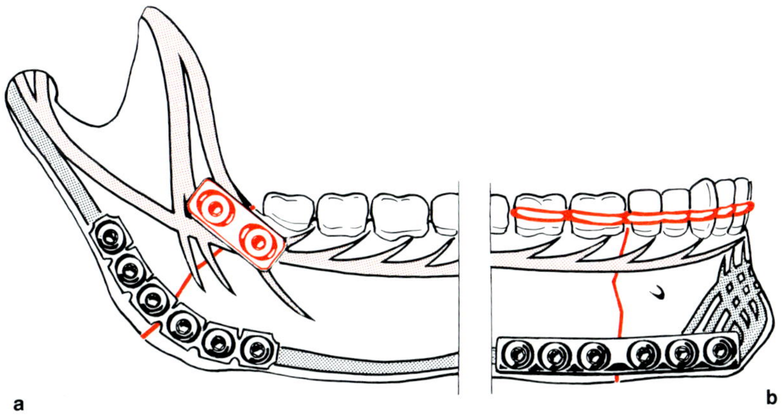

Fig. 15 a, b. The tension and pressure trajectories can be restored by a *plate and tension band system.* The tension band may consist of a small plate **(a)** or a dental splint **(b)** applied on the tension side of the bone. The compression side may be stabilized with a reconstruction plate **(a)** or a dynamic compression plate **(b)**

stances prohibit the use of a tension band. We characterize this mechanical principle as *buttressing away from the plate.* There are two ways in which the buttressing can be accomplished on the side of the pressure trajectory:

- with a *reconstruction plate* (see p. 63) that is substantially stronger than the tension band, or
- with an *eccentric dynamic compression plate* (*EDCP*) (see p. 60 ff.).

3.2 Biomechanics of Fracture Treatment: Experimental Background

(B. Rahn)

Internal fixation of mandibular fractures triggers an intense interaction between mechanics and biology. On one side there exists a series of purely mechanical influences upon the bony tissue, which in part may have biological implications. On the other side, changes of the mechanical situation are induced by biological reactions. Resorption of bone at the fragment ends or at the interface to the implants, for instance, may endanger the entire stabilization. In addition, the tissue formation in the fracture area is noticeably influenced by the mechanical situation. Surgical intervention and the incorporation of implants, by denudation of the bone and by drilling, can lead to an interference with the blood supply, which is then related to the subsequent remodelling pattern.

3.2.1 Mechanisms of Stabilization

Displaced fragments may present a bony union even if the fracture is not treated at all, but often the resulting function is not optimal. To avoid permanent malalignment, the fragments are reduced with the highest possible accuracy, and they are held in this position until bony union is secured. This requires the mechanical limitation of interfragmentary motion during the healing process.

3.2.1.1 Stabilization by Splinting

External splinting immobilizes a fracture without surgical intervention. Stabilizing forces provided by the splint do not act directly upon the fractured bone, but through an intermediate tissue layer, which includes periodontium and soft tissues. Inevitably, a certain amount of motion in the fracture gap remains.

Internal splinting requires a surgical procedure to introduce the means of stabilization. Pins, medullary nails, and flexible plates (the last again coming into fashion) belong in this category. The external fixator takes an intermediate position between internal and external splinting (see p. 69).

The various splinting techniques achieve different degrees of, but never complete, immobilization. One therefore has to accept that the initial reduction may not be maintained throughout the entire healing period. Many sites in the skeleton tolerate such a slight displacement without problems. An exact anatomical reduction, however, is necessary in intraarticular fractures, as arthrotic complications may result later on. Fractures within a dentulous area necessitate an exact realignment as well, otherwise a malocclusion results.

3.2.1.2 Stabilization by Compression

A higher degree of stability can be achieved by using inter-fragmentary compression. Dynamic compression originates from the combined action of an implant and of physiologically occurring forces, whereas static compression is primarily produced by the implant itself and by its application technique.

A fractured bone is still able to transmit compressive forces across the aligned fracture gap, while tensile forces have to be taken over by the implant. This tension band principle, as it is called, can be applied in situations in which mainly tensile forces are expected (see p. 51). Wire or very thin, flexible plates may fulfill this function as long as the force always acts in the same, defined direction. As soon as changing directions of the forces are to be expected, other mechanisms must be added to the tension band function to guarantee the immobilization of the fracture area (see p. 21).

Static forces produce a situation at the fracture site which no longer allows for any relative motion between the fragments. Thereby two separate mechanism supplement each other (Perren 1971). Firstly, compression leads to increased friction between the fragment ends. This helps to resist shearing and torsional forces. It is intensified by the interdigitation of the fragment ends. Secondly, the axial preload produced by compression counteracts the axial tensile forces (see p. 38 ff.). Technically, the preload is generated by means of plates and screws. Various techniques may be used to compress a fracture.

A removable tension device attached to one end of the plate (Fig. 16) will cover a long distance. Additionally, the screws are not extensively bent when high forces are applied, and the tension device can be removed as soon as the bone is compressed and the plate is fixed to the bone. There are several disadvantages: it requires a wider exposure, its force acts far from the fracture, and a certain loss of compression is observed upon removal of the device.

Tension devices which are incorporated into the plate design, such as built-in screws or moving parts with eccentric action, make the implant more difficult to handle and favor corrosion. Such implants, therefore, have never found a wide application.

If a screw is placed eccentrically in a plate hole, the screw head engages against one edge of this hole. The plate edge slides along the screw head in an oblique plane, and a movement of the plate on the bone surface results. Elongation of the originally conical holes in the long axis of the plate does not provide stabilization in the lateral direction. The cylindrically shaped oblique plane of the screw hole in the "dynamic compression plate" (DCP) provides lateral support to the spherical screw head (Perren et al. 1969 b) (see p. 39). Numerous copies of this design have been marketed since. Compromises in their design, like steeper or flatter sliding planes, or the sacrifice of the lateral guide, had to be performed to avoid patent problems.

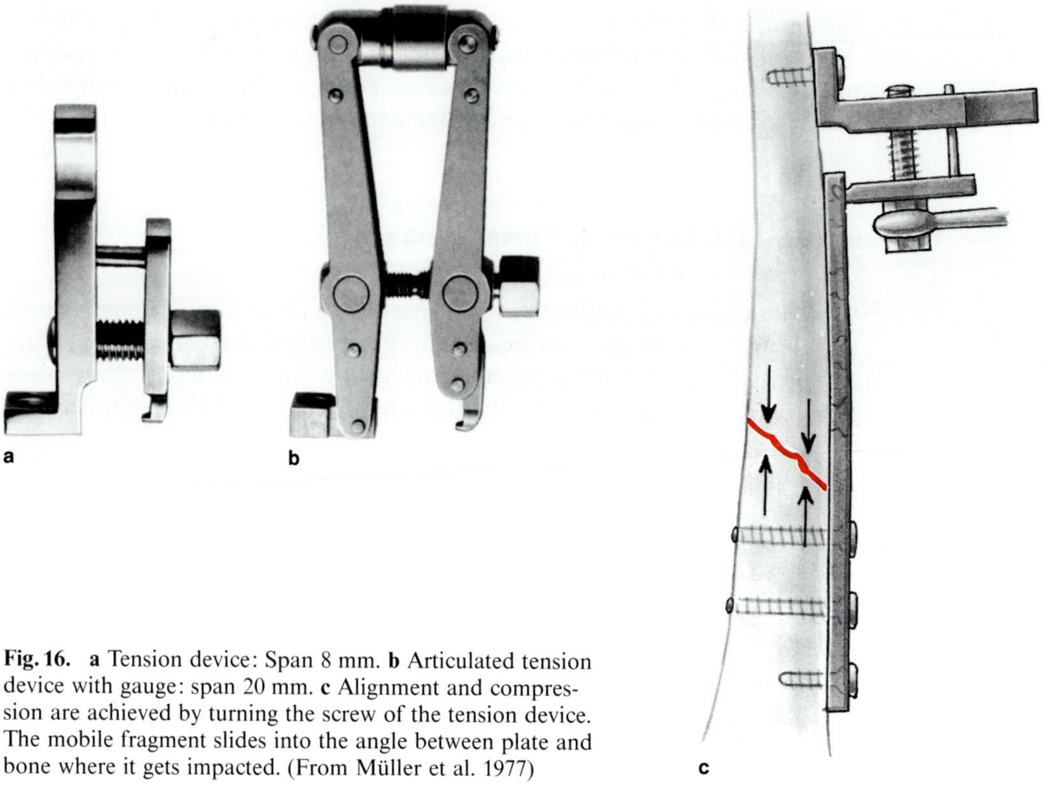

Fig. 16. **a** Tension device: Span 8 mm. **b** Articulated tension device with gauge: span 20 mm. **c** Alignment and compression are achieved by turning the screw of the tension device. The mobile fragment slides into the angle between plate and bone where it gets impacted. (From Müller et al. 1977)

Both removable tension devices and self-compressing plate designs produce an asymmetric distribution of compression across the fracture area, which is due to the asymmetric position of the plate (Fig. 17). A few technical tricks help to obtain a more homogenous force distribution. Knowledge of these mechanisms facilitates alignment and helps to avoid unintentional and unnoticed displacement of the fragments.

The selection of plate position can favorably influence the force distribution across the fracture. Muscle groups arranged eccentrically to the bone axis produce tensile forces on the opposite side of the bone. If the plate is placed on this opposite side, the muscle tonus, together with the tension band effect of the plate, leads to more uniform compression of the fracture.

Overbending of the plate is an additional mechanism to compress the fracture far from the implant (Perren et al. 1974). After perfect contouring of the plate to the bone surface, a bend is produced over the fracture site, which leads to a slight midspan deflection (see Figs. 18 and 32 a). Thus, the insertion of the screws in eccentric position compresses the fracture directly under the plate, while the spring effect of the plate compresses the opposite side. In plate fixation of mandibular fractures, this procedure is a useful technique to close a gap on the lingual side.

The use of lag screws is another possibility of compressing fragment ends (Claudi et al. 1979; Regazzoni 1982).

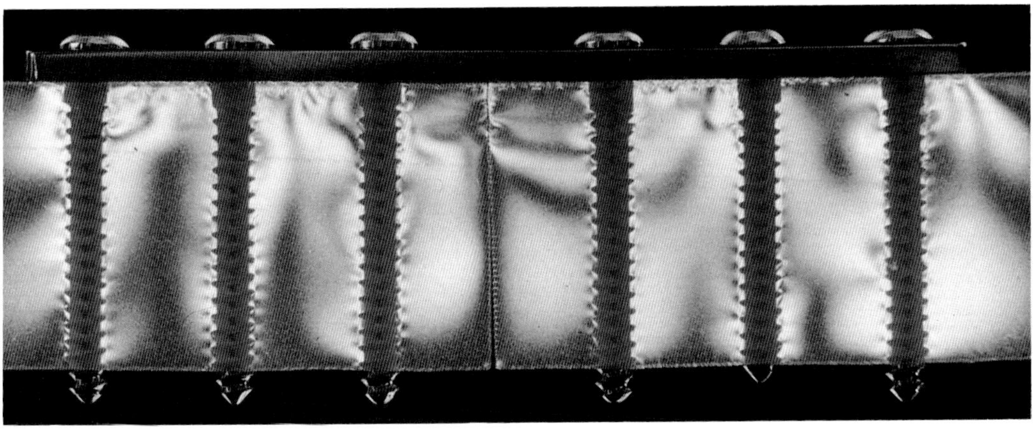

Fig. 17. Asymmetric stress distribution after compression by a plate which was exactly contoured to the bone surface: high pressure directly under the plate, gap on the opposite side (photoelastic model)

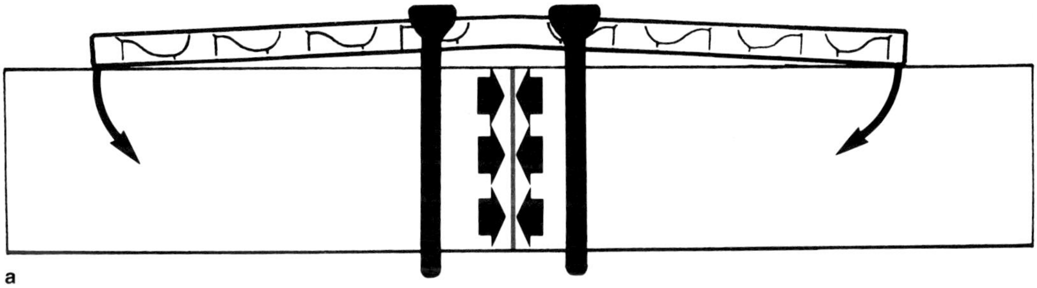

a

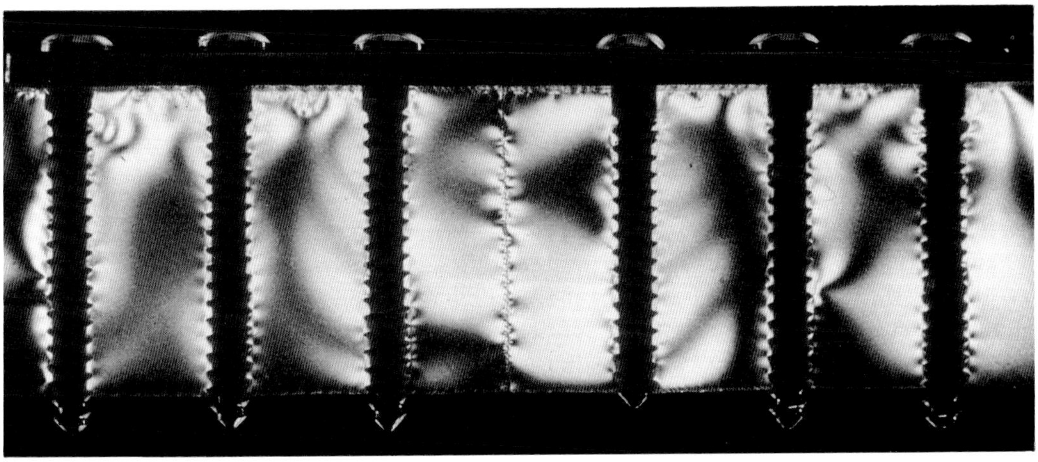

b

Fig. 18. a Effect of overbending: symmetric stress distribution in the fracture area; the spring function of the plate closes the fracture evenly far from the plate. **b** Effect of overbending in a photoelastic model (no gap on the opposite side)

Depending on the fracture type, lag screws can be combined with plates, either as separate lag screws or lag screws occupying a plate hole. Since interfragmentary compression is already provided by the lag screws, the plate is usually placed without any axial compression. Due to a longer lever arm, lag screws are especially efficient in bones of large diameter, but they may be useful in smaller bones, too (see Fig. 35).

3.2.2 Special Situation in the Mandible

In the mandible high forces may be applied. The maximum biting force, as determined in a group of male test persons, reaches values in the order of 750 N, in a group of females 500 N (Rahn et al. 1975). In the region of the premolars the corresponding values were 500 N and 300 N, in the incisor area 300 N and 250 N, respectively. In the case of a fracture in the mandibular angle a moment of approximately 20 Nm would result. Under these (normally unrealistic) extreme loads, an implant would have to withstand a force of 2000 N, if it were placed at a distance of 10 mm from the caudal edge of the mandible. An implant placed at the occlusal side would still be loaded to about 700 N. Wires of adequate dimensions could certainly withstand those forces, but under cyclic loading a loosening of the locking wire spiral has to be expected. In this respect plates with screw anchoring in the bone behave better.

It seems obvious, that the tension side, e.g., in a fracture of the mandibular angle, is found on the occlusal side, especially if a two-dimensional model is considered. A study using three-dimensional models (Kroon, manuscript in preparation) may demonstrate that this is true for most of the occlusal loading situations, but there are loading sites which shift the tension side to the caudal margin of the mandible. Loading contralaterally to an angular fracture or in the incisor region has no problems. The more the loading forces approach the fractured angle, the less the plate acts as a tension band. The inversion starts in the area of the first molar, and if the load moves further dorsally, an opening of the fracture gap in the angle results (Fig. 19). Since the tension side may vary, a pure tension band fixation, e.g., by one simple "mini"-plate alone, could not fulfill the complex biomechanical requirements of the mandible. An uncritical use of such plates in a contaminated wound may thus bear a higher risk of infection.

3.2.3 Bone Healing

Radiologically speaking, the morphology of fracture healing varies widely. Even without treatment, variations are visible: Fractures with high amounts of motion in the fracture area produce more callus than fractures with less motion. Depending on the method of treatment, only little callus or even no callus at all may be observed, the latter especially after operative fracture fixation. Mechanical influences seem to influence significantly the differentiation of the repair tissue.

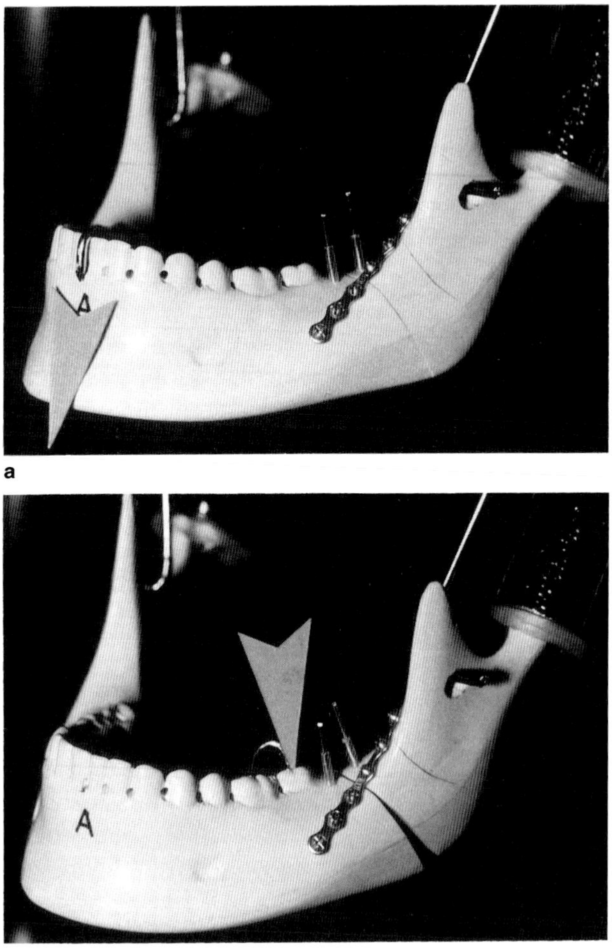

a

b

Fig. 19. **a** Stability testing after fixation of mandibular fractures by "mini plates". Under load in the frontal region the small plate in the linea obliqua acts as a tension band, and the fracture of the mandibular angle is closed. **b** Inversion of tension side and compression side when loading the mandible in the vicinity of the fracture: the stiffness of the "mini plate" is not sufficient to maintain the reduction under all loading conditions. A similar behavior can be observed clinically as well. (Kroon 1986)

3.2.3.1 Indirect Bone Healing

Fracture healing is classically characterized by the formation of periosteal callus, resorption of the fragment ends, and tissue formation which passes through various steps of differentiation (Coutelier 1969; see Sect. 2.3.1).

In the initial phase, the presence of interfragmentary motion, provides the most difficult conditions for bridging. The early repair tissue still has little strength. Periosteal callus formation increases the cross sectional area and thus provides more favorable lever arm conditions to counteract external forces. This increase, however, is still not sufficient to provide conditions which are comparable to the ones offered by cortical bone. Several times the length of the lever arms would be necessary for this purpose.

In the early phases of healing there is continuous interfragmentary motion present. Tissues between the fragments are squeezed and torn, conditions which interfere with tissue formation. Those tissues which are formed during the early phases of fracture healing tolerate deformation much better than cortical bone would do (Perren and Cordey 1977). While granulation tissue allows for stretching to double its length, cartilage tolerates a deformation of only 10%–20%, cortical bone of 2% only. During the healing process a step by step differentiation is observed which proceeds via granulation tissue, connective tissue, fibrocartilage, and mineralized cartilage to bone. This differentiation cascade permits the formation of tissues which are more and more sensitive to strain while their precursor tissues provide a protected environment. Bone will only be formed under strain conditions which do not endanger its existence.

Interfragmentary strain will be further reduced by a resorption of the fragment ends. The increased width of the fracture gap allows the distribution of the displacement over a longer distance. Thus, each single tissue element will undergo less deformation, which facilitates the differentiation process.

The structure of the repair tissue appears unorganized in the beginning. Callus is resorbed after bony union of the fragment ends, and the newly formed bone is remodelled comparable to the original shape.

3.2.3.2 Direct Bone Healing

Stable internal fixation may eliminate interfragmentary motion to a major extent. The implants take care of the tensile forces, while contact areas give the support to transmit compressive forces across the fracture. This immobilization of the interfragmentary zone allows the formation of cortical bone right at the beginning.

Following trauma, internal (Haversian) remodelling in the fracture area is intensified. Groups of osteoclasts resorb canals into the compact bone. Blood vessels grow into these canals, and osteoblasts deposit new bone into their lumen. In the absence of interfragmentary motion such newly formed bone structures, so-called osteons, may cross directly from one fragment into the other (Fig. 20) (Schenk and Willenegger 1964). This leads to a gradual replacement of the bone in the fracture-affected area. This remodelling process results in a transitional period of localized bone porosis, which means a temporary weakening of the bone. Depending on the site, the remodelling lasts several months; in a long tubular bone, substantially longer. For example, in a femur it takes approximately 2 years before the progress of remodelling allows the removal of a plate without risk.

On a microscopic level, an absolutely perfect realignment of the fracture fragments may rarely be reached. Gap zones between the fragments are neighbored by contact areas. If the contact areas give enough support to immobilize together with the implant the fracture area, then blood vessels may sprout into the immobilized gaps as early as in 1–2 weeks and lamellar bone is deposited onto the fragment ends (Fig. 21). Gaps up to a width of approximately half a millimeter are filled within a few weeks directly by lamellar bone. Wider gaps are subdivided into smaller compartments by woven bone trabeculae, followed by a deposition of lamellar bone into these compartments. This subdivision allows a more rapid filling even of larger gaps. Significantly wider gaps do not permit direct bone formation. There, regeneration will follow the indirect pattern.

Bone circulation is interrupted by the fracture trauma. Depending on the course of the fracture plane the intracortical circulation of the fragment ends is jeopardized over a distance of a few millimeters up to several centimeters (Fig. 22) (Gunst et al. 1982).

Surgical access to the bone means additional trauma and often leads to a certain denudation. It only seems justified to take the risks of surgery

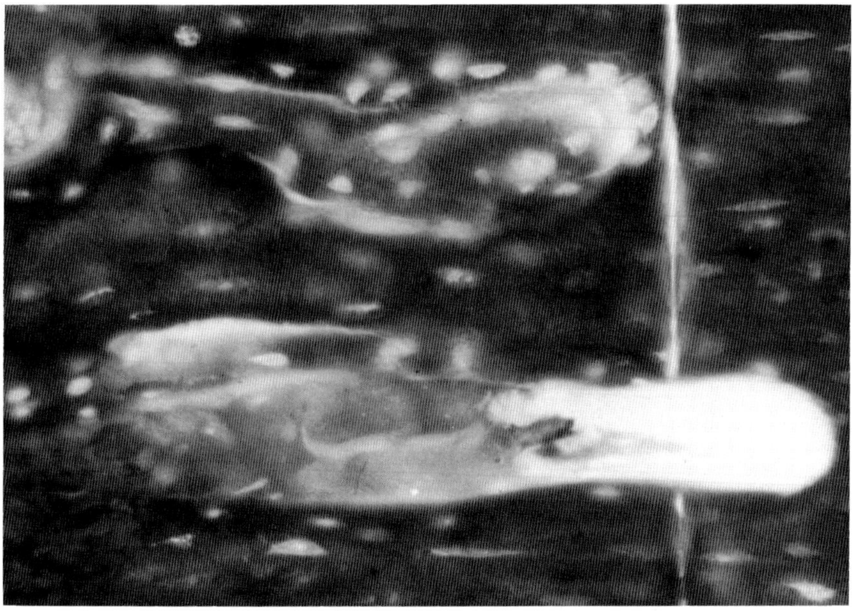

a

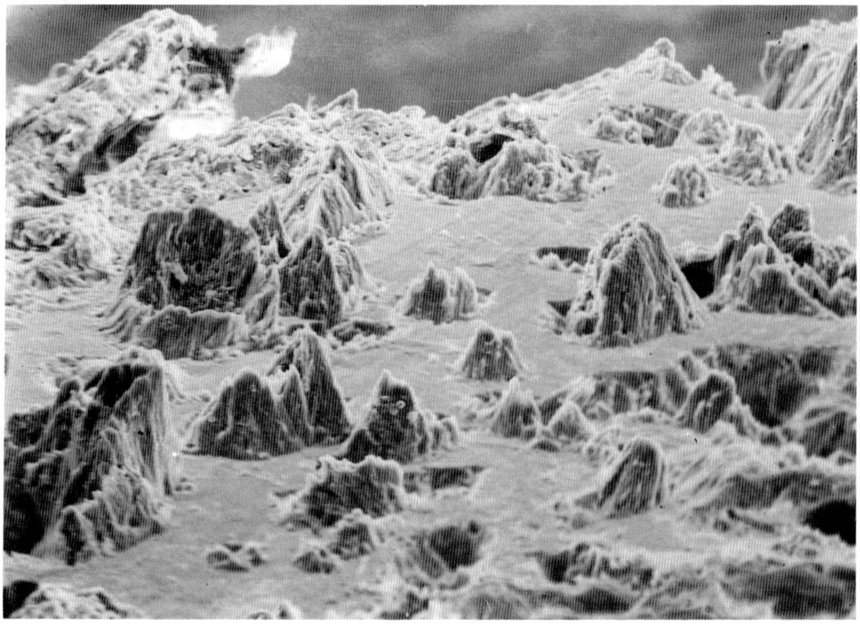

b

Fig. 20 a, b. Direct bone healing under stable fixation in a contact area. **a** Direct connection of both fragments by a newly formed osteon which is distinguished by its tetracycline labelling from the darker background. (From Rahn 1982). **b** View of a fracture plane under the scanning electron microscope (as exposed by a tensile test): The protruding osteons are the elements which have connected the two fragment ends

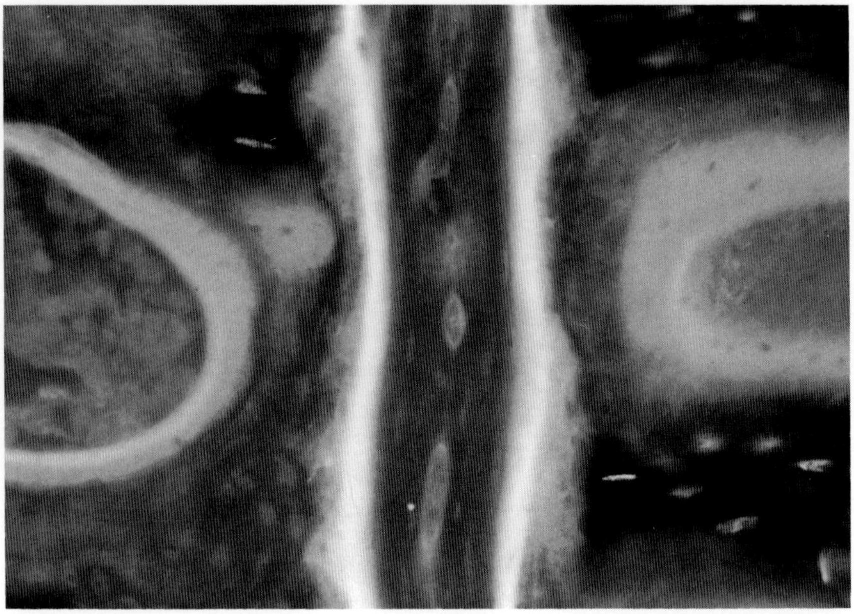

a

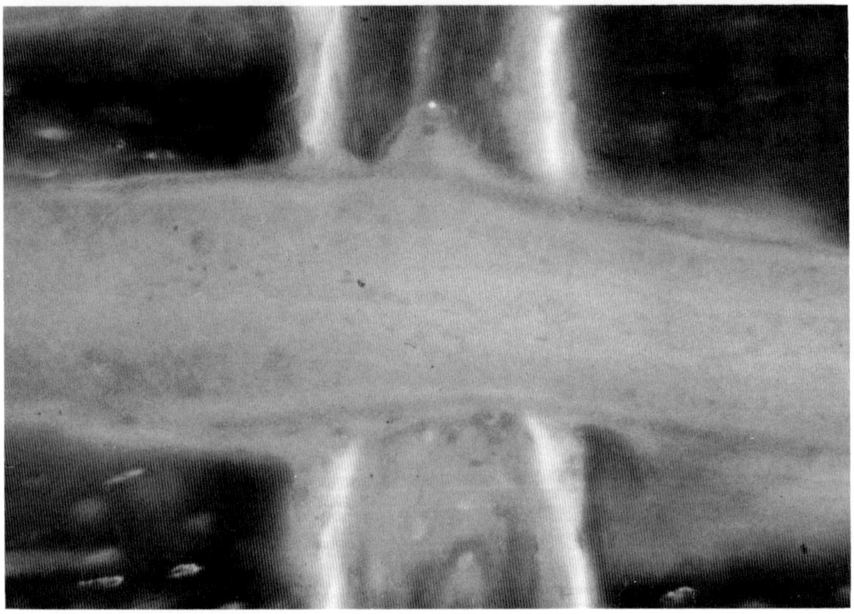

b

Fig. 21 a, b. Direct bone healing under stable fixation in a gap area. **a** The gap area is immobilized by support in neighbouring contact areas. This allows for direct bone formation in the gap. There is no need for tissue differentiation via a series of intermediate steps. **b** The gap between the fragment ends is primarily filled with bone, undergoing a secondary remodelling which reconstructs the original aspect of the bone structure. (From Rahn 1985)

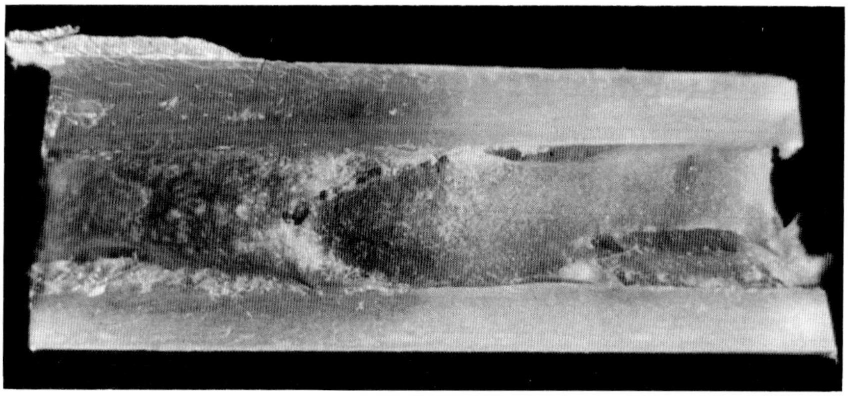

Fig. 22. Disturbed blood supply in a fragment end as a sequelae of fracture and denudation. Visualization by intravital staining with disulfine blue. (From Rahn 1982)

(anesthesia, infection, soft tissue damage) if a better starting point for healing can be expected. One has therefore to strive for the goal of surgical fracture treatment, the establishment of full stability in the fractured area, without any compromise. Maintenance of the anatomical reduction during the healing period and functional stability provide favorable preconditions for recovery of the circulation. An immobilized fracture with otherwise unrestricted mobility helps to improve soft tissue circulation in the neighborhood, and the elimination of interfragmentary motion favors a circulatory reconnection between the fragments. Optimal circulatory conditions clearly help to reduce the risk of infection.

A plate interferes with the circulation of the underlying bone cortex (Fig. 23) (Gunst 1980). The reason for this locally disturbed circulation cannot be found in a compression of intracortical vessels, since bone only tolerates minimal deformation, but rather in a blocked flow at the bone surface and eventually a retrograde thrombosing. The insertion of screws disturbs circulation in their environment, as does an intramedullary nail on the endosteal side of the cortex (Pfister et al. 1979). Reestablishing intracortical circulation is related to bone remodelling processes. In a first step, existing spaces in the bone are reconnected to the circulatory system. This is followed by widening of these spaces and refilling with lamellar bone, similar to Haversian remodelling. The vessels gradually enter the nonsupplied bone, and the remodelling zone migrates from the zone with intact circulation into the nonsupplied area.

3.2.3.3 Plate-Induced Porosis, "Stress Protection"

The principal function of a plate consists in immobilizing a fracture. Minimal implant dimensions are required to guarantee this task under the various conditions, which not only include tension band function but also tensile and torsional loads.

Forces produced by functional loads of a bone are in part absorbed by a plate fixed to that bone, resulting in a local unloading of the bone. This may have certain implications when using massive implants in the presence

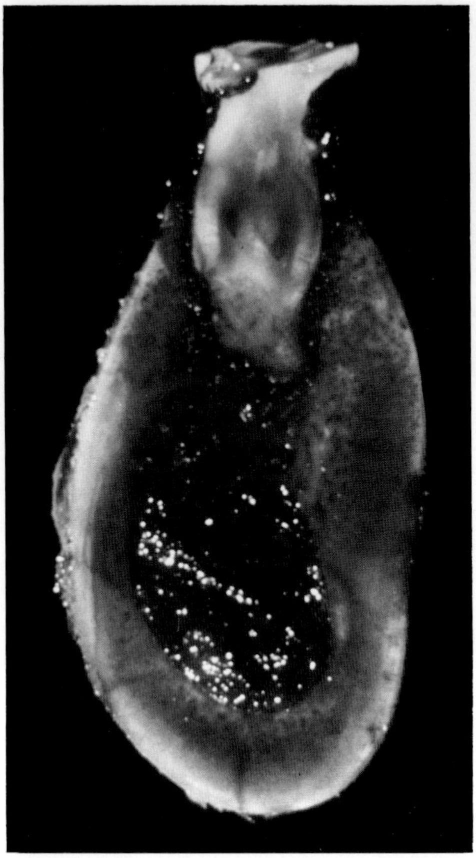

Fig. 23. Jeopardized blood supply in a sheeps mandible induced by fixation of a plate. Almost the entire thickness of the buccal cortex is affected. (From Rahn 1982)

of high functional loads, as is the case in the long bones of the lower extremity. A series of researchers attribute the porosis found regularly under plates contacting the bone to such a "stress protection."

The extent of bone porosis parallels the dimensions of the plates used (see Fig. 24, Matter et al. 1974). It can be demonstrated experimentally that this zone correlates with that in which intracortical circulation is jeopardized by the implant (Gunst 1980). It depends on the dimensions of the bone, whether only a part of the cortex is affected or whether the entire thickness of the cortex is involved, as may be the case in the relatively thin mandibular cortex (Fig. 23). The area of early porosis underneath the plate shows a direct relationship with the area of vascular damage, whereas a corresponding correlation cannot be established for the change in the pattern of unloading (Gautier et al. 1984). Many findings attributed to stress protection could be explained as sequelae of disturbed circulation. However, late structural changes in connection with extremely massive implants cannot be excluded.

In the mandible, the relatively small cross sectional area of the plate has to be compared with the much larger cross sectional area of the bone. In addition, the functional forces are much smaller than in the lower extremities. The unloading effect of a plate used for fracture fixation is minor, and if porosis occurs, it is more probable that it arises from the disturbed circulation.

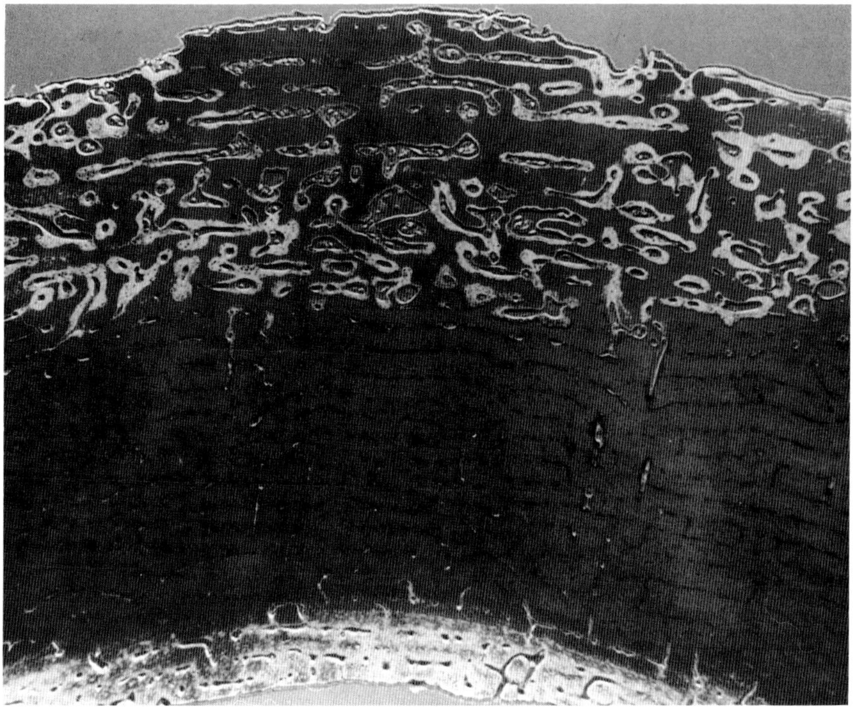

Fig. 24. Temporary bone porosis under a plate. The remodelling pattern matches exactly the pattern of disturbed blood supply as induced by the plate. (From Matter et al. 1974)

3.2.3.4 Disturbed Healing Process

The normal course of fracture healing can be severely troubled by infection. Open wounds practically always must be considered to be contaminated. The local defense conditions, closely related to the quality of the local circulation, may decide whether or not an infection starts. Full stabilization of the fracture with its beneficial effects on local soft tissue circulation does compensate, at least in part, for the circulatory shortcomings produced by the fracture and surgery.

In the presence of instability and bacterial contamination, a part of the initially nonsupplied areas will not undergo the regular remodelling process. Intense bone resorption takes place at the border between supplied and nonsupplied bone, which leads to a sequestration of nonsupplied parts (Fig. 25).

The treatment of an infection can be conducted more efficiently under stable conditions than under continuing motion in the injured area. Even in the presence of infection a bony union can be achieved if the stability of the fracture fixation is guaranteed (Rittmann and Perren 1974). It is therefore advisable to leave a solidly anchored implant in place until the bone has united.

A pseudarthrosis represents a standstill in the process of tissue differentiation (Fig. 26). Frequently, a mechanical origin can be found behind this

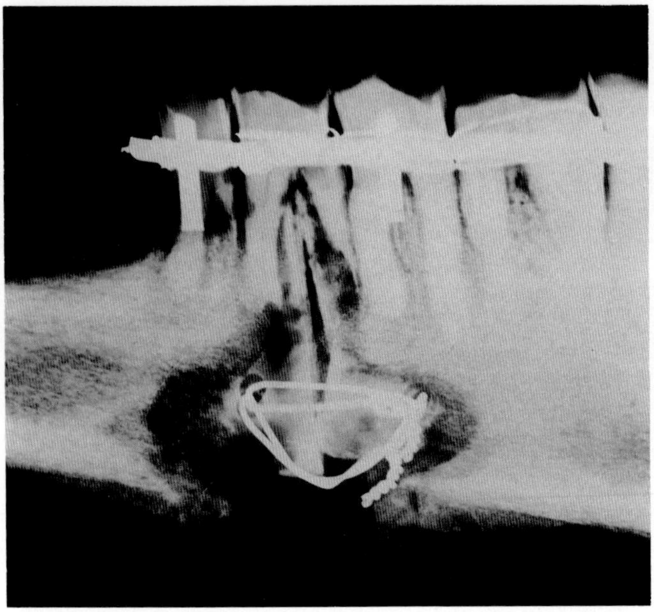

Fig. 25. Osteitis with sequestration after insufficient stabilization by wire sutures. Those bone areas are involved, in which circulation was interrupted by osteotomy, denudation, and drilling

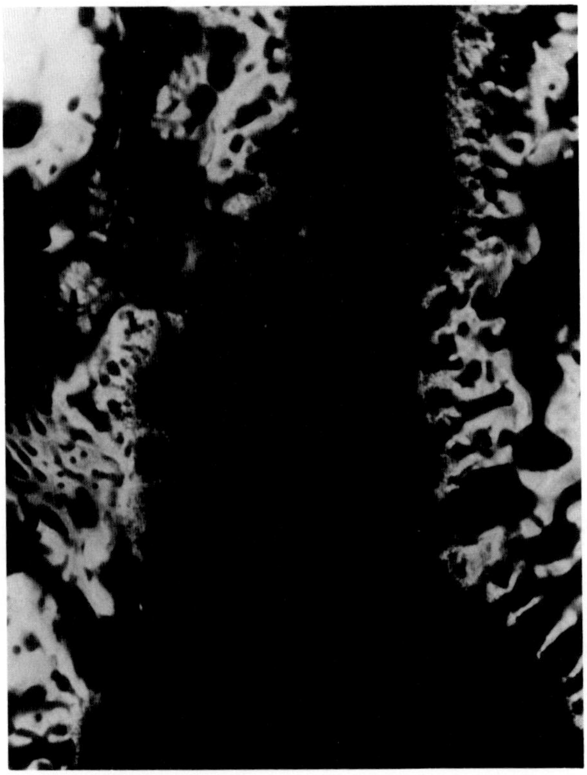

Fig. 26. Microradiography of a pseudarthrosis. The cascade of tissue differentiation has come to a standstill which results in a complete absence of bone formation in the fracture gap

disturbance. The tissues in a pseudarthrosis are identical to those which develop during the normal process of fracture healing. It seems as if insufficient immobilization of the fracture gap interferes with the course of the differentiation cascade and renders the formation of a successor tissue, especially a mineralized tissue, impossible. This tissue should not be removed, since the healing process has already started and has only come to an arrest. Additional stabilization is the only thing required for the resumption of the differentiation process and its continuation to the formation of a bony bridge.

3.2.4 Implant Design

The holding force of screws in bone is especially influenced by the width of the threads. Since bone is significantly weaker than the implant material, a thread design is chosen which gives the bone a larger share of the volume.

The pretapping of the thread into the bone means an additional working operation, but it offers some profits, especially in thicker bone. The flutes which are cut into the tap provide sufficient space for the removed bone pieces, allowing the use of a wider thread (see Fig. 141). At screw insertion the torque of the screwdriver corresponds directly to the axial screw force, and it is not absorbed by the friction due to cutting of the threads. A certain amount of heat drainage may be obtained by the removal of material warmed by the cutting process.

In self-tapping screws the flutes are restricted to the tip of the screw (see Fig. 141). Laboratory tests have shown that self-tapping screws may produce cracks in the cortical bone (Ansell and Scales 1968). The thread dimensions are limited due to the small capacity of the flutes for clearing away the cut off bone particles. The contouring of an implant to the local bone configuration often requires repeated insertion and removal of screws. Damage to the bony threads by the cutting flutes is not impossible, and a loss of holding capacity could then result. Furthermore, bone growth into the flutes renders screw removal more difficult.

The hexagonal drive in the screw head provides good force transmission from the screwdriver to the screw. In contrast to slotted or Phillips, the hexagonal drive does not require an axial force to apply torque to the screw. Thus, the danger of slipping and damaging the screw head is reduced, and screw removal, especially with soft metals like titanium, is not complicated.

The material used for plates has to allow a perfect contouring to the bone surface. It has to provide an implant stiffness sufficient to eliminate interfragmentary motion. In addition, fatigue properties are required which allow bony union to occur before the risk of fatigue failure of the implant arises (Pohler and Straumann 1975).

Titanium is an implant material which is very well suited for fracture fixation, in spite of its higher costs. Besides its mechanical properties it presents an excellent tissue compatibility. Steel has proven and still is considered to be a good compromise. It can be contoured without problems, has good strength, presents no compatibility problems in most cases, and is relatively inexpensive. Both materials can easily be machined. Implants made of chromium-cobalt-molybdenum alloys have high strength and can be contoured. The alloys present good compatibility characteristics, in spite of the lesser compatibility qualities of some of their components. Since implants made from these alloys are cast, the production is less flexible when changes and improvements of the implant shapes have to be considered.

The dimensions of the implants have a substantial influence upon the degree of immobilization of the fractured area, and thus upon the healing process. As long as an implant only has to fulfill tension band functions, thin plates may be used; if it has to guarantee the immobilization of a fracture under all physiologic loading conditions, larger dimensions are required.

Corrosion of the implants does not pose any problems as long as the passive layer, a dense oxide layer on the surface of the metal, remains intact (Contzen et al. 1967). A single scratch has no consequences, since the passive layer will regenerate in an electrolyte environment within a short time. In the case of instability, however, screw heads and plate fret against each other with each loading cycle. This destroys the passive layer before it has a chance to regenerate and results in a continuing corrosion process. Fretting of titanium implants leads to a grayish staining of the surrounding tissues, but no adverse tissue reactions result. Steel, even stainless steel, presents obvious signs of corrosion, when the passive layer is continuously destroyed. Under fretting conditions the chromium-cobalt--molybdenum alloys corrode too, but their corrosion products in the tissue are not as evident as the brown-red, rusty corrosion products of steel. These alloys and steel contain in part the same elements, e.g., chromium. A concentration of certain components of alloys in the tissue produces more or less localized tissue reactions (Dumbleton and Black 1975) (Graph 3). Additionally, some heavy metals present systemic effects. Nickel and chromium ions can lead to allergic reactions (Merrit and Brown 1980). At the occurrence of such symptoms the implants have to be removed. If fracture healing is of that time not yet finished replacement by titanium implants of identical dimensions is recommended.

After completion of healing, implants are routinely removed in bones with heavy mechanical loads. Differences in the mechanical properties of the implant and bone would always lead to minute relative motion between the two. Fretting between plate and screws might result, and corrosion products might be released over longer periods. It is not predictable whether a continuous influence over decades would not carry the risk of biological damage. Although there is no clear evidence for a deleterious effect of long-term implants, to stay on the safe side, it is recommended to remove them, especially in patients with a long life expectancy. Cosmetic considerations and temperature sensitivity of implants immediately underneath the skin could be further reasons for removal.

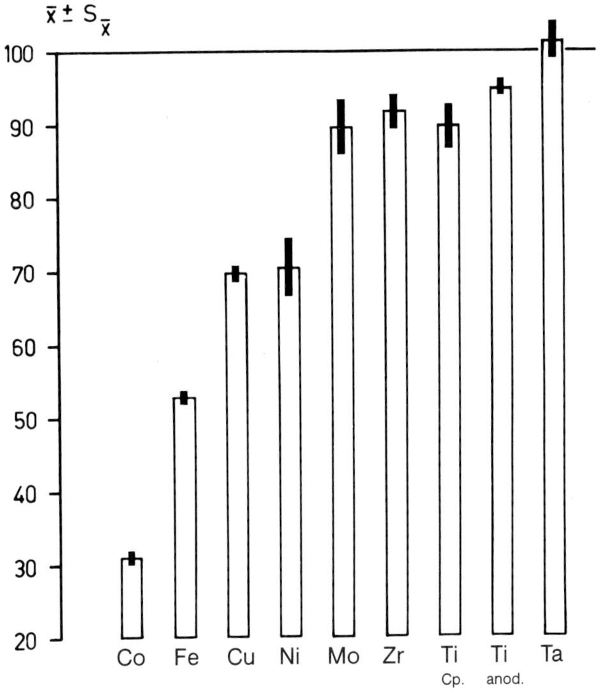

Graph 3. Relative growth inhibition of embryonic rat femurs as produced by metal ions added to the tissue culture medium. The metals cobalt, iron, and nickel, components of implant alloys, produce a significant effect on in vitro growth, whereas titanium shows little disturbing effects. (From Gerber and Perren 1980)

4 Principles of the ASIF Technique

4.1 Interfragmental Compression for Functionally Stable Internal Fixation

The next question to be addressed is how we can apply the principle of absolute stability to the mandible. Either of two basic types of fixation system may be employed: the system *with* intermaxillary fixation (IMF) and the system *without* IMF.

In the system *with* IMF, the affected jaw is immobilized by anchoring it to immobile portions of the skull by means of intra- and extraoral splints.

The system *without* IMF relies on stability as previously defined. Two mechanical principles are applied: *interfragmental compression* and *surgical splinting*. We already know the principle and effects of prestressing. Its practical application is interfragmental compression.

The ASIF has acquired more than 25 years of experimental and clinical experience with interfragmental compression (Matter 1986). The compression may be accomplished in either the *static* or *dynamic* form.

4.1.1 Static Compression

Two types of device are used to produce static interfragmental compression: the *self-compressing plate* and the *lag screw*.

Before discussing the instrumental aspects of static compression, we should consider the true purpose of compression: *The primary aim of interfragmental compression is the production of large frictional forces.*

Friction prevents gliding between the metal and bone. It enables a rigid fixation (with high bending strength) to be achieved that, with a minimum of material, can withstand all the forces that are imposed on the mandible during function. Bending, torsion, and shear forces associated with mastication are the major factors that disturb fracture healing. The complete neutralization of these forces obviates the need for intermaxillary fixation.

Even with immediate opening and movement of the jaw, the fracture will unite under functionally stable conditions. Interfragmental compression eliminates relative motion between the bone ends. The fracture is immobile (i.e., stable) and unites primarily with no intermediate fibrous stage. Thus the terms "prestressing" and "interfragmental compression" are equivalent. When sufficient interfragmental compression is applied at the time of internal fixation, the pressure between the bone ends *will not decrease to the "zero load" point,* and load cycling cannot occur (see p. 10). This is the manometrically defined criterion for stability sufficient to preclude implant loosening and bone resorption; hence it is a major prerequi-

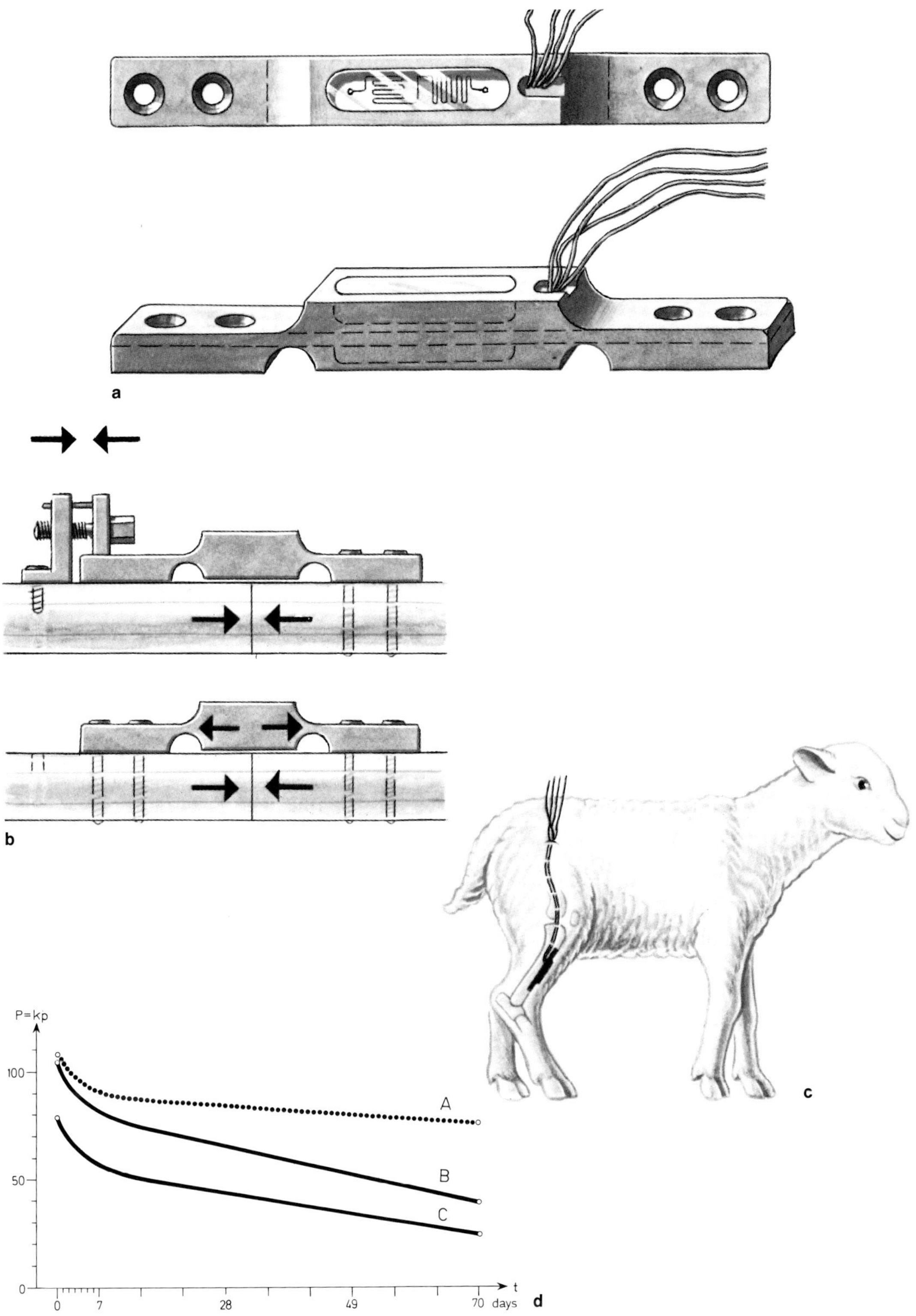

Fig. 27 a–d. Biomechanical experiments of Perren (1971). **a** The plate is fitted with strain gauges accurate to within 1.5 kg in the range of 300 kg. **b** The plate is prestressed using a tension device. The tension in the plate is directly proportional to the compression at the fracture site. **c** The plate is attached to the tibia of a sheep, and the leads from the strain gauges are brought out subcutaneously to the trochanteric area. **d** The standard curve plotted from dozens of measurements indicates a gradual decline of compression over a 4-month period. (From Müller et al. 1977)

site for uncomplicated fracture healing. It is this key discovery that forms the foundation of the ASIF method.

As for the traditional belief that pressure causes bone resorption, Perren and his colleagues (1969a) were able to show conclusively that bone will tolerate a static pressure of more than 300 kg/cm^2 without becoming necrotic.

But primary pressures of 50 to 100 kg are sufficient for a functionally stable internal fixation. By the end of two months these pressures decrease by approximately 50% and then remain fairly constant ("static compression") until fracture healing is complete (Fig. 27). The distribution of interfragmental pressure should be as uniform as possible during this time - a difficult condition to fulfill in mandibular fractures, as we shall see below. For now we shall consider the instrumental aspects of interfragmental compression.

4.1.1.1 Static Compression with a Prestressed Plate (DCP)

The ASIF has designed a self-compressing plate called the "dynamic compression plate" (DCP) (Perren et al. 1969b). It generates interfragmental pressure through a mechanism known as the "spherical gliding principle" - so named because it can be explained in terms of the movement of a sphere inside an angled cylinder (Fig. 28). If a screw with a spherical head is driven into a plate hole having the same geometric shape as the hollow cylinder, the hole will provide a track that compels and constrains the movement of the screw, as the cylinder does the sphere. It is this action from which the "dynamic compression plate" (DCP) derives its name. Lateral movement is impossible, hence there is minimal friction between the screw head and the hole.

The horizontal movement eliminates undesired locking between the screw and plate and prevents distraction of the fragments. As the screw is tightened, the shape of the plate hole adds a horizontal component to the vertical movement of the screw head. It ist this horizontal component that approximates the fractures surfaces and creates interfragmental pressure (Fig. 29). The distance traveled by the screw head (the compressive displacement) is predetermined by the geometry of the hole. The final position of the screw head is at the point where the inclined and horizontal portions of the "cylinder" meet. In that position the screw has optimum contact with the plate hole, and optimum stability is achieved. The compressive displacement of the 2.7-mm cortex screw is 0.8 mm (Fig. 30). Once the screw head has traveled that distance, reaching its definitive position in the plate hole, the interfragmental pressure is maximal, and no additional tightening will increase it. Hence, great importance is placed on a precise anatomic reduction and a standardized technique (use of the 0.8-mm DCP drill guide) so that the available compressive displacement can be fully utilized for axial compression (Fig. 31; see also Fig. 114).

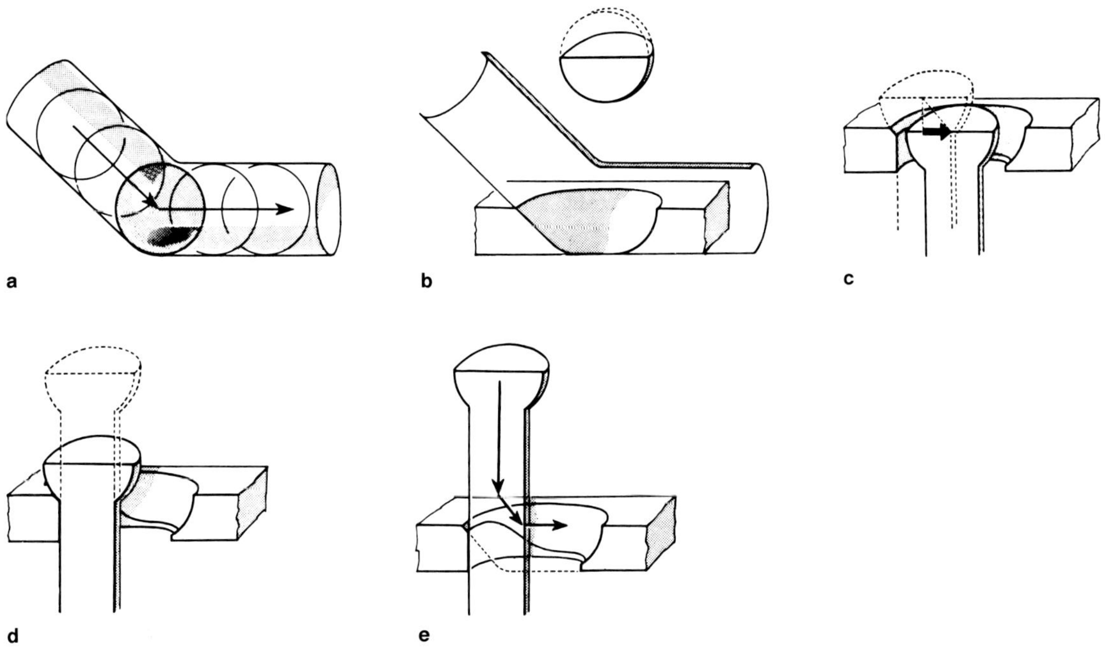

Fig. 28 a–e. Spherical gliding principle of the DCP as described by Allgöwer, Perren, and Matter. **a** Motion of a sphere in an angled cylinder. The sphere moves downward and then horizontally, the directional change occurring at the intersection of the inclined and horizontal cylinders. Lateral movement is prohibited. **b** The screw hole in the DCP is shaped basically like the middle segment of the angled cylinder, and the screw head is shaped like a sphere. Thus, when the screw is inserted, the motion of its head in the hole recapitulates the downward and then horizontal motion of the sphere in the cylinder, producing a corresponding movement of the bone fragment relative to the plate. The horizontal component prevents a "locking" action between the screw and plate. **c** DC plate hole, representing a combination of two hemicylinders, with matching screw head and neck. **d** Screw head on the gliding plane of the oblique hemicylinder. **e** Vertical and horizontal path taken by the screw during insertion. (From Spiessl 1976b)

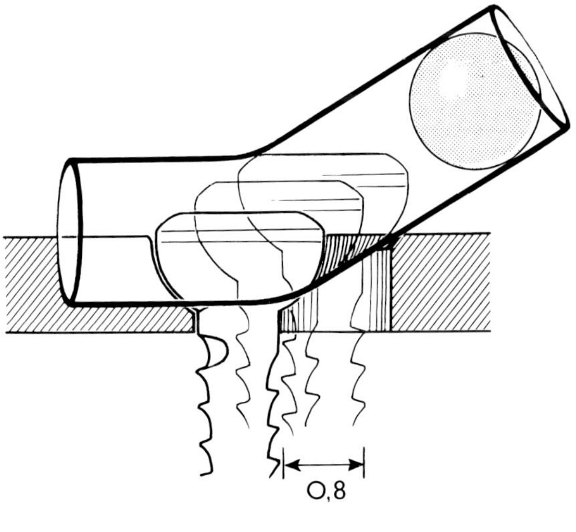

Fig. 29. Maximum stability of the plate and screw is achieved when the screw has traveled 0.8 mm to its definitive position

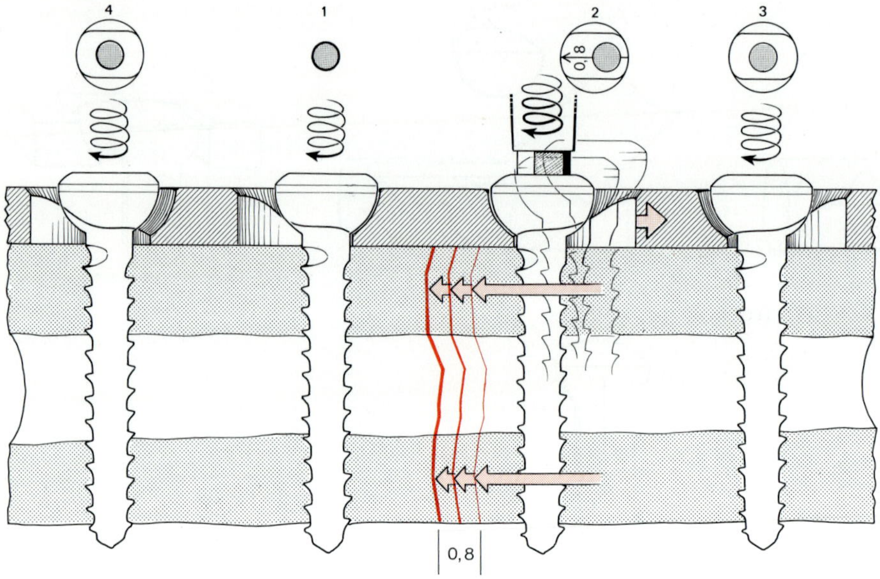

Fig. 30. The DCP acts by transforming the downward force of screw insertion into a longitudinally directed compressive force. This action displaces the screw and its fragment in the direction of the opposite fragment, resulting in static compression between the bone ends (= interfragmental compression). The interrelationship between the tension on the plate side and the pressure on the bone side is indicated by *arrows*. The *circle* marked with 0.8 and an eccentric inner circle symbolizes the 2.7-mm eccentric drill guide; 0.8 indicates the compressive displacement in mm that is produced by the DC hole of the plate

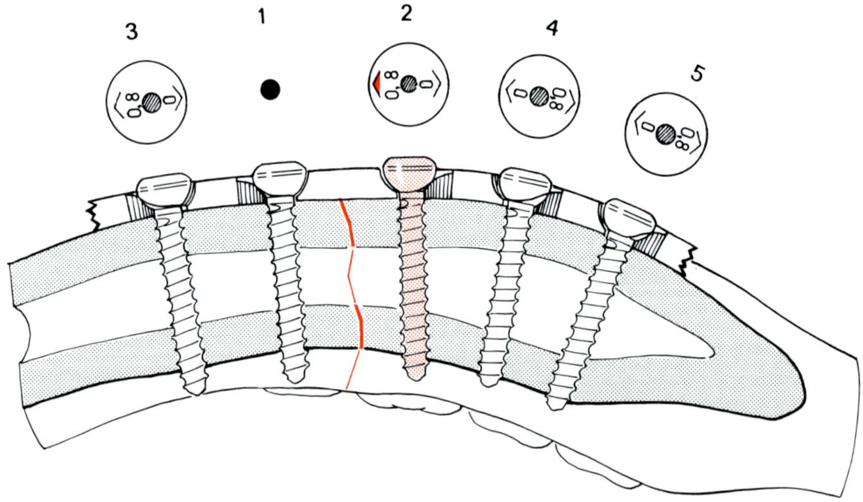

Fig. 31. Use of the DCP drill guide. After optimum reduction of the fragments, the contoured plate is fixed on one side of the fracture with a screw in the neutral position (*1*) so that the center of the plate is over the fracture line. The hole in the opposite plate hole is drilled using the DCP drill guide. The *arrow* marked 0.8 points toward the fracture line (*2*). With optimum reduction of the fragments, this will yield a compressive force of 60 kg or more. The remaining screws (sequentially numbered *3, 4,* and *5*) are inserted in the neutral position (*arrow* marked 0)

4.1.1.2 Eccentric Dynamic Compression Plate (EDCP) for Creating Uniform Pressure on the Oral Side

Clearly, it is desirable for the static compression to be distributed as evenly as possible over the fracture surfaces. But this is difficult to achieve in the mandible. The plate screws must not encroach upon the roots of the teeth or the mandibular canal, so we are limited to plating the narrow zone along the basal border. Peripheral fixation of this kind tends to produce an uneven pressure distribution at the oral or alveolar side of the fracture.

In vitro experiments (Vogel 1984) have shown that the pressure is greatest in the immediate zone of influence of the plate. In the mandible, then, the pressure is concentrated basally and diminishes in the oral direction (Graph 4), with associated distraction of the upper part of the fracture. This unstable situation can be avoided by use of the EDCP (Schmoker and Spiessl 1973). The two outer holes of the EDCP are oriented transversely or obliquely relative to the long axis of the plate (see p. 60). Even when applied basally, this device can produce uniform static compression at all points along the fracture line. The eccentric pressures measured for the 45° 4-hole EDCP are significantly greater than those produced by the 90° 4-hole EDCP (Graph 5; compare also p. 96, pressure roller prestressing).

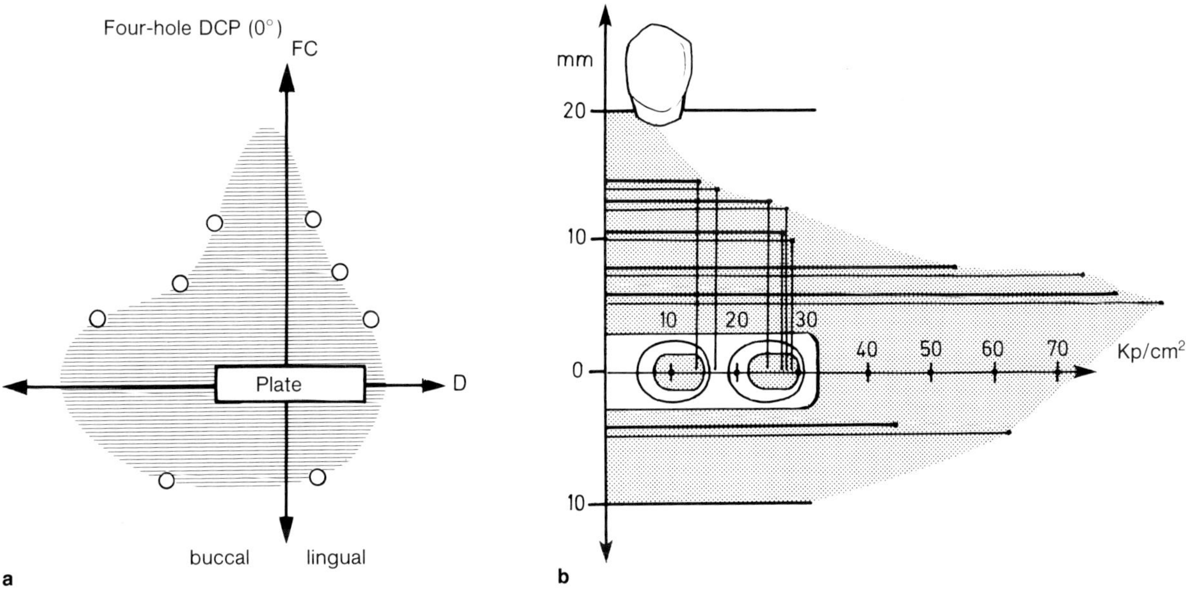

a b

Graph 4. Distribution of interfragmental pressure oral (superior), basal (inferior), buccal, and lingual to a *four-hole DCP* (extrapolated curves). *FC* Fragment contact oral and basal to the plate, *D* measured pressure values, *o* measured points. **b** Distribution of interfragmental pressure oral (superior) and basal (inferior) to a four-hole DCP. The pressures are highest in the immediate vicinity of the basally applied plate (from 60 to 80 kP/cm²) and fall off sharply in the oral direction

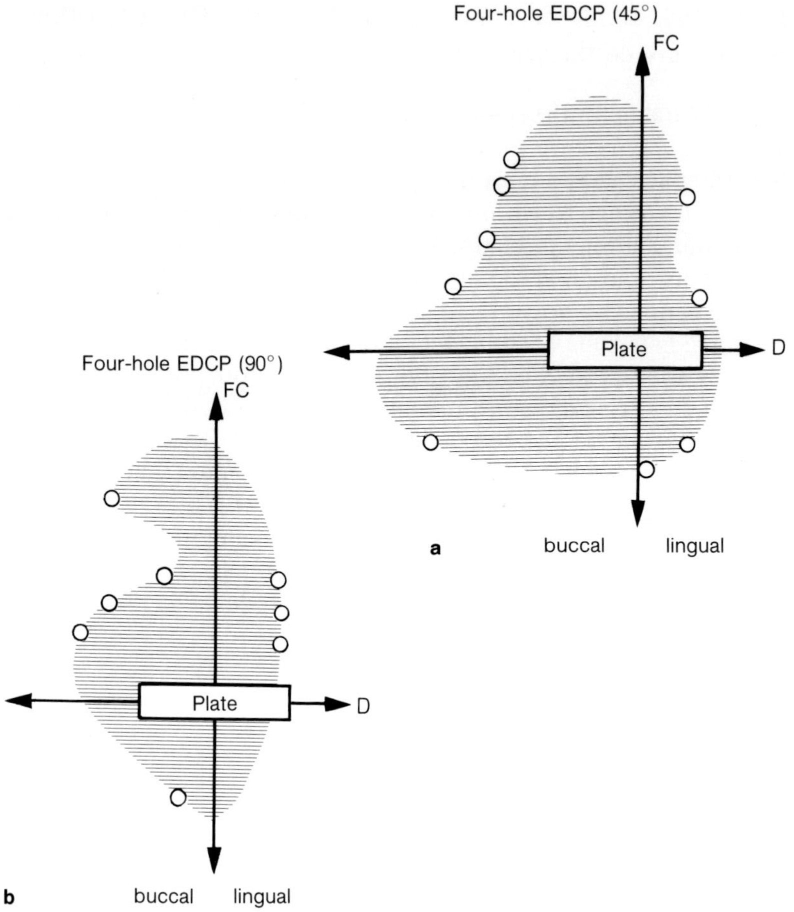

Graph 5. a Distribution of interfragmental pressure oral (superior), basal (inferior), buccal, and lingual to a *four-hole EDCP (45°)* (extrapolated curves). **b** Distribution of interfragmental pressure oral (superior), basal (inferior), buccal, and lingual to a *four-hole EDCP (90°)* (extrapolated curves)

4.1.1.3 Overbending the Plate to Improve Compression on the Lingual Side

A compression plate applied to the buccal aspect of the mandible tends to produce substantially higher pressures on that side than lingually (see Graph 4). This can result in lingual gaping of the fracture line with associated instability and malocclusion (see Fig. 17).

The in vitro measurements of Vogel (1984, see above) clearly indicate that a rise of pressure on the buccal side of the mandible leads to a fall of pressure on the lingual side. However, an optimum distribution of static pressure can be achieved by routinely "overbending" the plate by 1–2 mm. This imparts a spring action to the plate effectively apposes the lingual cortex (Figs. 32 and 18).

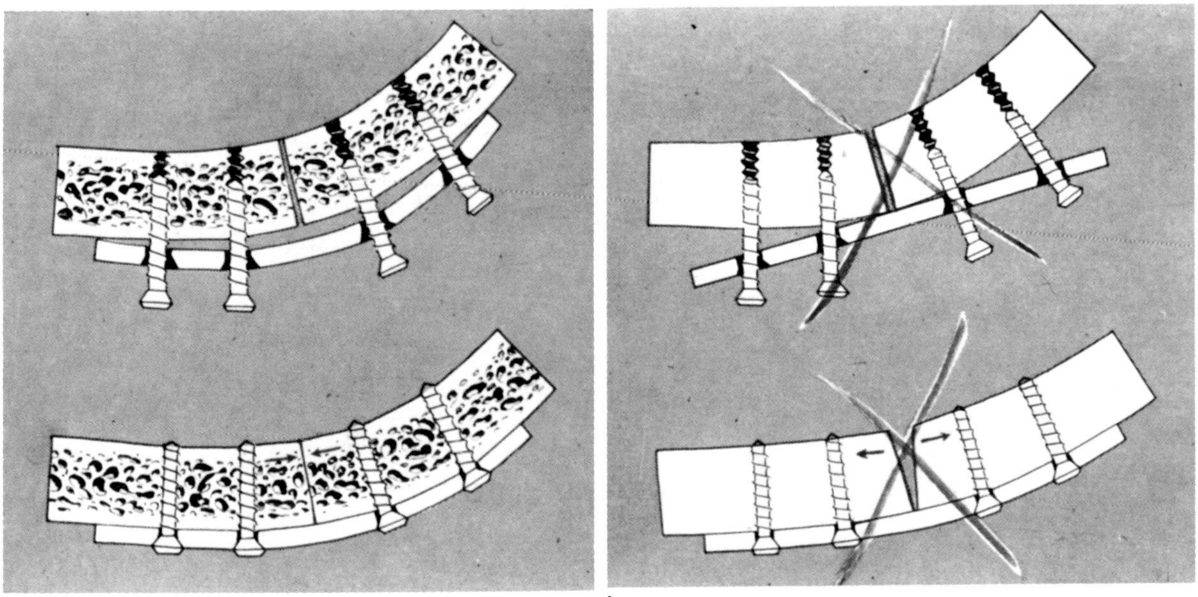

a

b

Fig. 32. **a** Effect of a slightly overbent plate (1–2 mm): closure of the gap on the lingual side. **b** Effect of a straight plate: widening of the gap on the lingual side

4.1.1.4 Static Compression with a Lag Screw

Even without a plate, interfragmental compression can be produced by means of lag screws. This technique, applied by Danis in 1949 for the fixation of oblique fractures in long bones, has become widely utilized. The principle is well known: A screw that glides through the cortex of one fragment and engages the cortex of the opposite fragment with its threads will, when tightened, draw the fragments together and compress their surfaces.
Several technical points must be borne in mind:

1) The gliding hole and thread hole must be coaxial.
2) When a cortex screw is used (Fig. 33 a), the gliding hole should match the outer diameter of the thread (2.7 mm), while the thread hole matches the diameter of the shank (2 mm) (Fig. 33 b). Otherwise the screw will transfix the fragments without approximating and compressing them (Fig. 33 c).
3) The screw should be placed so that it *bisects* the angle formed by lines perpendicular to the fracture line and to the long axis of the bone.

The applications for lag screws in the mandible are quite limited. Unlike the long bones, the mandible is a flat bone whose medullary space is occupied by the inferior alveolar nerve coursing between the mandibular and mental foramina. (Most fractures in this region run transversely or obliquely relative to the mandibular axis, the fracture surfaces occupying the fron-

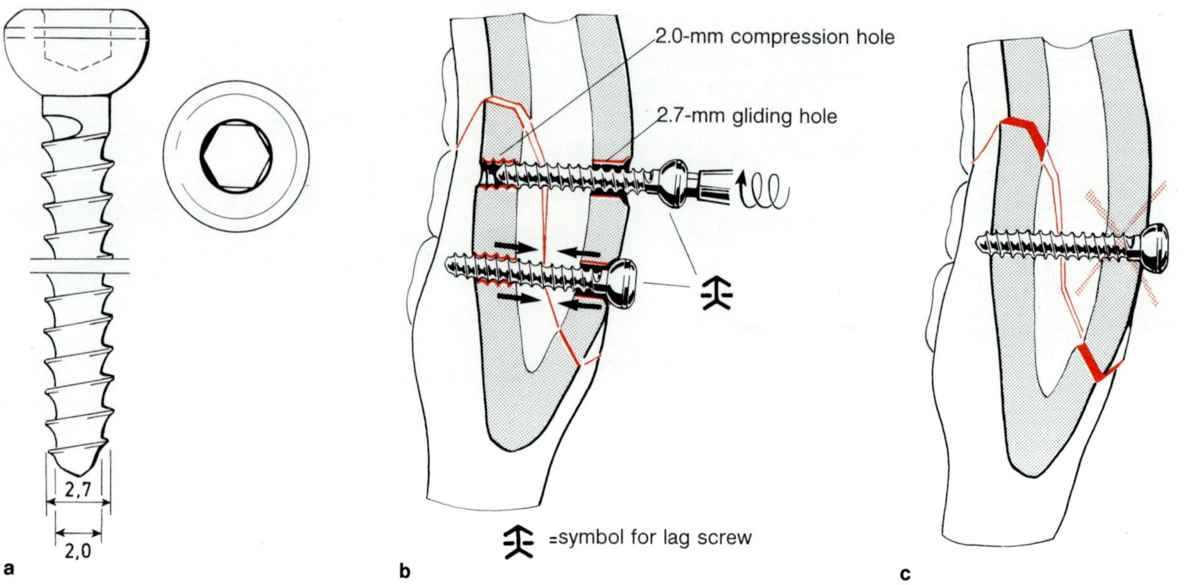

Fig. 33. **a** The 2.7-mm cortex screw: thread diameter 2.7 mm, core diameter 1.9 mm, spherical head diameters: 5.0 mm horizontal, 2.5 mm vertical, hex socket 2.7 mm; pitch 1.0 mm. **b** *Axiom:* Interfragmental compression is obtained only if the screw glides freely through the near fragment and grips the far fragment. The gliding hole is cut with the 2.7-mm drill bit; the compression (thread) hole is cut with the 2.0-mm bit and threaded with the 2.7-mm tap. The rounded tip of the screw projects about 2 mm from the bone to ensure that the last thread completely engages the far cortex. ⚹ Symbol for *lag screw.* **c** Without a gliding hole, the fragments are transfixed but not compressed

tal plane.) Because correct application of the lag screw principle requires that the implant be inserted across the fracture site, there is a potential for damage to the nerve and to the roots of adjacent teeth. Thus, lag screw fixation is appropriate only for "oblique-surface" fractures that exhibit a more sagittal than frontal orientation (see p. 154). A lag screw can be placed across a fracture surface on the sagittal plane without causing nerve or dental injury.

It is important to note that lag screws can produce a functionally stable fixation of the mandible only if the fracture surfaces are large enough to accommodate at least two and preferably three screws. The general rule states that the length of the fracture surface should at least equal the height of the mandible and should be twice the height of the atrophic mandible. This condition is satisfied in the oblique-surface fracture (Fig. 34a; see examples in Fig. 34c, 132b, and 216ff.).

In other oblique fractures that have a more transverse orientation, the lag screw can be used to supplement plate fixation, space permitting. The lag screw can greatly augment the rigidity of the plate fixation when used in this way. It should be considered that as the obliquity of the fracture surfaces increases, some of the primary tension in the plate becomes converted into a shearing force that is operative in the direction of the fracture line. Unless neutralized by interfragmental compression, this shearing force can cause displacement at the fracture site. In a 45° oblique fracture, for example, approximately 30% of the primary axial plate tension may be convert-

Fig. 34. **a** Rules for the use of lag screw fixation:
1) Ideal for the oblique-*surface* fracture: a ≥ b. The length of the fracture surface a should be greater than or equal to the mandibular height b.
2) Ideal number of lag screws: 3 or more in order to neutralize the functional forces in all directions (2 screws are an absolute minimum).

b Detail from a preoperative AP roentgenogram demonstrates the oblique fracture, which is found to be an oblique-*surface* fracture at operation. The fracture length is sufficient for the placement of 4 lag crews.
c Status after healing and prosthetic reconstruction of the anterior mandible

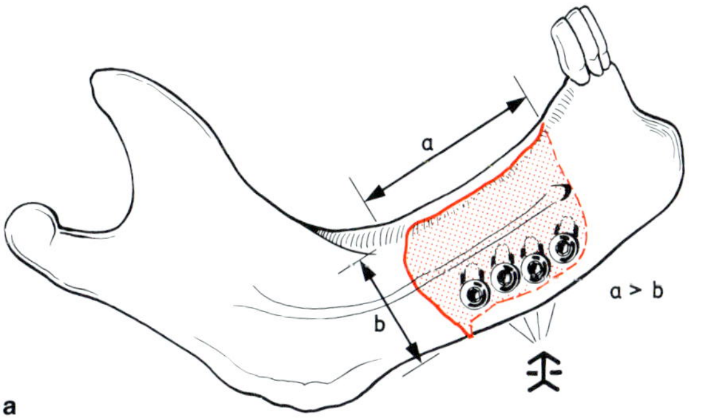

a

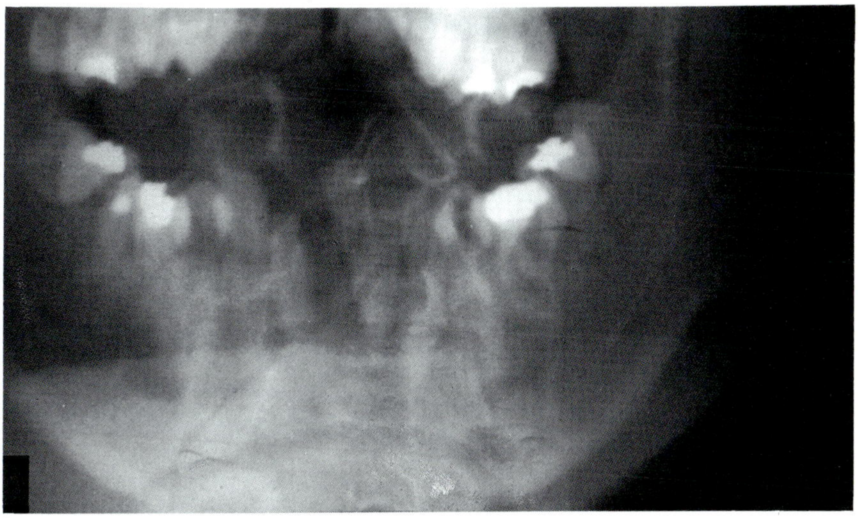

b

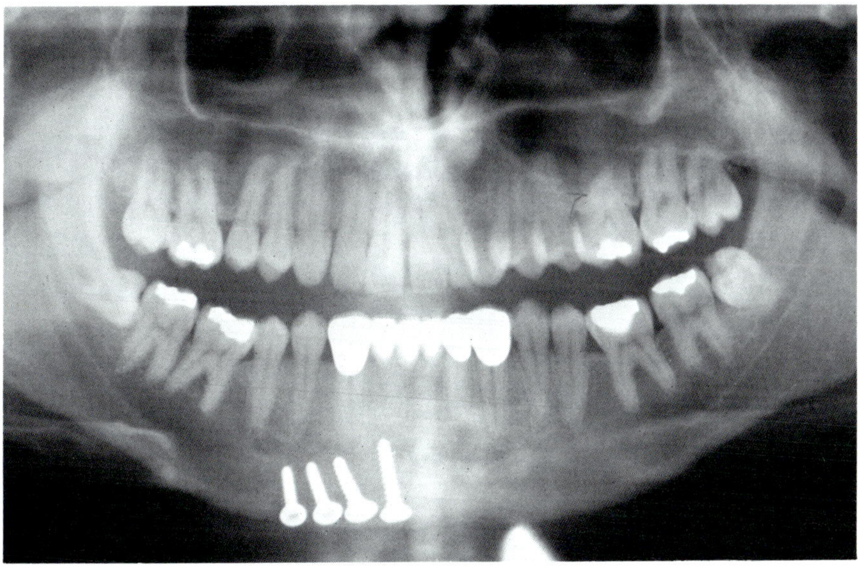

c

ed to shear. The shear forces can be eliminated by supplementing the compression plate with an interfragmental lag screw. The lag screw will also reduce the shear load on the plate itself.

The use of a lag screw as an adjunct to plate fixation may be planned from the outset, or the necessity of placing a screw across the fracture may become apparent when the plate is applied. In that case the plate hole over the fracture site may be left vacant, or a lag screw may be placed obliquely through the hole (see p. 107) so that it traverses the fracture at an optimum angle without causing nerve or dental injury (Fig. 35).

The lag screw can function as a retention screw to maintain the position of a wedge-shaped fragment in a segmental fracture. Not infrequently, the loose fragment will have to be fixed to a main fragment with a lag screw before the plate is applied to make sure that the small fragment will not slip out of alignment – the "antiglide" principle (Fig. 36).

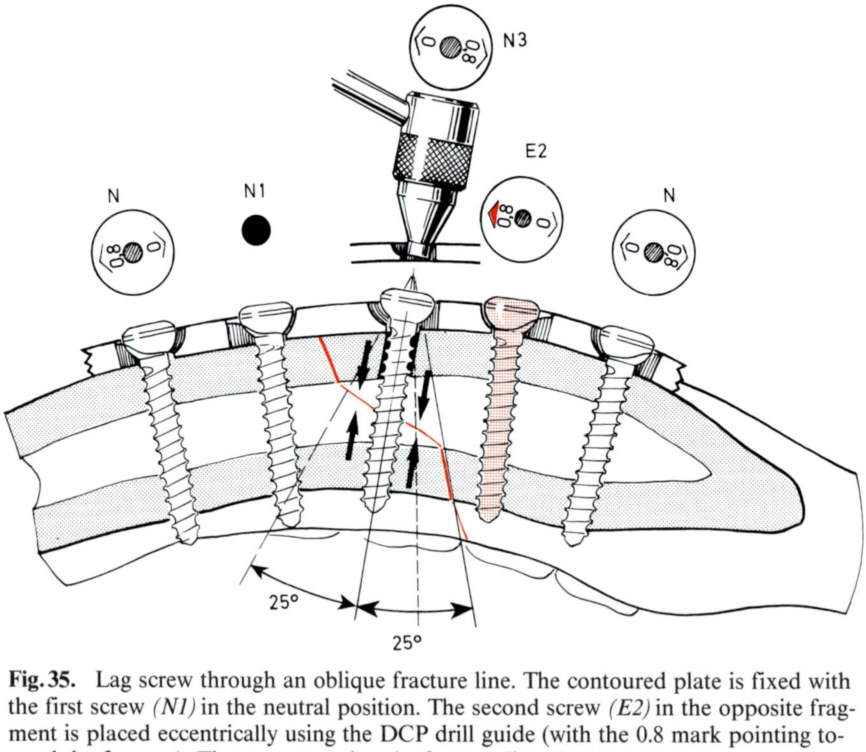

Fig. 35. Lag screw through an oblique fracture line. The contoured plate is fixed with the first screw *(N1)* in the neutral position. The second screw *(E2)* in the opposite fragment is placed eccentrically using the DCP drill guide (with the 0.8 mark pointing toward the fracture). The screw crossing the fracture line *(N3)* is a lag screw inserted through the plate. The spherical screw head in the round gliding hole makes it possible to angle the screw as needed to cross the fracture line at approximately right angles. The hole is drilled by positioning the drill guide at the appropriate angle (±25° in the axial direction, ±7° transversely). The remaining screws are inserted in the neutral position *(N)*

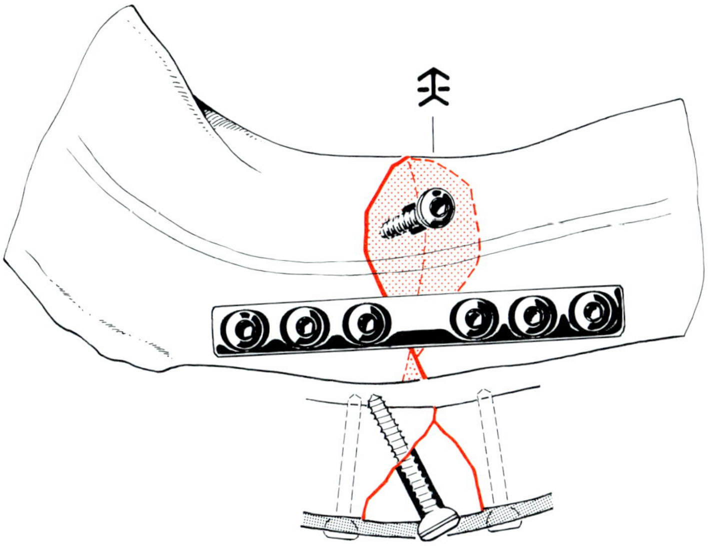

Fig. 36. Antiglide principle: The fragments are kept from slipping by applying axial forces to augment interfragmental compression. Lag screw fixation of the loose wedge fragment before the plate is applied prevents 1) redisplacement of the small fragment and 2) overriding of the main fragments at the jaw base when the 6-hole DCP is attached

Another application of the lag screw is for the refixation of a temporary mandibular osteotomy. Figure 37 illustrates the repair of an oblique mandibulotomy performed for the resection of an oral floor carcinoma.

Very good functional results have been achieved with a single lag screw for the internal fixation of angle fractures. This method, practiced by Niederdellmann (1980), offers the advantages of minimal implant material and an intraoral approach. With the fracture reduced, the gliding and thread holes for the lag screw are made using the percutaneous drill guide and

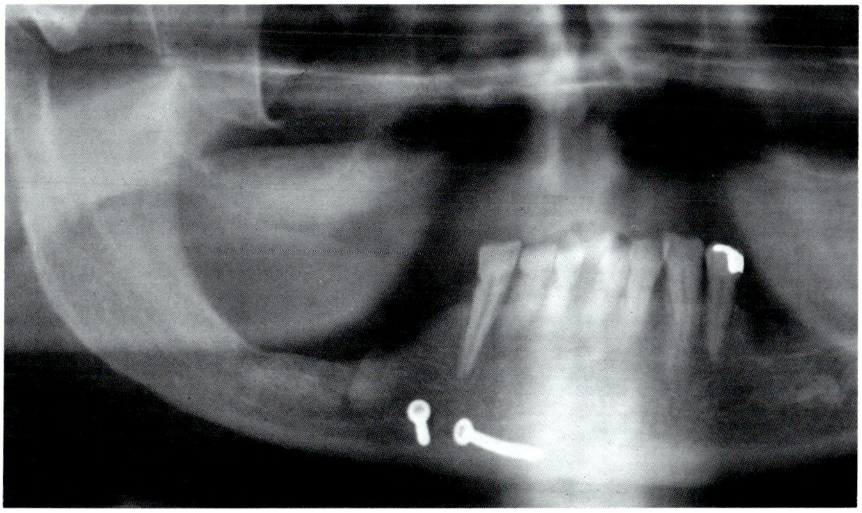

Fig. 37. Functionally stable refixation of a temporary oblique osteotomy of the mandible for removal of a carcinoma of the floor of the mouth

special countersink, and the screw is introduced by the same route (Figs. 38 and 39).

Though this method seems appealing at first sight, it requires specialized experience in determining the proper drilling angle and also in patient selection, since the technique should be limited to fractures involving only the mandibular angle (see p. 202). With this type of fracture there is a signifi-

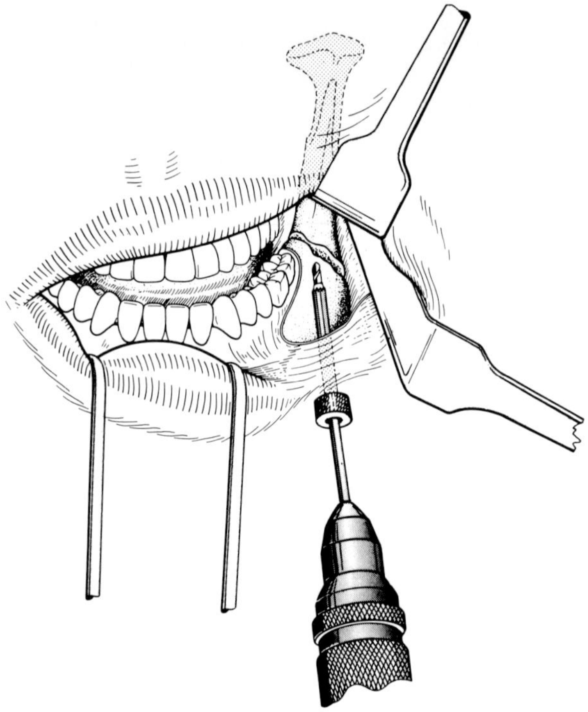

Fig. 38. Technique of single lag screw fixation of an angle fracture. A tap sleeve is used as a perfacial guide for drilling the 2.7-mm gliding hole and 2.0-mm compression hole. The tip of the drill bit is applied at the level of the third molar and oblique line (tension side), the bit forming a shallow angle with the oblique line. (Drawing courtesy of Prof. Niederdellmann, Regensburg)

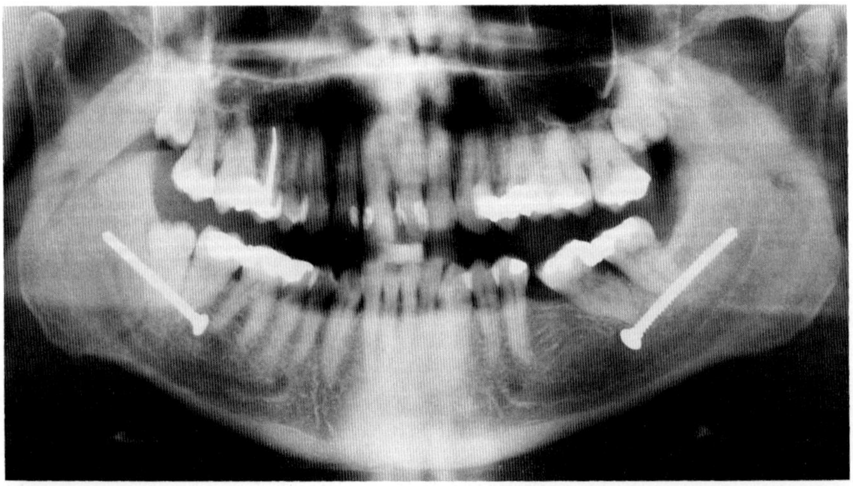

Fig. 39. Single lag screw fixation of bilateral angle fractures. Note that the third molar on the *right* side was retained to avoid iatrogenic displacement and preserve the bony buttress. (Roentgenogram courtesy of Prof. Niederdellmann, Regensburg)

cant danger of aligning the fragments improperly, leading to malocclusion, or of inserting the lag screw at a faulty angle to the fracture plane. The latter circumstance can complicate revisionary fixation and necessitate an extraoral exposure, assuming that intermaxillary fixation is not planned.

4.1.2 Dynamic Compression

The methods of static compression alone are not sufficient to cope with all fracture situations that may arise. The biomechanics of the mandibular motor apparatus and the special anatomy of the mandible frequently make it necessary to apply the principle of the tension band. Very simply, this principle utilizes *tension to counteract bending stresses.* With the bending stress neutralized, the total stress on the fixation system is drastically reduced. Pauwels (1935, 1965) was the first to make practical use of this principle. His classic schematic drawings (Fig. 40 a–d) show how effective the tension band can be in improving the relationship of load and stress in a mechanical system.

Practical application of the tension band principle is illustrated in the design of the tower crane. The load at the end of the cross-boom will cause

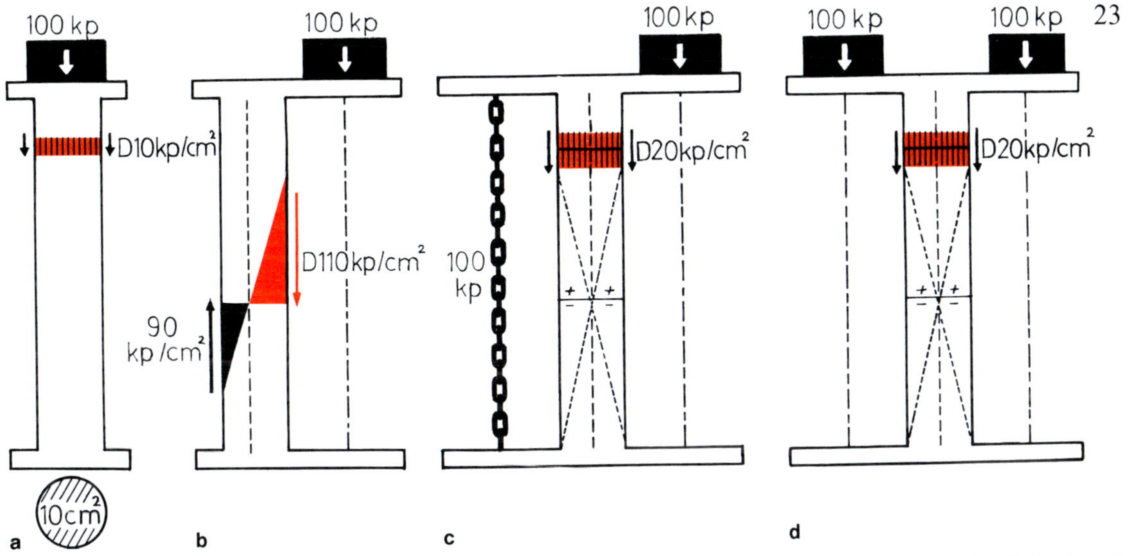

Fig. 40 a–d. Pauwels' schematic diagram illustrating the difference between load and stress and demonstrating the principle of tension band fixation. **a** If a column with a cross-sectional area of 10 cm^2 is loaded axially with a weight of 100 kg, it is subjected to a pure axial compression of D = 10 kg/cm^2. **b** Placing the weight eccentrically subjects the column to a bending load, which gives rise to new *compressive* and *tensile* stresses. In our example, the resultant compressive stress on the medial side equals 110 kg/cm^2, and the tensile stress on the lateral side is 90 kg/cm^2. These bending stresses can be neutralized by a *tension band* in the form of a chain (or wire). **c** The resultant compression equals the pressure exerted by a second weight placed on the opposite side of the column. **d** Although this increases the total load (200 kg), the total stress is reduced to one-fifth (D = 20 kg/cm^2) because the bending stress has been neutralized.
If we wish to use the tension band principle in internal fixation to increase interfragmental compression and neutralize bending forces, we must place the implant (wire or plate) at the site where tensile forces are greatest, i.e., farthest from the load axis. (From Müller et al. 1977)

the crane to collapse (Fig. 41 a) unless an effective counterload is present. This counterload is provided by a cable passed over the mast of the crane and down along its tension side. The cable brings the eccentric load into an axial alignment so that only compressive forces act upon the vertical mast (Fig. 41 b). This stabilizes the system and restores its load-bearing capacity using a minimum of material.

The same principle can be applied to internal fixation of the mandible. The tensile forces are absorbed by a tension band and transformed into compression both by the action of the compression-reduction forceps (Fig. 42) and by muscular pulls (Fig. 43), with the result that the ends of the fragments are pressed together. We call this process "dynamic compression" (not to be confused with the "dynamic compression plate," which is self-compressing).

Two conditions must be met in order for this principle to function: a bony buttress must be present, and there must be sufficient space to apply the tension band.

A bony buttress is necessary because the bone must absorb the functional loads that are transformed into compression; i.e., the shape and strength of the fragments must be such that they are able to transmit compression effectively. This is essential for a stable bone-metal composite system, because the true function of compression is to enable the implant to sustain a functionally stable internal fixation, and not to create it. If the integrity of the fixation relied solely on the implant, a high incidence of fatigue failure would result. An ideal bony buttress is present in all single and multiple transverse fractures that are anatomically reduced. An effective buttress is lacking, however, in comminuted fractures and fractures with a bone defect. These types of fracture require a reinforced implant that can bear the functional loads by itself (see p. 64 ff.).

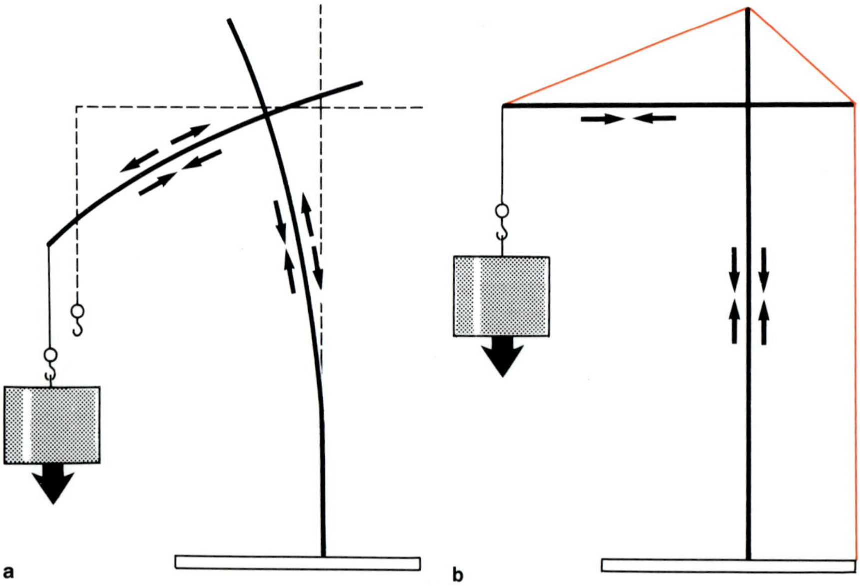

Fig. 41 a, b. Practical utilization of the tension band principle

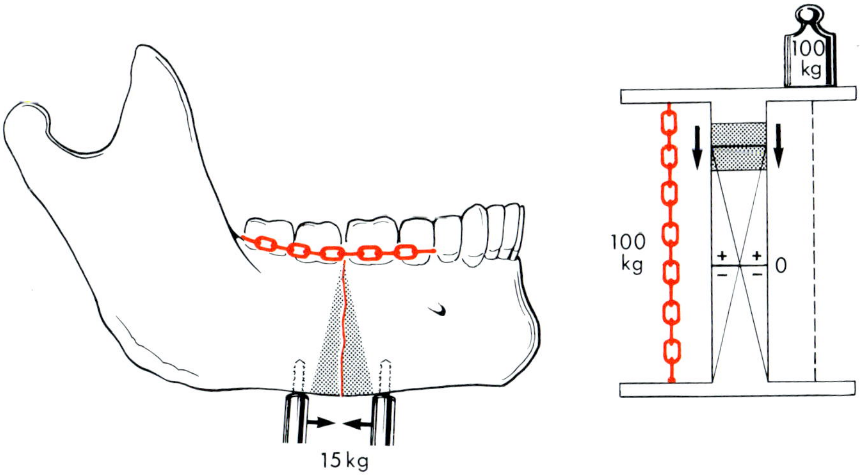

Fig. 42. Dynamic compression of the mandible, analogous to Pauwels' scheme. The bending stresses can be neutralized by a "chain," such as a dental splint, or converted to interfragmental pressure by applying a force of 15 kg across the basal side of the fracture with the reduction-compression forceps. [The stiffer the tension band (e.g., a wire acrylic splint), the more favorable the distribution of axial compression]

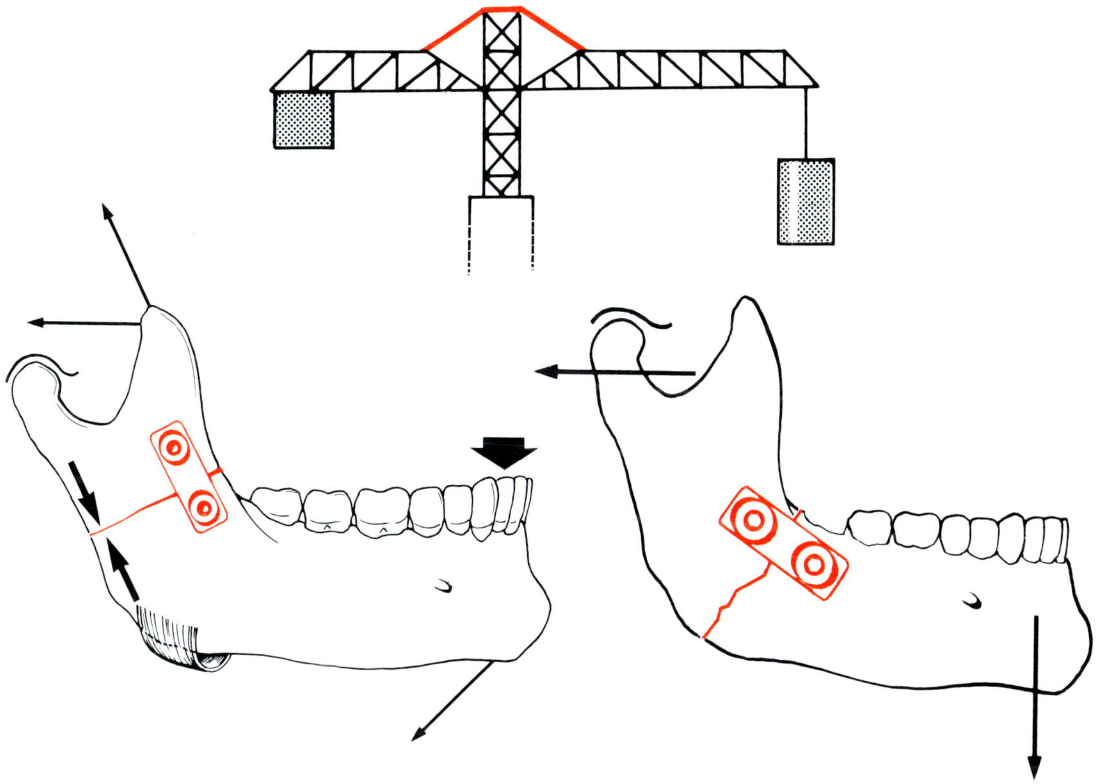

Fig. 43. *Left:* Internal fixation with a tension band alone eliminates the bending stress. The two-hole DCP (tension band plate) applied strictly on the tension side of the bone (= maximum distance from the load axis) neutralizes the tensile forces of the mandibular muscles and causes pure compression to act across the fracture site (= dynamic compression). *Right:* Here the tension band as the *one* component of a *plate and tension band system* (see p. 58 ff. and Fig. 50)

4.1.2.1 Application of the Tension Band Principle in the Mandible

In ideal situations, such as fractures of the femur, the tension band principle can be implemented with a single plate. But the special anatomy of the mandible limits its applications there, because the majority of fractures involve the body and angle of the mandible, where plating is made difficult by the presence of the teeth or mandibular canal. Thus, a classic application of the tension band principle is possible only in the relatively uncommon fractures of the supra-angular region (see Fig. 43, left).

4.1.2.2 Tension Band Plate and Tension Band Splint

The tension band principle involves not only the transformation of bending forces into compression but also the elimination of these forces. Therein lies its great value in the stabilization of mandibular fractures.

The typical mandibular fracture is unstable and will show varying degrees of abnormal motion and displacement according to the location, intensity, and direction of the imposed forces and muscular pulls.

We shall illustrate the tension band technique for the simple case of an axially displaced fracture. The pulls of the muscles that elevate and depress the jaw cause tension forces to develop on the oral side of the mandible and compressive forces on the basal side, causing the fracture to gape superiorly (Fig. 44 a). This gaping or distraction increases by a factor of 10 to 65 (Spiessl and Schroll 1972, p. 85) when a DCP is applied to what is often the only site available for plating - the inferior border (Fig. 44 b).

This a fundamental problem that cannot be solved without taking the tension side of the mandible into consideration. The DCP needs to be applied in conjunction with a tension band, which may take the form of a *dental splint* or *bone plate,* depending on the location of the fracture and the status of the teeth. The tension band need not be large. For example, a rigid splint anchored to a minimum of two sound teeth on each side of the fracture is adequate within the dental arch, and a two-hole plate is satisfactory for retromolar fractures (see Fig. 198 a, b). This minimal use of material is made possible by the fact that, as the height of the mandible increases in the direction of the ascending ramus, the resistance to bending forces increases geometrically (Küppers 1971, p. 14) while the vertical dimension of the bony buttress expands; finally the total stress is diminished due to reduction of the bending stress (see Fig. 40). Therefore the tension band does not require great strength. The farther the tension band is placed from the center of rotation of the fragments (Fig. 45), the lower are the stresses to which it will be subjected (up to 100 times lower). Conditions are most favorable in the dentulous mandible with an intact alveolar process, where the distance D between the inferior border and the splint or plate (3-4 cm) is maximal. Consequently a small splint will be adequate on the tension side. Behind the dental arch the distance between the retromolar trigone and the inferior border of the angle mandibular tends to be even greater, and a two-hole plate is satisfactory (see Fig. 43).

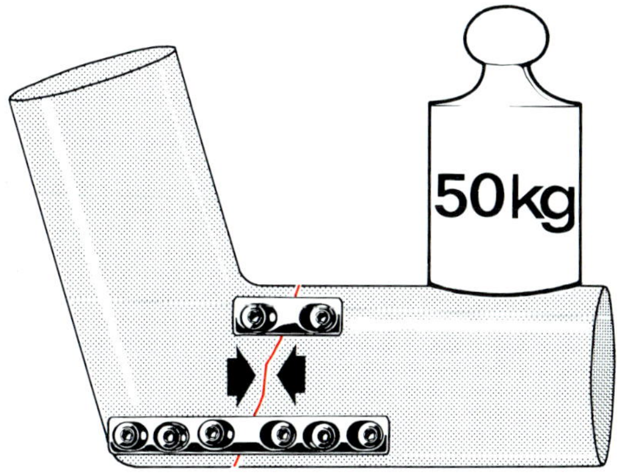

Fig. 50. *Plate and tension band system* comprising a two-hole tension band plate and a six-hole stabilization plate

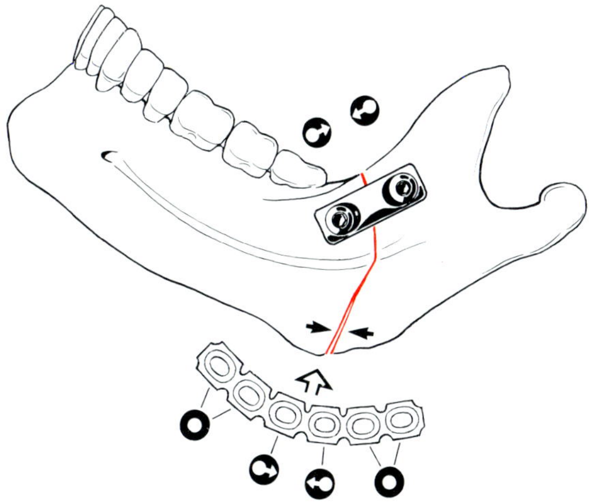

Fig. 51. Plate and tension band system in a central angle fracture, the angled reconstruction plate is used to comply with the three screw rule

4.1.2.6 Interfragmental Compression Without a Tension Band

Three factors contraindicate use of the plate and tension band system:

- lack of space,
- absence of teeth,
- lack of need.

In the great majority of fractures of the dentulous and edentulous mandible and in angle fractures, there will be insufficient space to apply a tension band plate. Moreover, gaps in the dentition often will preclude the use of a tension band splint for fractures within the dental arch. Then there is a category of fractures that can be adequately managed without a tension band: the isolated, reducible transverse fracture.

Thus, an EDCP or reconstruction plate *without* a tension band is indicated for:

- angle fractures,
- edentulous fractures,
- isolated transverse fractures.

4.1.2.7 Applications of the EDCP

The EDCP (eccentric dynamic compression plate) has longitudinal inner holes for producing interfragmental compression on the basal side and oblique outer holes for compression on the alveolar side (Fig. 52; see p. 109). The eccentric action of the plate obviates the need for a tension band, especially when a reduction forceps with pressure rollers is used initially to reduce and compress the fragments (Fig. 53). Especially in transverse fractures, this technique provides an ideal reduction and interfragmental pressure distribution. It is not easily applied to angle fractures, where the distal roller may not appose well to the bone. The need for extended exposure of the fracture may be seen as another disadvantage. Nevertheless, the pressure roller principle is an ideal adjunct. The EDCP, with or without pressure rollers, is generally indicated for smooth transverse fractures in the molar region. The transverse fracture of the edentulous mandible is an ideal indication (Fig. 54). The EDCP is not appropriate for central fractures of the mandibular angle (Fig. 55), as there is not enough space to insert the necessary number of screws. These cases should be managed with a recon-

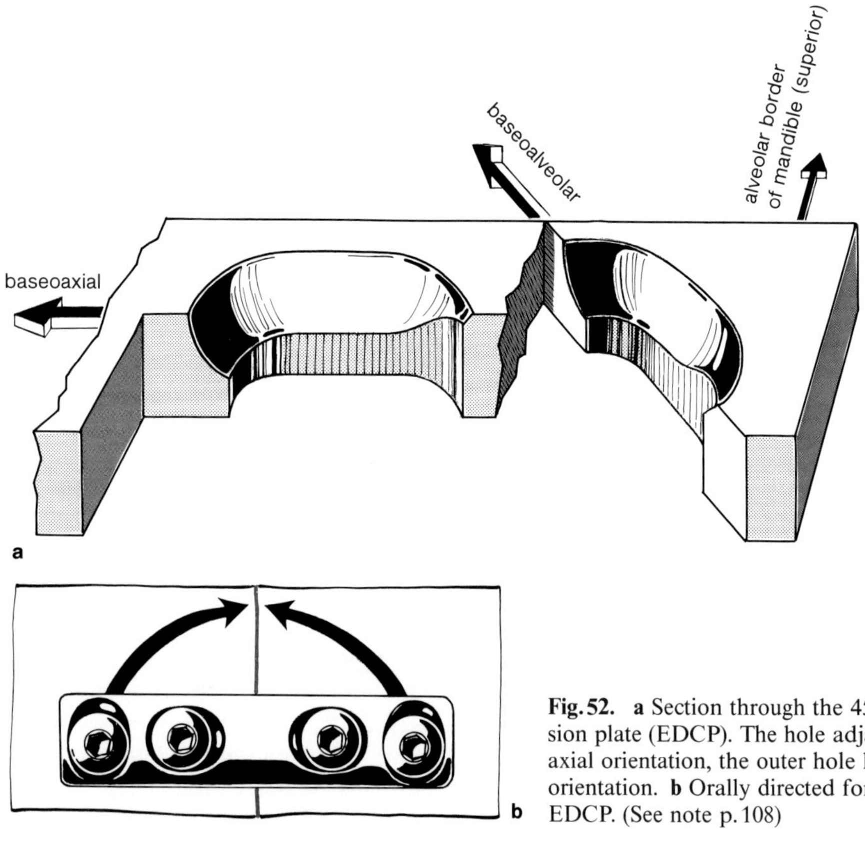

Fig. 52. **a** Section through the 45° eccentric dynamic compression plate (EDCP). The hole adjacent to the fracture has a baseoaxial orientation, the outer hole has an oblique, baseoalveolar orientation. **b** Orally directed force component with a 90° EDCP. (See note p. 108)

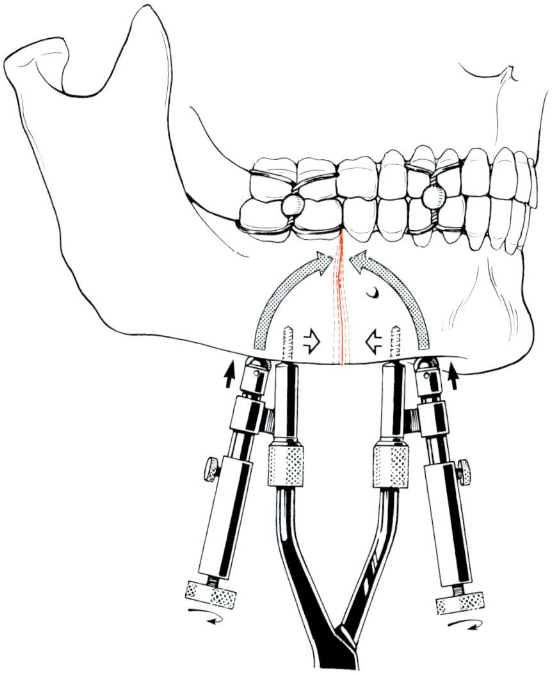

Fig. 53. Effect of pressure rollers on the compressive action of the reduction-compression forceps. Both baseoaxial and baseoalveolar compression are obtained (occlusal reduction is maintained with *Ernst ligatures*, which consist of V2A steel wire 0.5. The twisted maxillary and mandibular wire ends are surrounded with self-curing resin to protect the mucosal surface of cheeks)

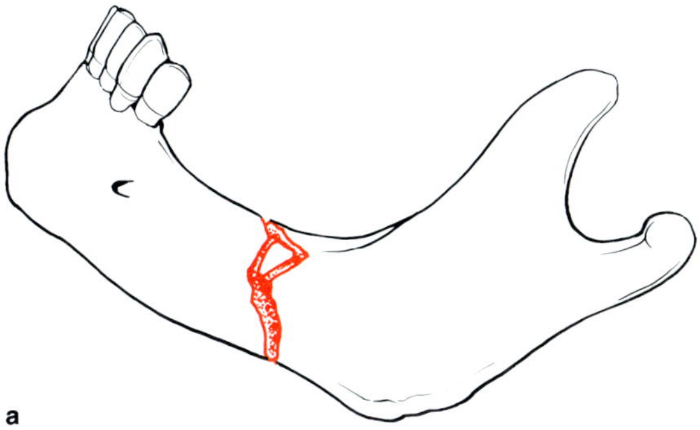

a

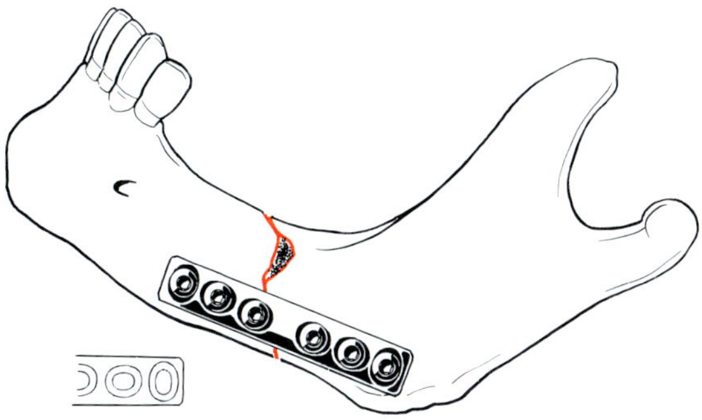

b

Fig. 54. **a** Ideal indication for the EDCP: fracture located between the canine tooth and mandibular angle, with no teeth available for splinting. **b** Mode of application of the six-hole EDCP (the four-hole EDCP may not give adequate stability)

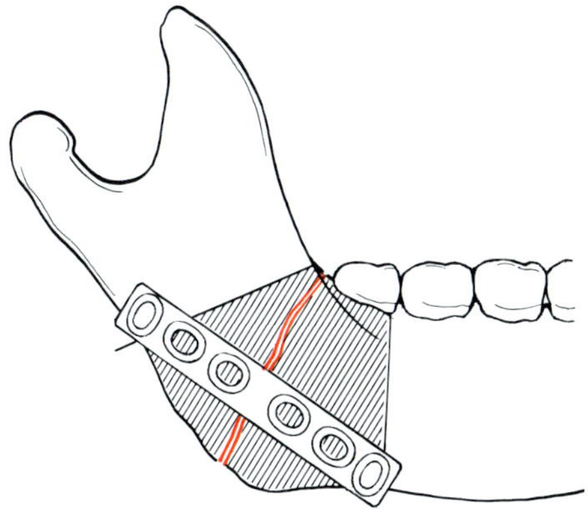

Fig. 55. The EDCP is contraindicated for a central angle fracture, as there is not enough space for a *third* (eccentric) screw on each side (see p. 191)

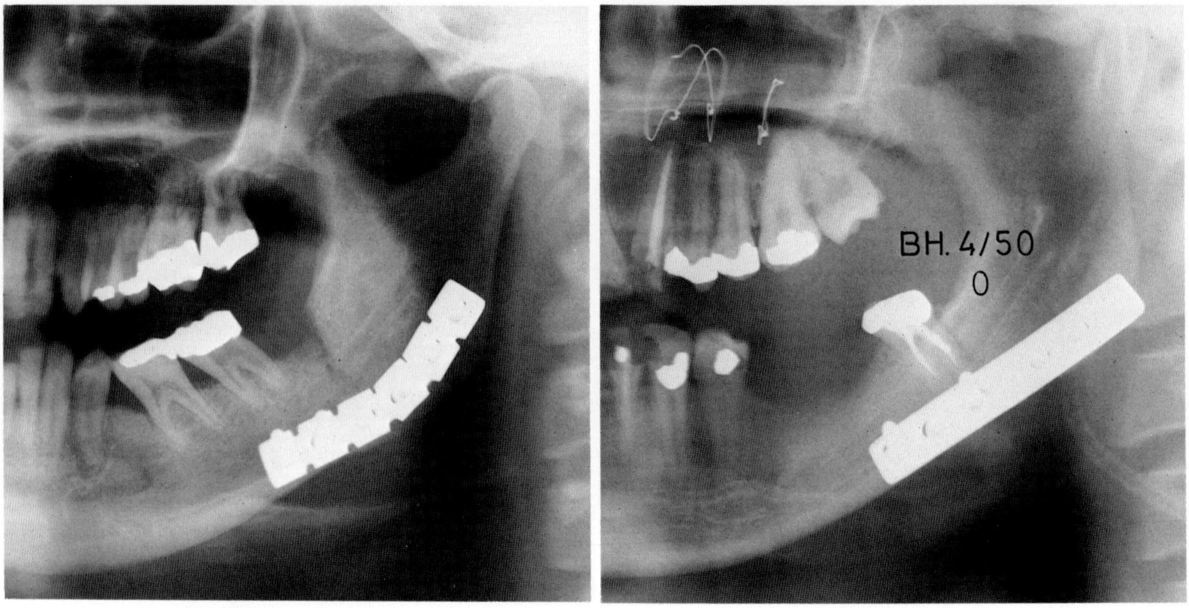

a b

Fig. 56. **a** A *central* angle fracture is stabilized with the reconstruction plate instead of the EDCP. The contoured plate permits the use of three screws per fragment. **b** The EDCP can be used on a marginal angle fracture, as there is room for placement of a third (eccentric) screw in the proximal fragment (see p. 197). However, the eccentric compression in this fragment is occasionally uncertain because of the angulation of the fragment and its termination at the joint

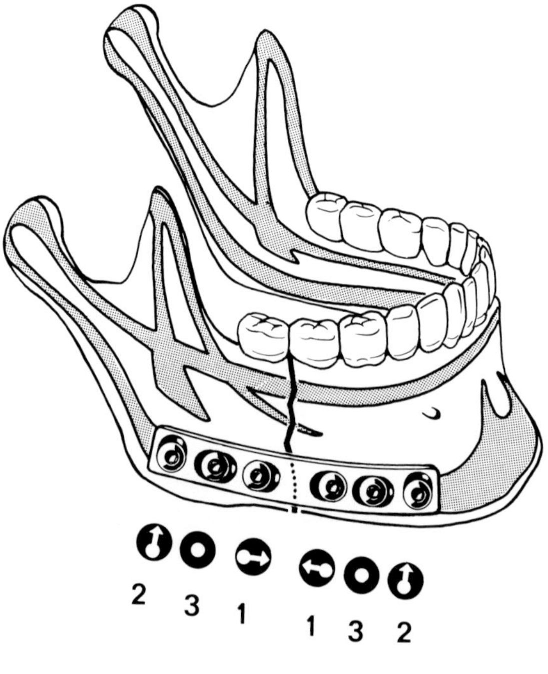

Fig. 57. The functional reconstruction of the tension trajectory depends on the efficacy of the gliding mechanism in the eccentric screw hole. Besides the transverse holes, *the holes adjacent to the fracture play a key role in the generation of interfragmental pressure.* A stripped screw hole in this area often leads to instability and infection

struction plate that conforms to the shape of the mandibular angle (Fig. 56a). An EDCP can be used for marginal angle fractures where there is space for the placement of three or four screws on the angle side of the fracture line (Fig. 56b). Experience has shown that, as in other types of fracture, a four-hole EDCP is too weak. The EDCP may be used only if the "three-screw rule" is satisfied (Fig. 57; see also p. 191).

4.1.2.8 Applications of the Reconstruction Plate (see Fig. 137a–e)

There are other types of fractures that are difficult or impossible to manage with the devices and techniques described thus far. This problem led to the development of the reconstruction plate – a longer, reinforced version of the basal stabilization plate designed for use without a tension band.

The reconstruction plate is twice as thick as the DCP and EDCP. It comes in 6- to 24-hole lengths, and preshaped models are available for use in the angle region. The plate is malleable and can be adapted to local bony contours. In addition, the plate has two-way DC holes that enable compression to be applied in either longitudinal direction, depending in the placement of the drill hole (Fig. 58).

The reconstruction plate is indicated for all difficult fractures of the mandible that require a plate with special contouring capabilities, especially angle and supra-angular fractures and multiple fractures.

In apical angle fractures (see p. 191 ff.), care should be taken that a minimum of three holes are active in each fragment. This provides maximum static strength that ensures uncomplicated bone healing even if interfragmental compression cannot be produced. It is recommended that standard preshaped reconstruction plates be used on the mandibular angle, since overbending a straight plate can deform the holes, thus degrading the compressive action of the plate and interfering with the seating of the screw head.

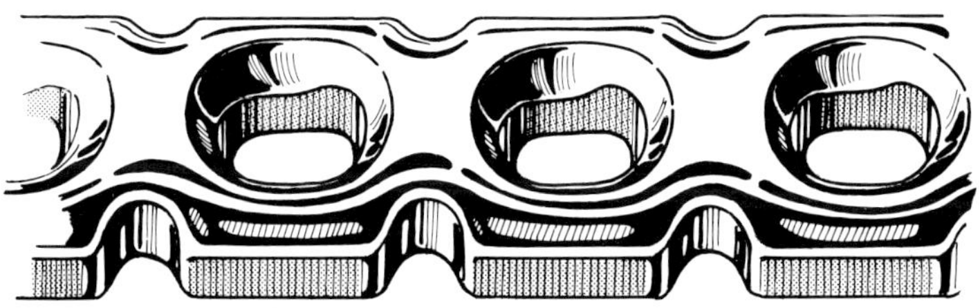

Fig. 58. The reconstruction plate has two-way DC holes or applying compression in either longitudinal direction

4.2 Principle of Surgical Splinting

Surgical splinting should not be confused with dental splinting. The surgical splint is a high-strength, stainless steel device that is applied directly to the bone.

The strength or rigidity of the splint is not as high as that of a system that functions by interfragmental compression (DCP or EDCP). But the purpose of the splint is to immobilize the fragments, not compress them, so that the fracture can go on to union. The only difference with respect to interfragmental compression ist that the splinted fracture may show some degree of callus formation on radiographs.

In accordance with the general principle of internal fixation that the functional load at the fracture site must be offset by a counterload of equal magnitude, the splinting device must have a correspondingly stronger anchorage than the DCP. This condition is satisfied by the reconstruction plate, whose practical importance derives from the universal scope of its applications (see p. 110).

It is clear that interfragmental compression is not a workable principle in comminuted fractures and fractures with bone loss, since the bone generally is incapable of significant stress transfer (see p. 240). Interfragmental compression is replaced by the reconstruction plate, which *buttresses* the fragments against displacement and angulation while absorbing all functional loads to restore continuity and permit early mobilization despite extensive fragmentation of the bone.

Unlike the dental splint, the surgical splint attaches directly to the bone to give ridigity to the main fragments. This principle can be applied in two forms: *internal* splinting an *external* splinting.

4.2.1 Internal Splinting

4.2.1.1 Buttressing

The chief function of the internal splint is to buttress large fragments which are separated by an area of comminution that cannot absorb or transmit stabilizing forces effectively. The reconstruction plate spans the comminuted area (see p. 254 ff.) to preserve or restore the original shape, length, and strength of the mandibular arch (Fig. 59 a). Intervening fragments of sufficient size may be fixed with a separate screw (Fig. 59 b). Another indication for buttressing besides the comminuted fracture is a fracture of the atrophic mandible (Fig. 60 a). Most of these injuries are shear fractures occurring secondary to osteoporosis. The obliquity of the fracture contraindicates fixation with a DCP or EDCP, because slippage of the oblique fracture surface would spoil the self-compressing mechanism of the plate. The fracture area is insufficient for fixation with lag screws (minimum of two), and the cortex is so thinned by atrophy and osteoporosis that the bone would be likely to shatter during drilling or screw insertion, even with the use of a countersink.

The best solution in these cases is to buttress the thin fragments with a reconstruction plate (Fig. 60 b). Dentures, if present, will aid the reduction. Retention of the mandible in correct occlusal relation to the maxilla is ac-

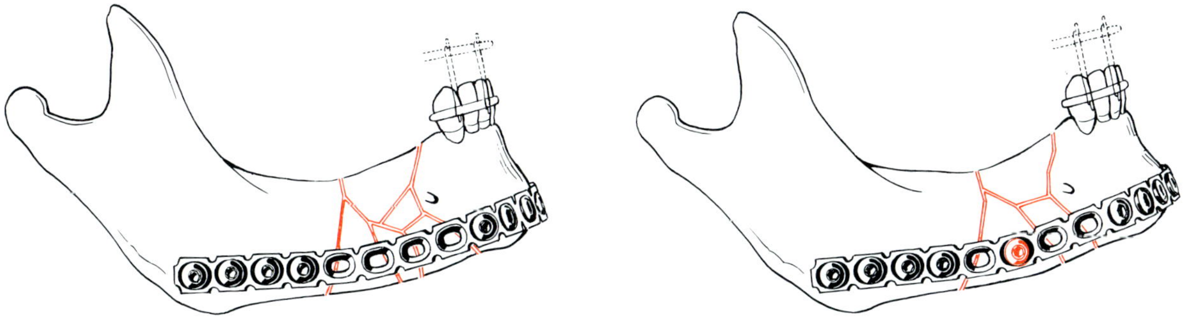

a b

Fig. 59. **a** Principle of internal splinting: The comminuted area is buttressed and supported by spanning it with the reconstruction plate. **b** Separate fixation of a relatively large individual fragment in the comminuted area that retains a periosteal attachment

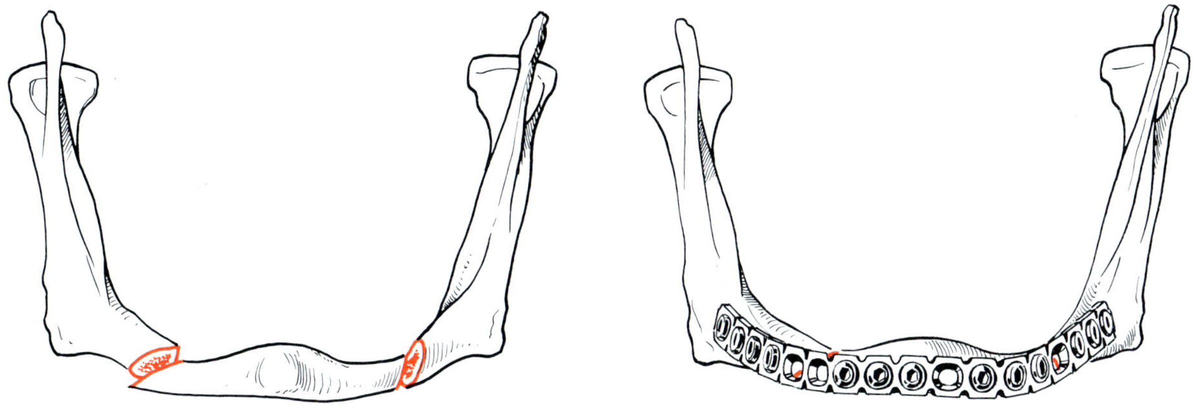

a b

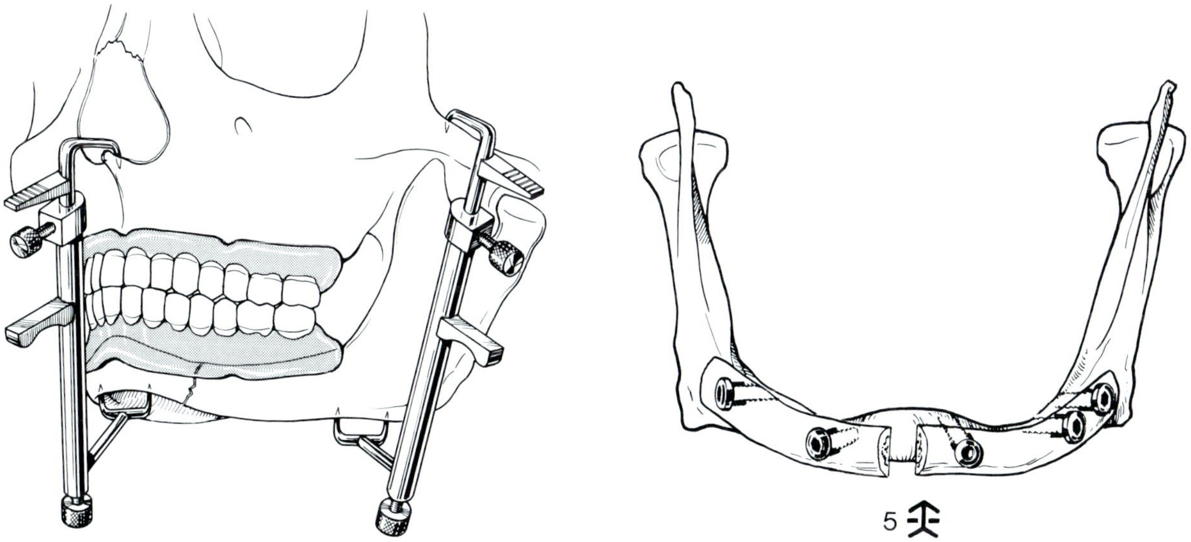

c d

Fig. 60. **a, b.** A common type of bilateral fracture in the atrophic mandible is stably bridged with the reconstruction plate. **c** Intra- and extraoral retention of the reduced fragments with existing dentures and intermaxillary clamps. The anterior clamp engages the nasal floor through the nares, and the lateral clamp engages the zygomatic arch through the soft tissues. **d** Lag screw fixation of autologous rib grafts placed at the time of plate removal to augment the atrophic mandible complished with intermaxillary clamps (Fig. 60c). A year or so later, at the time of plate removal, the atrophic mandible can be augmented by bone grafting. This can be done with rib grafts held in place by lag screws (Fig. 60d).

4.2.1.2 Bridging

"Bridging" means the creation of a stable connection between the bone ends in cases where a bony buttress is absent or deficient. The bony buttress is absent in comminuted fractures and fractures with a segmental defect (see pp. 255 and 262).

The goal of bridging is the primary restoration of the basic form and function of the jaw. The process begins by positioning the mandibular stumps in correct relation to the maxilla and securing them by temporary intermaxillary fixation. Any existing teeth are utilized to support the fixation. Then the defect is bridged with a reconstruction plate attached to the mandibular stumps with at least four screws per side ("four-screw rule") to permit immediate function.

This procedure greatly facilitates intensive care and minimizes late posttraumatic sequelae. Later, after reconstruction of the soft tissues, bone grafting can be performed under the stable conditions afforded by the bridge plate.

Besides fractures with bone loss and gunshot fractures, bridging is appropriate for the mandibular defects created by tumor resections. Benefits are a significant lowering of morbidity through early function and reduced mutilation through primary soft-tissue reconstruction. Restoring the jaw contour with a bridge plate is especially useful as a prelude to the reconstruction of external defects in the wall of the oral cavity (see p. 264).

4.2.1.3 Internal Bone Splinting Combined with Interfragmental Compression

Some oblique-surface fractures may allow the placement of no more than one lag screw. It is necessary in such cases to "protect" the single lag screw with a plate. Torsion and shear forces can be effectively neutralized with a bridge plate, also called a "neutralization" plate (Fig. 61).

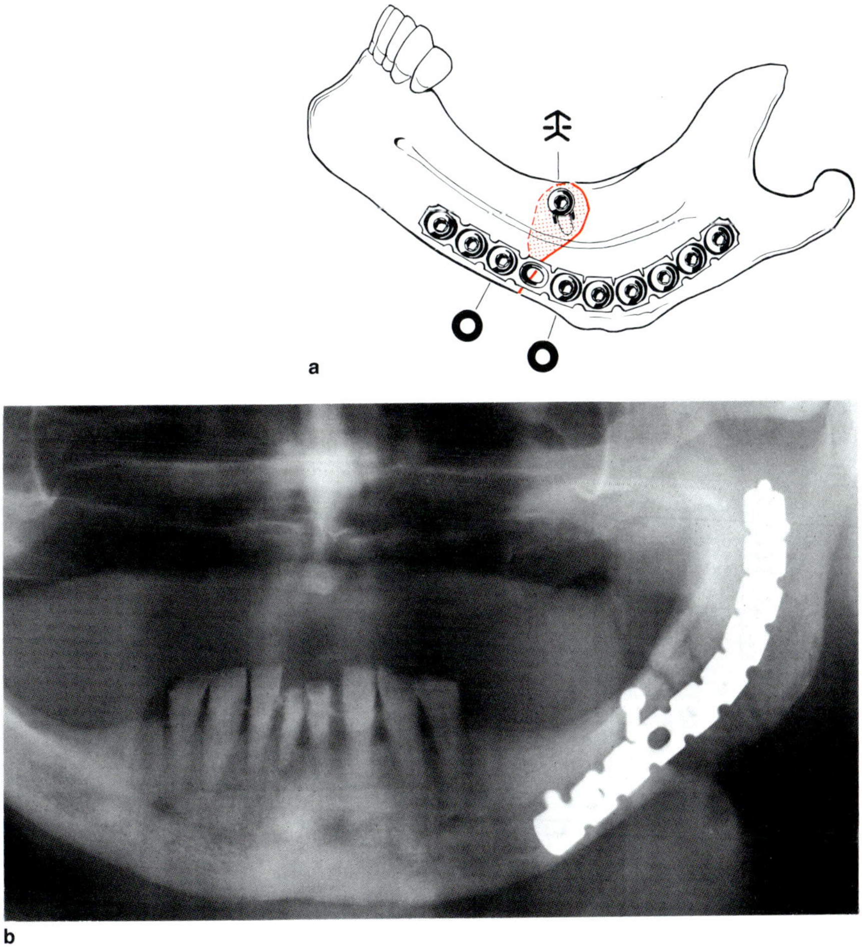

Fig. 61. **a** "Neutralization plate" protecting the lag screw in an oblique preangular margin fracture. Principle: The static compression produced by the lag screw is maintained during fracture healing by using a reconstruction plate to neutralize torsion and shear forces during function. The screw holes for the plate are drilled in the neutral position (the "O" arrow on the eccentric drill guide; see Fig. 31) so that the plate screws will not disrupt the placement of the lag screw. **b** Illustrative roentgenogram

4.2.2 External Splinting: External Fixator

Finding the optimum solution for a particular fracture problem depends on more than asepsis, anesthesia, and instrumentation. It requires a mastery of various modes of therapy. Each mode has its ideal and poor indications. It would be futile to attempt to apply a single treatment method to all types of fracture. For this reason it is appropriate to consider a form of treatment that has been widely regarded as outmoded, but which provides an option for cases where internal fixation would be disadvantageous: external skeletal fixation.

4.2.2.1 Principle, Design, and Advantages

The external fixation device offers an alternative to the buttress or bridge plate as a medium for stress transfer in the deficient mandible. External fixation is a *biologically* oriented modality that involves *no periosteal stripping* of bone, yet serves the same operative goal as internal fixation: reduction and functionally stable fixation of the fragments and the bridging of discontinuities. Thus, external fixation differs from internal plating in that it is a *closed* technique that *preserves or only minimally disrupts the nutritive milieu of the traumatized bone.* The external fixation device consists of skeletal fixation pins interconnected by external elements to form a single, stable framework. The frame is assembled by means of clamps.

The mandibular fixation device that will be described below is a two-dimensional, one-bar type of system. The use of two or three pins (Schanz screws) per main fragment and the proximity of the connecting bar to the bone afford optimum stability with a minimum of soft-tissue disruption and implanted foreign material. Additional advantages are the small time expenditure at the start of treatment, the ability to make adjustments during treatment, and the ease of removal at the conclusion of treatment.

4.2.2.2 Clinical Significance

There are several reasons why, despite these advantages, external fixation is not widely viewed as an acceptable alternative to functionally stable internal fixation. One is the lack of development in the technique and application of external fixation in the mandible. The horseshoe shape of the mandible makes it necessary to erect the pins and frame in a horizontal, one-plane configuration. This arrangement, along with deficient techniques for anchoring the pins in the bone, has resulted in high rates of failure. Another problem is that patients find the external hardware objectionable, especially because of its exposed location. This objection goes beyond cosmesis, for the device interferes with natural head movements during gait, restricts flexion of the head, and can be cumbersome during rest or sleep. Pin fixation of the extremities, by contrast, is associated with considerably less physical and emotional discomfort.

Another factor is that the effects of soft-tissue damage have much less biologic significance in maxillofacial surgery than in surgery of the extremities. Wounds with contusion of the surrounding skin and damage to the underlying muscles, vessels, or nerves, representing a Grade 2 or Grade 3 injury in general traumatology, do occur in the head region, but their local consequences are far less severe. (Indeed, an entire limb may be lost due to the severity of soft-tissue injuries.) This explains why external fixation has assumed greater importance in general traumatology and orthopedic surgery. In those fields growing interest is centering on the application of two principles: the ring-like frame of Wittmoser and Ilisarov (Schewior and Schewior 1984; Hierholzer et al. 1985) and designs such as the unilateral frame, bilateral frame, and polygonal frame. Here the *primary goal of external fixation is the management of soft-tissue problems in the immediate post-injury or postoperative period.*

Nevertheless, external fixation has a legitimate role in the management of certain problem cases in mandibular surgery. It does not compete with internal fixation in this capacity, but rather extends the range of available treatment options. When the technique of mandibular external fixation is more fully mastered and understood, it will provide a third treatment modality with its own indications. The design of the fixation device should be as simple as possible, and its external dimensions should be acceptable to the patient. Its rigidity is implicitly associated with a certain "instability". It should be stated at the outset that the only realistic goal of external fixation is secondary bone healing with the formation of a fixation callus. The lack of absolute immobility compared with functionally stable internal fixation leads to the formation of an irritation callus that undergoes remodeling in response to functional loads - a process normal in bone healing. But therein lies the advantage of external fixation: In only 6-8 weeks the irritation callus attains a strength that permits safe removal of the fixation device. With primary bone healing, by contrast, the plate and screws must remain in the body for an average of one year. External fixation must be maintained for a comparable period only in the presence of certain bone diseases such as osteoradionecrosis (see p. 88).

Thus, external fixation is closer to conservative fracture therapy in its biologic effect (callus formation), but unlike conservative methods it permits *immediate oral opening*, analogous to a functionally stable internal fixation. This function is comparable to "exercise stability" in the internally fixed limb, and a soft diet may be consumed during the first two weeks after the frame is applied.

4.2.2.3 Indications

The indications for external fixation of the mandible are limited to:

- *infected* open comminuted fractures, fractures with bone loss, and gunshot fractures (Grade 4 and 5);
- open fractures in multiply injured patients;
- pathologic fractures;
- osteomyelitis in the presence of unstable internal fixation;
- preliminary fixation after a mandibular resection;
- in exceptional cases, repositioning of the ascending ramus following a sagittal split osteotomy.

For these indications external fixation offers a genuine alternative to rigid internal fixation. The application of a plate invariably produces some degree of vascular insult. This is associated with a transient lowering of resistance to infection, especially on the side adjacent to the implant. Reoperation and implant removal for early infection frequently disclose an avascular, nonreactive cortical surface. This compromise of cortical viability explains why the initial weeks after plating represent a critical phase in terms of fracture healing.

It also explains why the plating of an open fracture is always a high-risk procedure, even if there are no overt signs of infection. On the other hand, experimental and clinical experience underscore the need for the operative stabilization of problem fractures with impending or presenting complications. Immobilization of the lesion is a necessary prelude to early revascularization and proper differentiation of the pluripotent mesenchymal cells at the fracture site. When these conditions are met, it has been found that healing consistently progresses well despite the initial critical phase.

In summary, the true purpose of operative fixation is to prevent complications by preserving natural barriers to infection and protecting the bone healing process. External skeletal fixation fulfills this purpose by bridging the endangered area.

4.2.2.4 Historical Aspects of External Fixation

Lambotte (1913) and Anderson (1936, quoted in Rowe and Killey 1955) initiated the use of percutaneous half pins in fracture therapy. Converse and Warnitz (1942) later applied the method to the treatment of mandibular fractures. The authors called their modified apparatus the "Frac-Sure" appliance.

Converse cautioned that the method, known then as pin fixation, was not "everyday surgery for everybody". There were major problems relating to infection, aseptic necrosis of bone, as well as to the instability, size, and weight of the hardware. Metal rods or polymeric materials were used to interconnect the skeletal pins and hold them in place.

A number of authors (Mathis 1956; Ullik 1953; Lorenz 1953; Schüle 1957; Harnisch and Gabka 1962; Frenkel 1961) advocated pin fixation of mandibular fractures on the grounds that it was a relatively simple procedure that enabled the patient to move the jaw while the fracture was healing. The procedure was mainly reserved for displaced fractures of the edentulous mandible, comminuted fractures, and fractures with a bone defect. Schüle cited the infected fracture as an additional indication.

Technical refinements were made in the Anderson device by Converse and Warnitz (1942) and later by Schüle (1957). The system consisted of Roger-Anderson pins with a self-tapping thread and a square end. Potential early complications included facial nerve injury, malalignment, and redisplacement (Birke 1972). Finally the high incidence of osteitis, soft-tissue infection, and nonunion caused pin fixation, which had been universally accepted for nearly tow decades, to be all but forgotten.

In 1984 Janecka of the U.S. published a case report on the external stabilization of the mandible with a "mini-H fixator" employing bicortical fixation pins, a prebent connecting bar, and compression clamps (Janecka 1984).

4.2.2.5 Biomechanics of External Fixation

By its nature, the mandible is not well suited for external splinting. The only sites available for the placement of fixation material are biomechanically unfavorable. Yet the external fixation device should be stable enough to neutralize disruptive forces and should also be acceptable to the patient. The latter requirement has led to a preference for a monoplanar assembly over a three-dimensional frame. However, this arrangement provides only a marginal type of fixation similar to that of a dental splint. This prompted Baumann (1973), in cooperation with the Mathys Co. of Bettlach, Switzerland, to develop a three-dimensional external fixation device. The fixation pins are arranged in horizonal and vertical rows (Fig. 62) and are linked by connecting bars to form a polygonal frame (Fig. 63). In experiments on dogs the system yielded a stability comparable to that of functionally stable

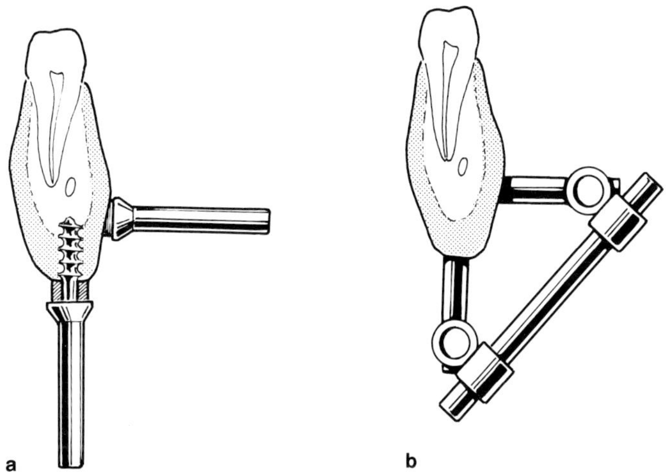

Fig. 62. **a** Each Schanz screw is supported by a shoulder and washer. **b** Polygonal external frame designed by Baumann (1973) (tested on the mandible)

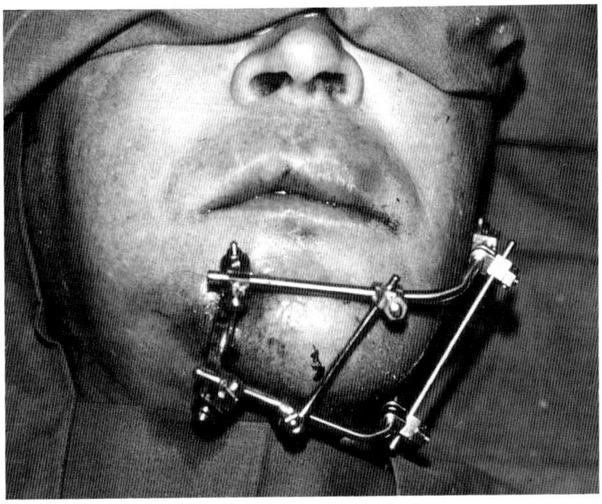

Fig. 63. Polygonal external frame (see text)

internal plating. However, this design did not gain wide acceptance because of its bulkiness and the potential for nerve injury during pin insertion.

Unless "humanized," external fixation of the mandible is simply not an acceptable mode of treatment, a compromise must be made in favor of a less stable but more easily tolerated two-dimensional type of assembly.

4.2.2.6 One-Bar External Fixator[2]

4.2.2.6.1 Three Components

The tow-dimensional or "one-bar" external fixator is well suited for bridging and stabilization of the mandible. In contrast to other designs, the device has only three components.

The *first* component is the metal connecting bar, which is 4 mm in diameter and preshaped to match the contour of the mandible. The bars are available in complete, three-quarter, and half-arch lengths (Fig. 64), depending on the location and configuration of the fracture. This results in a smaller, easier-to-handle device that simplifies the placement and removal of pin clamps. It also permits the use of a *drill guide system* which makes it easy to insert all the fixation pins on one plane. The shape of the connecting bar can be finely adjusted without kinking by using the special anvil of the plate bending pliers (see Fig. 126 c).

[2] I gratefully acknowledge the assistance of Dr. S. Winter (1987), Dr. C. Eicke, the Basel Dental Institute, and the Straumann AG Institute of Waldenburg in the development of this device.

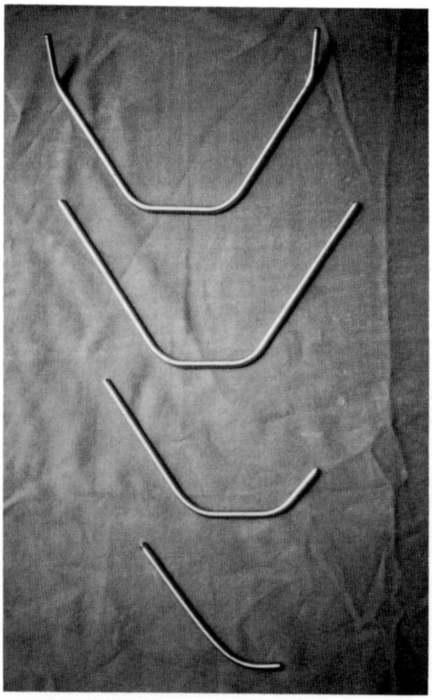

Fig. 64. Preshaped bars for the mandibular external fixation device. From *top* to *bottom:* complete arch with and without an ascending ramus, three-quarter arch, half arch

The following *bending technique* is recommended: For example, to make an individually contoured bar from a piece of straight stock, the bending should be started at one end of the bar and progress toward the other end. Any excess that remains is cut off.

Bending through a large angle should be performed in multiple small steps so that a curved shape is obtained rather than a sharp angulation. Otherwise the bar may be weakened excessively. The closer the successive bends are placed together, the sharper the curve. Any tracks or ridges left by the bending process should be polished smooth so that the clamps can slide easily on the bar.

The *second* component is the fixation pin, which consists of a Schanz screw with a "short thread" (Fig. 65). The short thread embodies a new technical principle that significantly enhances the stability of the screw in the bone. Sequin (1985, quoted in Hierholzer, Allgöwer, Rüedi) was able to show that Schanz screws which grip the inner cortex with a short thread have much greater rigidity than screws with a longer thread that grip both cortices. This is true only if the tubular shank of the screw fits snugly within the unthreaded drill hole in the outer cortex (Fig. 66), the diameter of the shank being 1.5 mm larger than the 2.0-mm core of the short thread. Besides giving improved bending stiffness and torsional stability, this arrangement permits the use of standard ASIF drill bits (2.0/3.5 mm) for pin insertion (see Figs. 69 and 72).

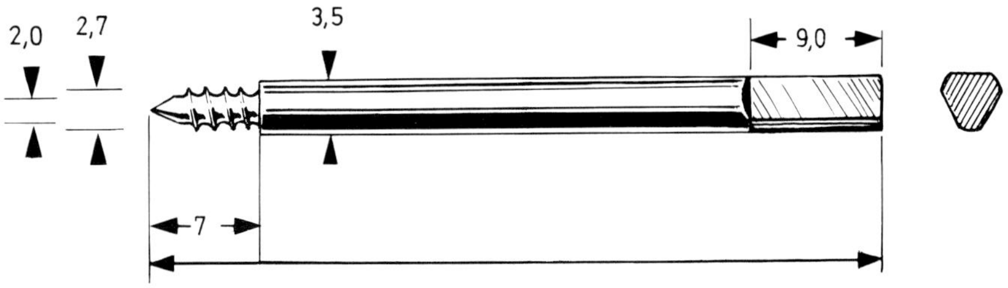

Fig. 65. Schanz screw for the mandibular external fixation device, available in lengths of 50, 60, and 70 mm to accommodate soft tissue swelling

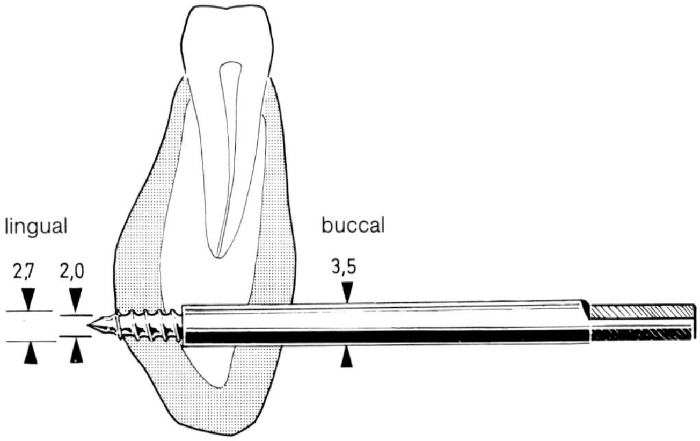

Fig. 66. Stiffness is increased by anchoring the thread in the far cortex and the shank in the near cortex (see text)

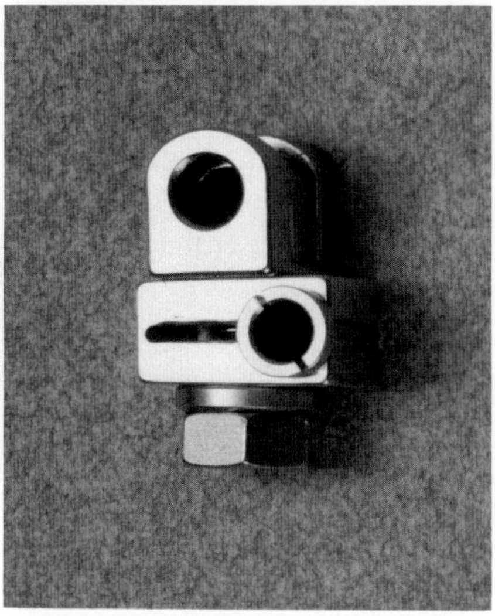

◁ **Fig. 67.** *Closed* swivel clamp for connecting the Schanz screw to the metal bar. The top clamp fits over the bar; the bottom clamp, with the slotted collar, holds the Schanz screw

▽ **Fig. 68.** *Left:* The *open* swivel clamp can be placed anywhere on the erected bar. *Center:* Guide clamp; can be substituted for the pin clamp to provide a drilling aperture. *Right:* Open swivel clamp in combination with the guide clamp for the "Troika" (Fig. 69)

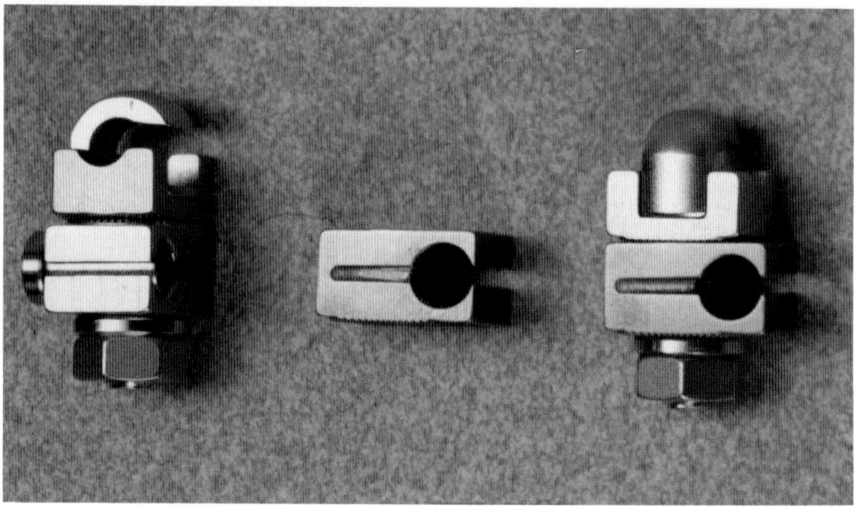

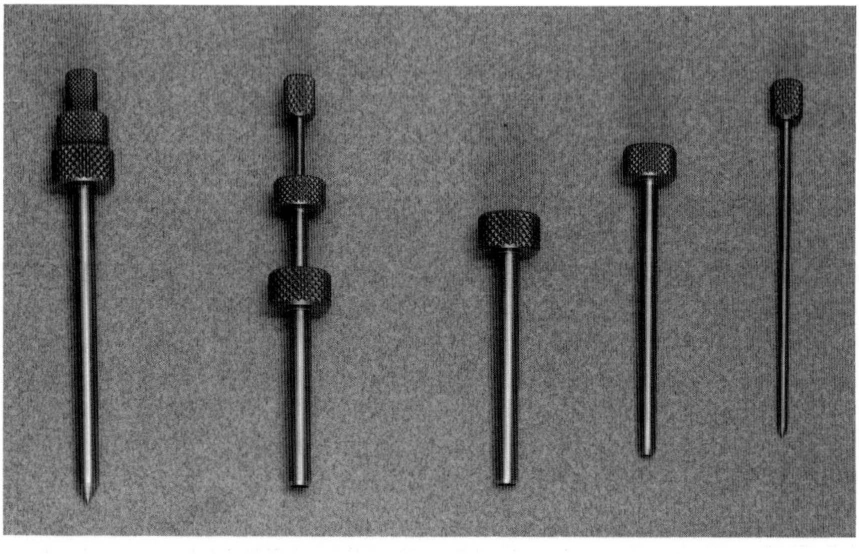

Fig. 69. Legend see page 75

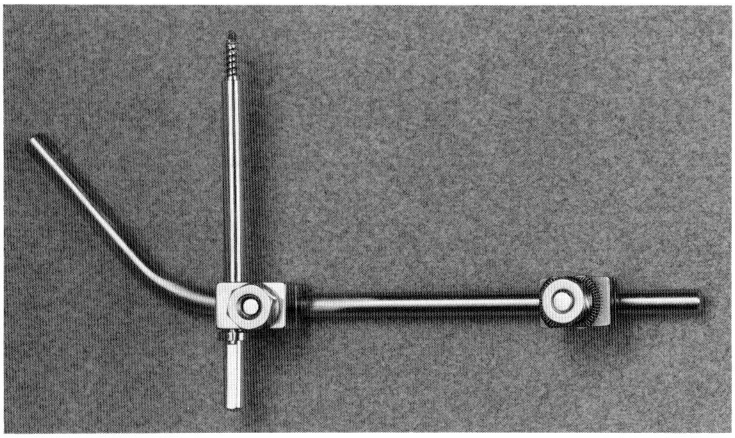

Fig. 70. The assembled components of the mandibular fixation device. A bar clamp and a pin clamp with Schanz screw are mounted on the *left* side of the bar. A bar clamp and a guide clamp are mounted on the *right* side of the bar

The *third* component is the *closed* (Fig. 67) or *open* swivel clamp[3] (Fig. 68), which forms the link between the Schank screw and connecting bar.

The advantage of the open clamp it that it can be hooked over the bar, even its curved portion, after the frame has been erected. Additionally, the open clamp has been shown to be more stable than the closed clamp. Both types can accommodate the three-part "troika" drill guide system (tissue protector, drill sleeve, trocar) used for the parallel insertion of additional Schanz screws (Fig. 69).

When assembled, the three components form an external frame (Fig. 70) that is strong enough to keep the mandible stable under functional loading. A soft diet can be consumed immediately after the frame is erected.

[3] Closed clamp 4.0/4.0 mm (order no. 395.57); open clamp 4.0/4.0 mm (order no. 395.55), matching socket wrench (order no. 395.36), open-end wrench (order no. 395.35).

◁ **Fig. 69.** "Troika" three-part trocar and drill guide system. The system fits into the guide clamp (see Fig. 68 center and right) and allows parallel screw holes to be drilled along the base of the mandible. The system consists of a *tissue protector, drill sleeve and trocar.* The outer tissue protector comes in 6-, 5-, and 4-cm lengths, corresponding to the lengths of the Schanz screws. *Left:* Nested together, the three parts from a smooth point at the front. *Center* and *right:* The parts are shown partially and completely disassembled: 1) *Tissue protector* (length 5 cm), which also serves as a guide for the 3.5-mm drill bit and 2.7-mm tap. 2) *Drill sleeve* for the 2.0-mm drill bit. 3) *Trocar*

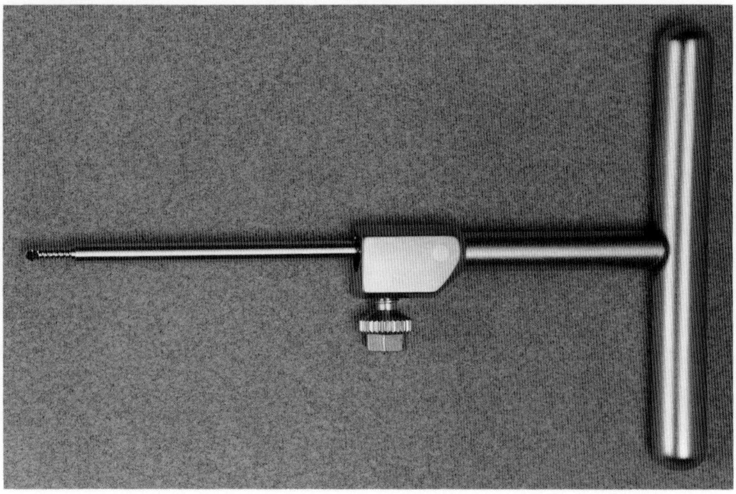

Fig. 71. Hand chuck with Schanz screw

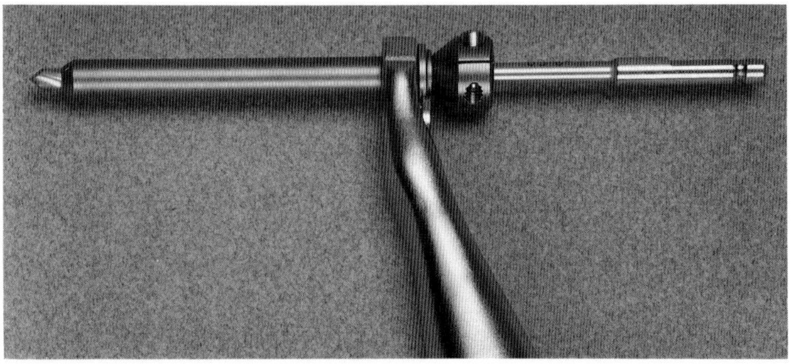

a

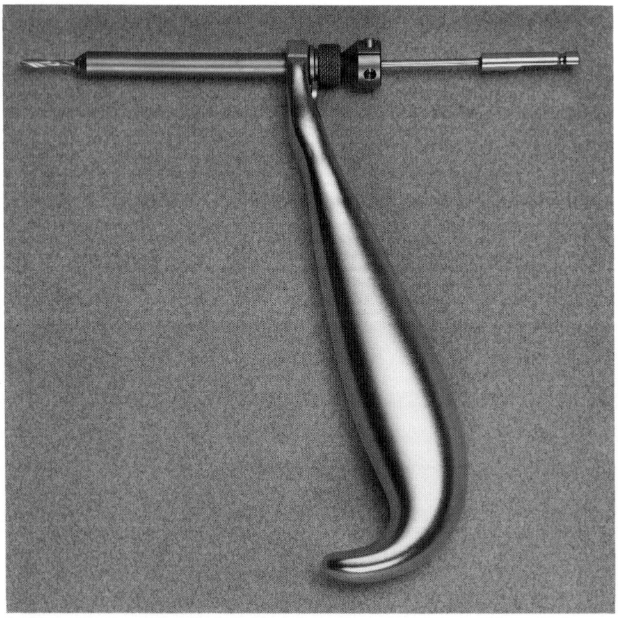

b

Fig. 72. **a** Transbuccal 3.5-mm drill sleeve, which also serves as a tissue protector and tap sleeve. The 3.5-mm drill bit is in place and carries a depth stop on its shaft (set to 4 mm for drilling the near cortex). **b** Transbuccal drill guide with handle ("door latch"), with the 2.0-mm drill sleeve in place. It contains the 2.0-mm drill bit with depth stop set to 16 mm

4.2.2.6.2 Auxillary Instruments

- Hand chuck (Fig. 71)
- Transbuccal drill guide (Fig. 72a, b).

4.2.2.6.3 Principles of Application

4.2.2.6.3.1 Basic Rules

The mandibular external fixator will provide stability adequate for its specific range of indications when the following basic rules are observed:

1) The Schanz screws *in one fragment* should be spaced a maximum distance apart.
2) The connecting bar should be positioned as close to the bone as possible.
3) The outer two Schanz screws are applied first, placing the *first* screw in the distal fragment and the *second* screw in the proximal fragment as far from the fracture line as possible (see Figs. 75 and 77).
4) The preshaped bar is attached to the outer screws using one clamp per side.
5) The second screw in the main fragment is placed as close to the fracture as possible. The open swivel clamp is used to connect it to the bar and to combine with the guide clamp (see Fig. 68).
6) If desired, the screws adjacent to the fracture may be manually prestressed relative to each other as a precaution against distraction.
7) Stability should be augmented if necessary by the insertion of additional Schanz screws.

4.2.2.6.3.2 Explanations

Biomechanics
Distraction of the fragments on the tension side under loading is an important criterion for evaluating the stability of the external fixation device. In tensile experiments, Winter (1987) measured the distraction on the tension side of the fracture for various fracture types and locations. He found that the fracture began to open when the tension force reached 5–10 kg (Fig. 73).

When the mandible is subjected to eccentric loading, as normally occurs on the tension side during function, a torque develops which tends to displace the fragment ends vertically relative to each other. When there is one Schanz screw in each main fragment, that screw forms the axis of rotation. With two screws per fragment, the rotational axis is midway between the screws. When the fragment is loaded, a countertorque is created that increases with the distance between the two screws. *Therefore the two screws in each fragment should be spaced a maximum distance apart,* with one screw placed as close to the fracture site as local circumstances permit (generally 8–10 mm).

The stability of the external fixation additionally depends on the free bending length of the Schanz screw. The shorter this length, the smaller the deflection of the fragment ends. *Therefore the connecting bar should be mounted as close to the bone as possible.*

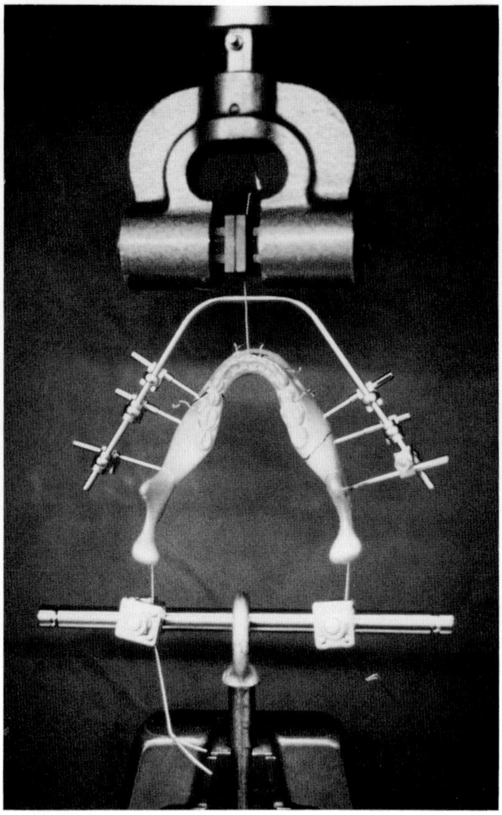

Fig. 73. The external fixation device on a double mandibular fracture: sagittal distraction test at the level of the occlusal plane. (Free test length 150 mm, distance between the two upper traction wires 90 mm). See text

Concept

Figures 74–83 illustrate the basic steps involved in erecting the external fixation device on the mandible. They are as follows:

1) The jaws are reduced in correct occlusion and secured by intermaxillary fixation.
2) The two outer Schanz screws are inserted as far from the fracture as possible.
3) The two screws are loosely interconnected on one plane with the external bar.

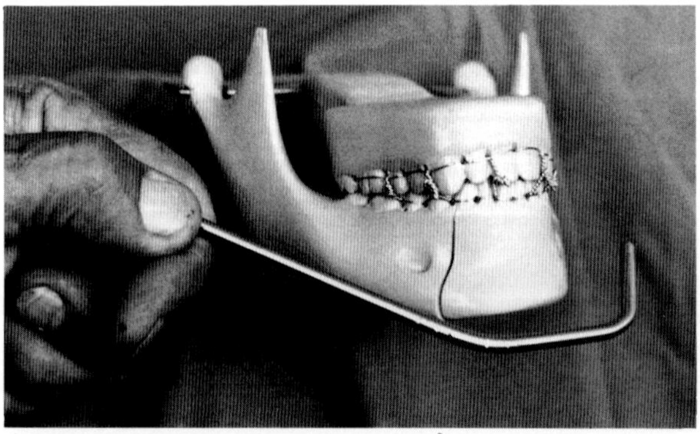

Fig. 74. 1) The jaws are retained in occlusion with Ernst ligatures (see Fig. 53). 2) The preshaped three-quarter-length bar is adapted to the mandible. 3) The stab incisions are marked on the skin

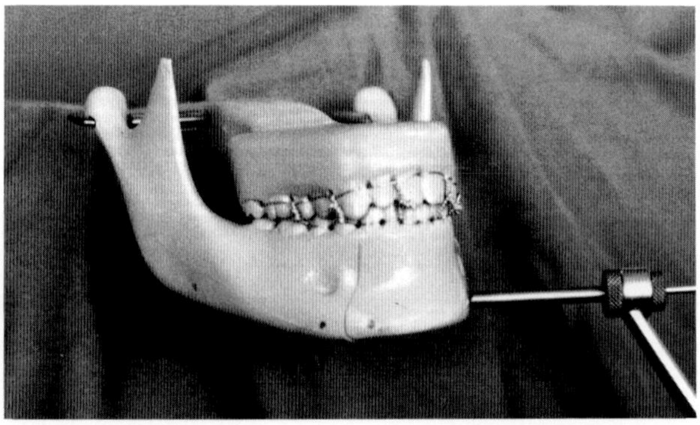

Fig. 75. The *first* hole is drilled on the unfractured side, *distant from the fractue,* parallel to the tangential plane of the inferior mandibular border and orthogonal to the bone surface

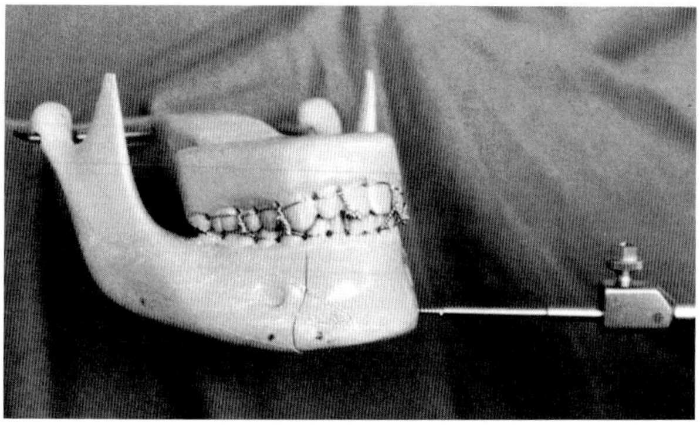

Fig. 76. The Schanz screw is inserted

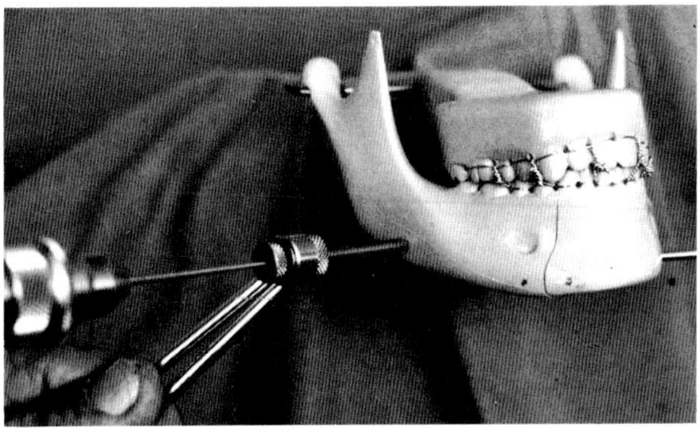

Fig. 77. The *second* hole for the contralateral Schanz screw is drilled on the fractured side, also *distant from the fracture*

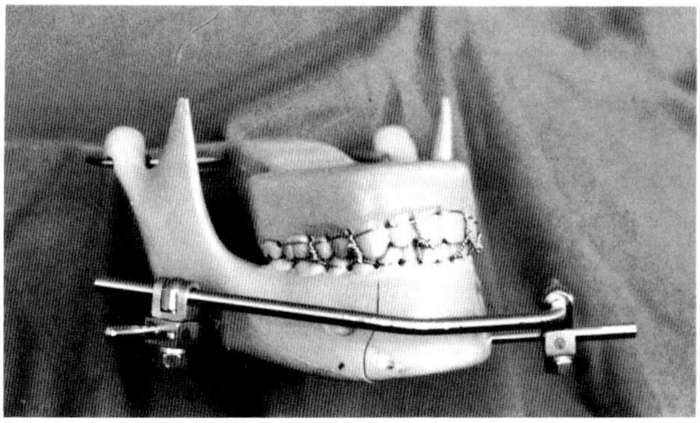

Fig. 78. The three-quarter arch is locked loosely in place with the closed clamps. The clamps that hold the Schanz screws are finger tightened

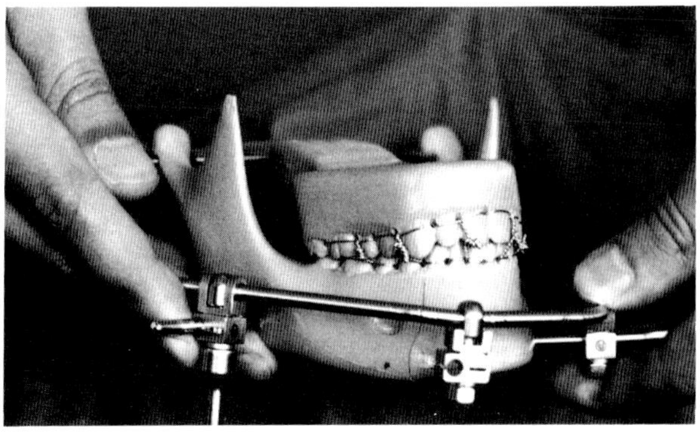

Fig. 79. Basal reduction is carried out, and the position is manually retained with the aid of the Schanz screws while the nuts are tightened with the socket wrench. The third clamp *(open)* with the *guide* clamp is mounted to the right of the fracture

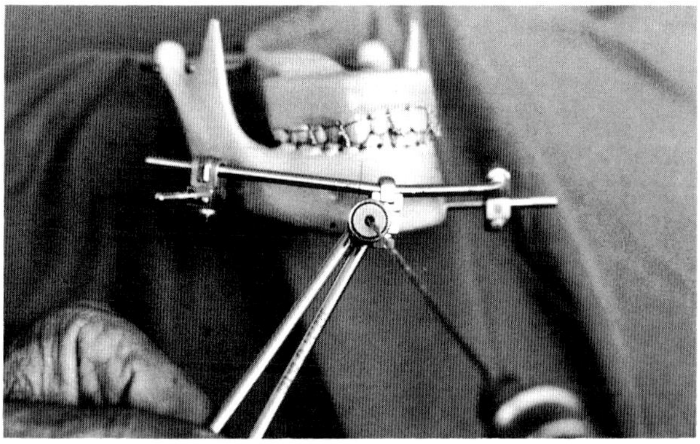

Fig. 80. The first hole adjacent to the fracture is drilled through the "troika" assembly inserted through the guide clamp

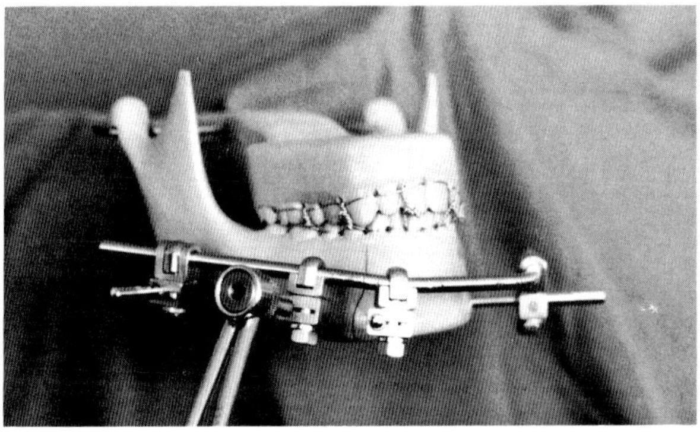

Fig. 81. After provisional adjustment of the third Schanz screw, the second open clamp is mounted on the rod, and the guide clamp is used as before to drill a second hole adjacent to the fracture

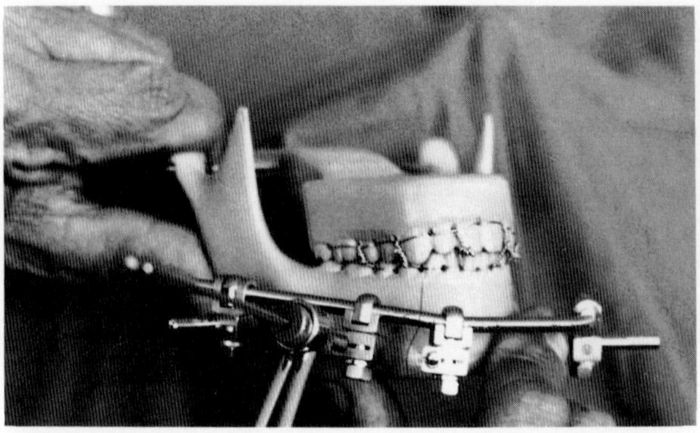

Fig. 82. The reduction is checked by loosening and retightening individual screws while manually compressing the Schanz screws adjacent to the fracture

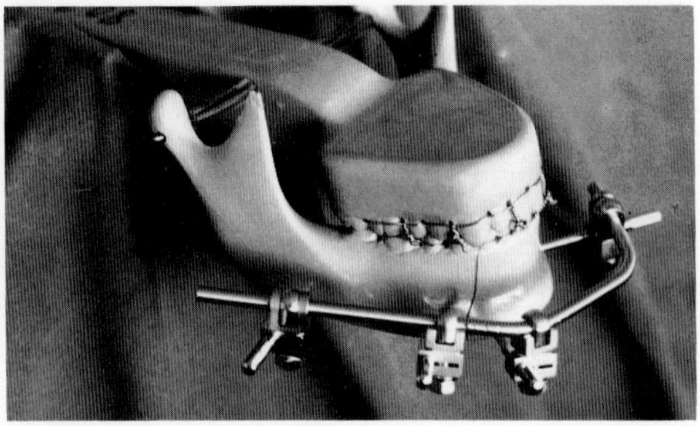

Fig. 83. The external fixation device in situ

4) Basal reduction is checked and adjusted with the pin clamps finger tightened.
5) The pin clamps are definitively tightened.
6) Schanz screws are inserted adjacent to the fracture using the "troika" guide system.
7) The reduction is checked, and all the pin clamps are tightened while manually compressing the Schanz screws adjacent to the fracture.

Practical Details

Intraoral Procedure

Manual reduction and retention of the occlusion with Ernst ligatures (see Fig. 53) or a wire acrylic splint (see Fig. 155) both facilitates and enhances the percutaneous stabilization.

Extraoral Procedure

Two Kirschner wires (1 mm diam.) are inserted tangential to the inferior border of the mandible (Fig. 84a, b). This will aid the less experienced operator in placing the stab incision and drill hole 8–10 mm above the mandibular border and arranging the Schanz screws in a straight line with proper spacing between them.

In accordance with the steps listed above, we determine the two end points of the external fixation on the basis of radiographic and local findings (see Figs. 75 and 77). The Schanz screws farthest away from the fracture should be positioned optimally in terms of bone thickness and *intra*-fragmental screw spacing. In our illustrative model, the distal end point would be just anterior to the mental foramen on the unfractured side of the mandible, and the proximal end point would be just in front of the angle on the fractured side (see Figs. 75 and 77). The appropriate connecting bar for this case is a preshaped three-quarter arch (see Figs. 67 and 74). Locked at its ends to the outer Schanz screws, the bar provides a solid base (fixation plane) for the rest of the screws. Four Schanz screws (50 mm long) are enough to create a stable assembly for a single fracture with minimal soft-tissue swelling.

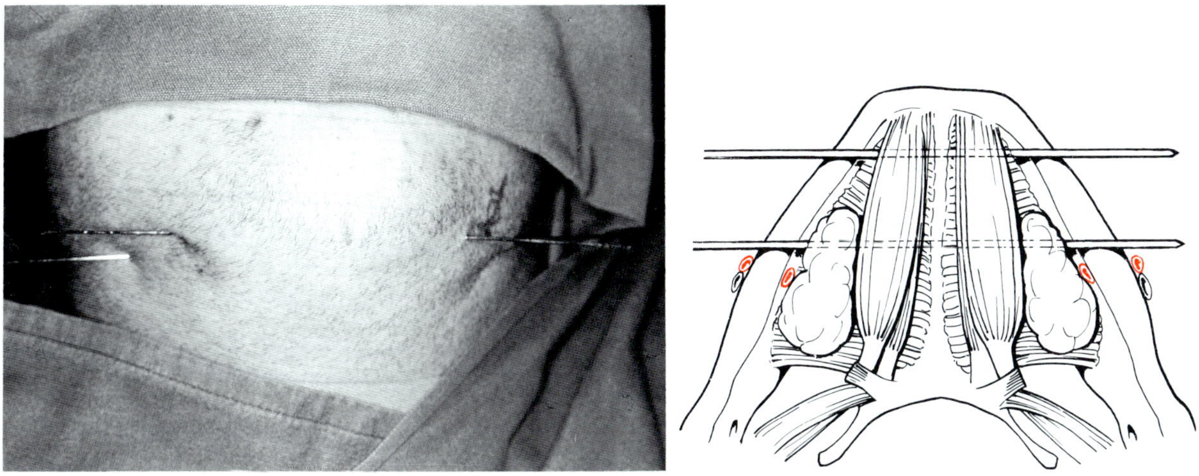

a b

Fig. 84. **a** The inferior border of the mandible is marked with Kirschner wires (1 mm diam.) as an aid to determining the correct placement of the drill holes. **b** Topographic drawing

Before any more of the frame is erected on the *edentulous* mandible, the alignment of the fragments is checked manually unless the reduction has already been secured with dentures and intermaxillary clamps (see Fig. 60). This is unlikely, however, since most of these cases present as emergencies.

In the *dentulous* mandible, on the other hand, a wide bony buttress exists, and the reduction is satisfactorily maintained by rigid intermaxillary fixation. There is no need to check the reduction intraorally, so there is no need to redrape before inserting the third and fourth Schanz screws.

All the pin clamps may be placed on the bar initially, before attaching it to the terminal screws, or open clamps may be hooked over the bar after it is in place. The holes adjacent to the fracture are drilled through the dark-colored guide clamps, which accommodate the "troika" system. When the 3.5-mm drill sleeve is locked in the guide clamp, care is taken not to over-tighten the lock nut so that the sleeve is not deformed.

Technique and Outlook

Repositioning of the ramus after a sagittal split osteotomy (see p. 335) is another potential application of the external fixation device. Figures 85–92 illustrate the basic techniques of handling the "door latch" and "troika" systems for repositioning the ramus after a sagittal osteotomy (with the mastoid as the fixed point).

Repositioning is a recurring problem. In mandibular resections, this problem can be solved by applying a reconstruction plate before the resection is carried out (see p. 292). Another option is external fixation. A good technique for midsegment resections of the mandible is to bridge the proposed defect with a perifacial bar anchored to Schanz screws placed in the sides of the mandible. Following the resection the frame is left in place for definitive fixation (see Fig. 93 a, b).

Such measures are appropriate for tumorous expansion of the mandible that prevents the preliminary attachment of a reconstruction plate. One day

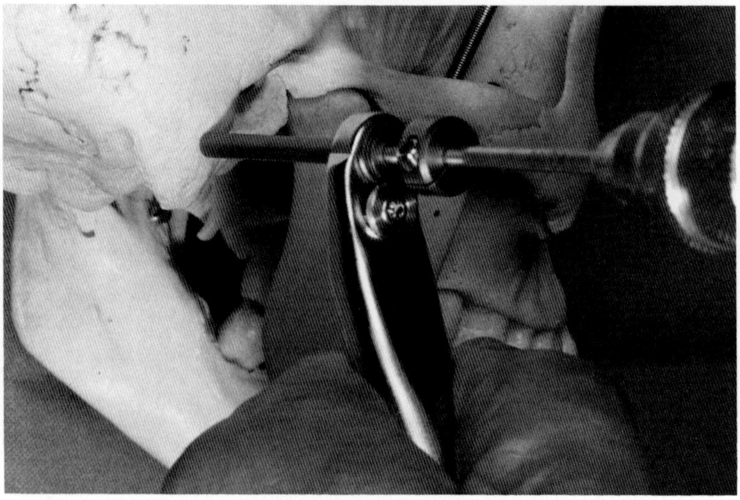

Fig. 85. The trocar (3.5-mm drill sleeve with handle) held against the mastoid in orthogonal position provides a stable guide for insertion of the screw shank into the near cortex. Drilling of the near cortex is initiated with the 3.5-mm bit, fitted with a depth stop. The drilling depth is 2–5 mm, depending on the estimated thickness of the cortex

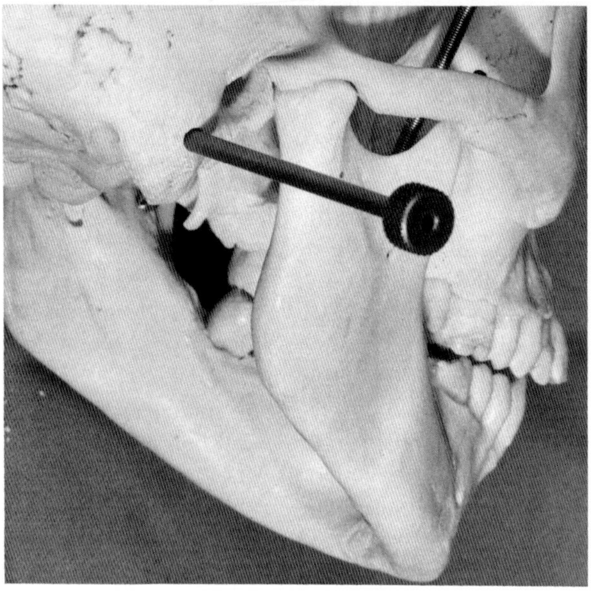

Fig. 86. For demonstration purposes the 2.0-mm drill sleeve with conical taper is shown inserted into the 3.5-mm hole in the outer cortex

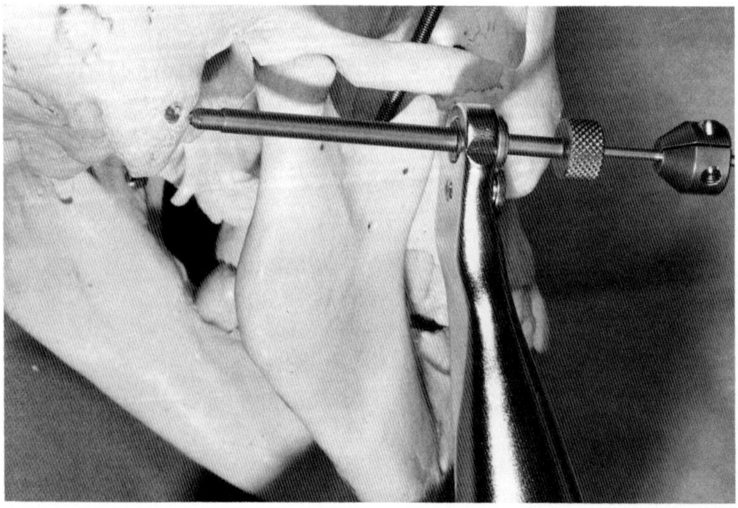

Fig. 87. The far cortex is drilled through the "door latch" using the 2.0-mm insert drill sleeve. The stop on the 2.0-mm bit is set to a depth of approximately 6 mm (see also Fig. 72a)

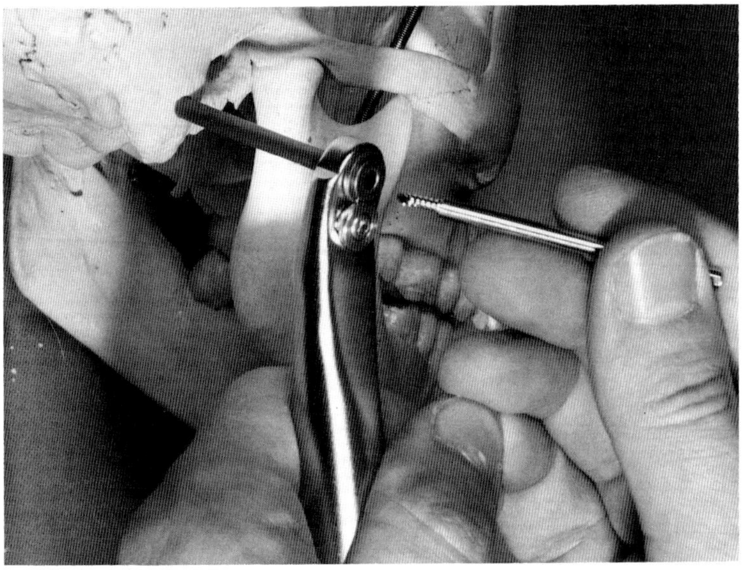

Fig. 88. After removal of the 2.0-mm drill sleeve, the Schanz screw is introduced by hand via the "door latch" until the screw shank is seated within the outer cortex

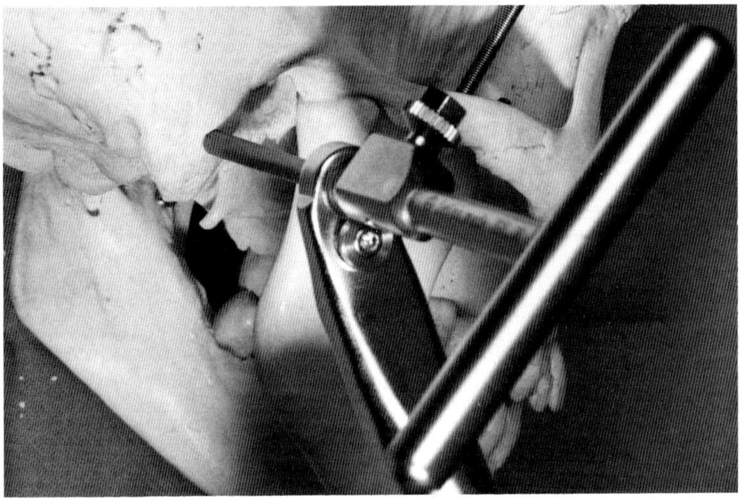

Fig. 89. The hand chuck is attached to the screw end, and the self-tapping thread (2.7 mm) of the Schanz screw is driven into the 2-mm hole in the far cortex

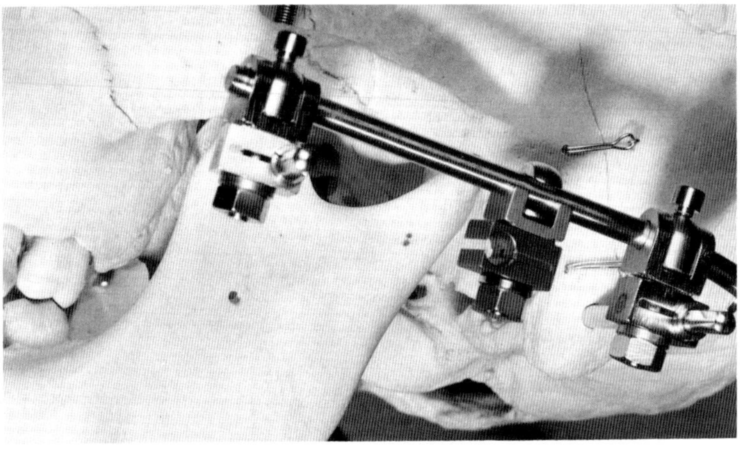

Fig. 90. Mandibula in central occlusion connected with the mastoid by means of the second Schanz screw. The open clamp with guide clamp for the "troika" has been mounted on the connecting bar for placement of the third drill hole. (The second Schanz screw is anchored in the base of the coronoid process)

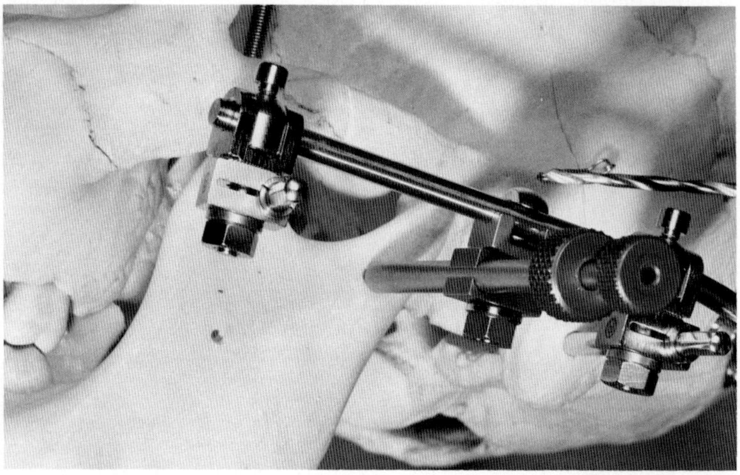

Fig. 91. The "troika" assembly has been locked in the guide clamp parallel to both Schanz screws. The trocar has been removed, the 3.5-mm hole has been drilled through the near cortex, and the 2.0-mm drill sleeve has been inserted in preparation for drilling the far cortex

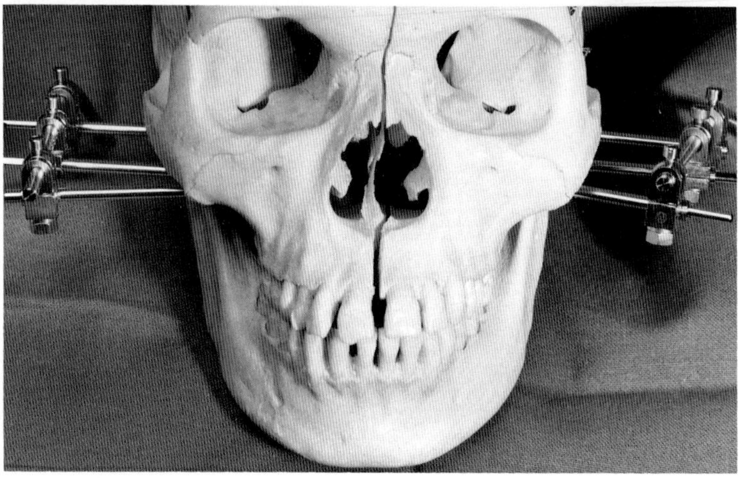

Fig. 92. The connecting bars and fixation clamps (with set screws) can be removed in one piece. Reapplied, they are used to reposition the ascending ramus after a sagittal split osteotomy. The mastoid provides the posterior anchoring point for the fixation

it may be possible, through immunosuppression, to replace entire segments of the mandible with alloplastic grafts. In that case external fixation would have a major role in stabilizing the graft and aiding its vascularization. This requirement already exists whenever the capacity of the graft bed for revascularization is compromised. In all cases where the soft-tissue bed is damaged by radiation or a covered soft-tissue defect is poorly perfused, it is desirable to keep foreign material away from the bone graft. The potential of the graft for revascularization is already diminished in these cases, and a plate would compromise it further. In the future, it is expected that external fixation will have a role in the transplantation of bone grafts with a vascular pedicle.

Fig. 96. **a** Mandibular external fixation device in the early phase of its development. The device was rigidly connected to a halo frame to immobilize the mandible and alleviate pain; perbuccal lidocaine was also infused (note the venous catheter). **b** The same fixation device 1.5 years later. Prolonged external fixation was necessitated by the very slow progression of bone and ulcer healing. There was no evidence of screw loosening during that period. **c** External fixation was used in this patient to stabilize a spontaneous fracture and relieve pain. **d** Spontaneous fracture on the left side. The patient had received cobalt irradiation (6500 rad) 12 years previously for a carcinoma of the tongue. **e** Follow-up radiograph at 3 months: Despite extensive necrosis, osteoprosis, and decalcification, the Schanz screws are seated well enough to stabilize the fracture owing to their thread and shank mode of anchorage. The fixation device provided immediate pain relief and reestablished oral opening

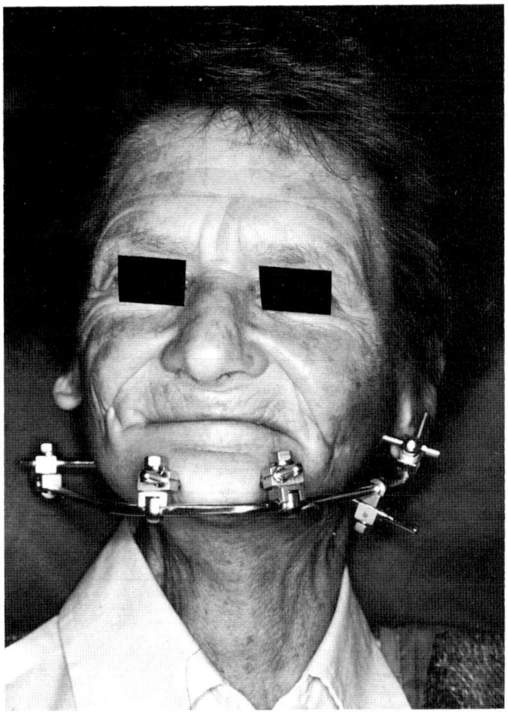

c

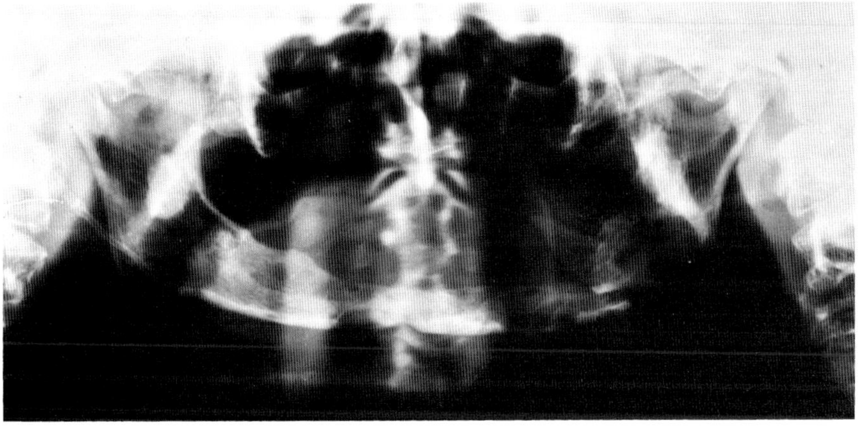

d

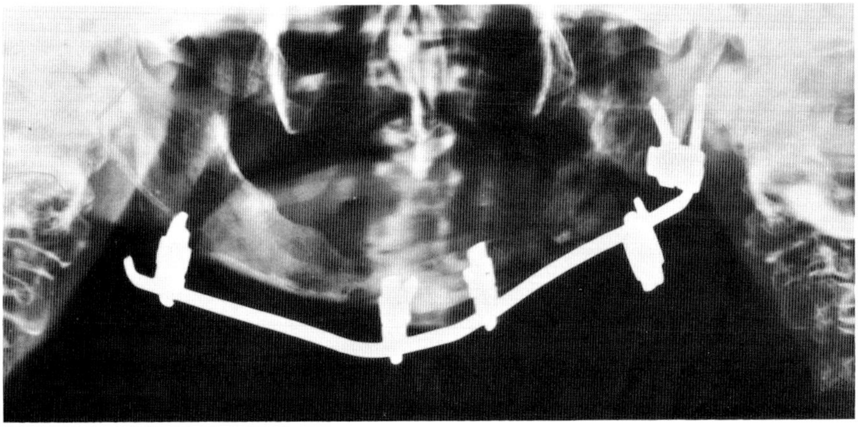

e

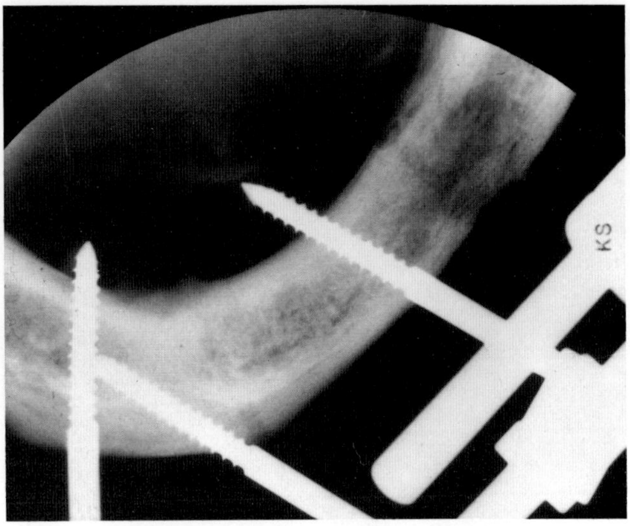

Fig. 97. Osteomyelitis with demarcation of a bony sequestrum in an untreated transverse fracture of an atrophic mandible. Although the second screw is poorly seated, the stability was sufficient for rapid healing. (The threaded portion of the new Schanz screw is shorter)

4.2.2.7.2.3 Clinically Overt Fracture Line Infection

Senile atrophy of the mandible, often seen in association with postmenopausal osteoporosis, becomes a problem of traumatology when, for example, osteitis develops in a neglected fracture line. Percutaneous stabilization is ideally suited for cases of this type, as it causes the least disruption in the blood supply to the bone. Figure 97 shows extensive bone destruction in the area around the fracture. The smooth shanks of the Schanz screws fit snugly in the outer cortex, and the threaded ends solidly engage the rest of the bone. With this method all portions of the cortex retain their periosteal covering.

External fixation is also appropriate for a primarily infected angle fracture communicating with the alveolus of a partially erupted third molar, as illustrated by the case in Fig. 98 a, where there is a coexisting oblique anterior fracture. External fixation was applied on the day of hospitalization to stabilize both fractures (Fig. 98 b, c). With the blood supply preserved and the mandible stabilized, primary union was obtained despite the infection (Fig. 98 d).

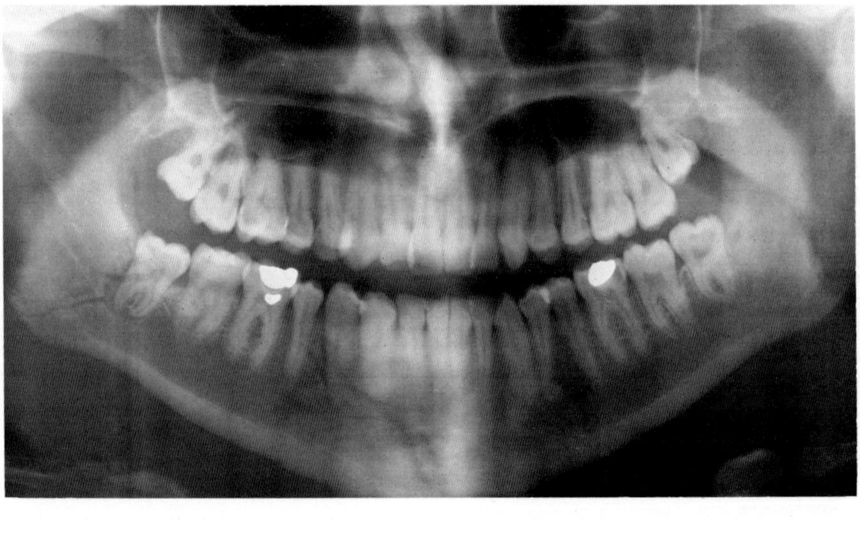

Fig. 98 a. Legend see page 91

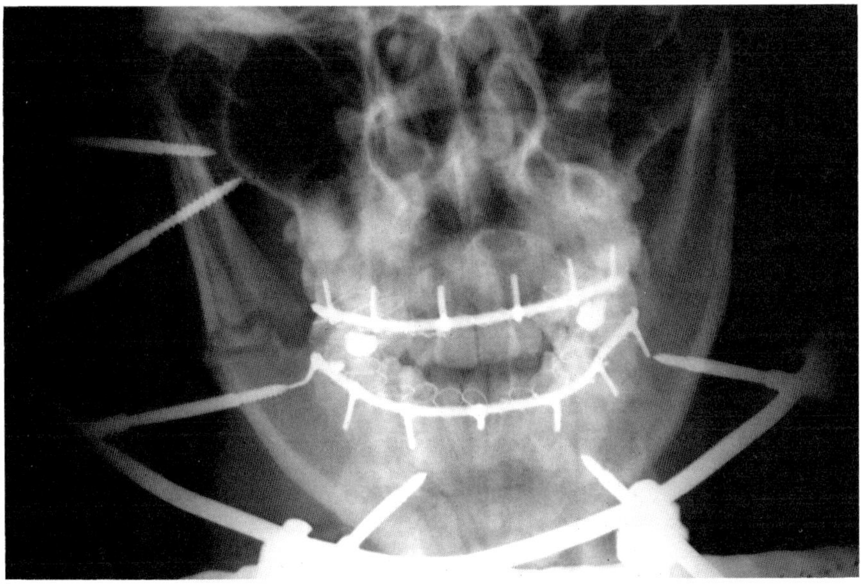

b

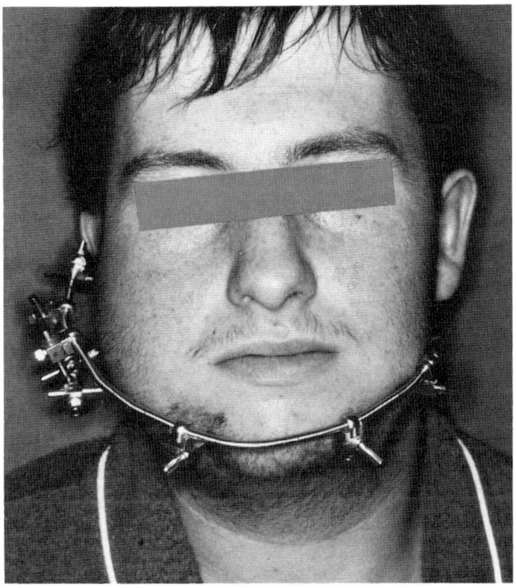

c

Fig. 98. **a** Primarily infected angle fracture communicating with the alveolus of a partially erupted third molar. There is a coexisting precanine fracture. **b** The mandibular fixation device was applied at once, without preliminary treatment of the infection; only the source of the infection was removed. **c** Appearance of the external fixation device immediately after treatment. **d** Status after removal of the fixation device

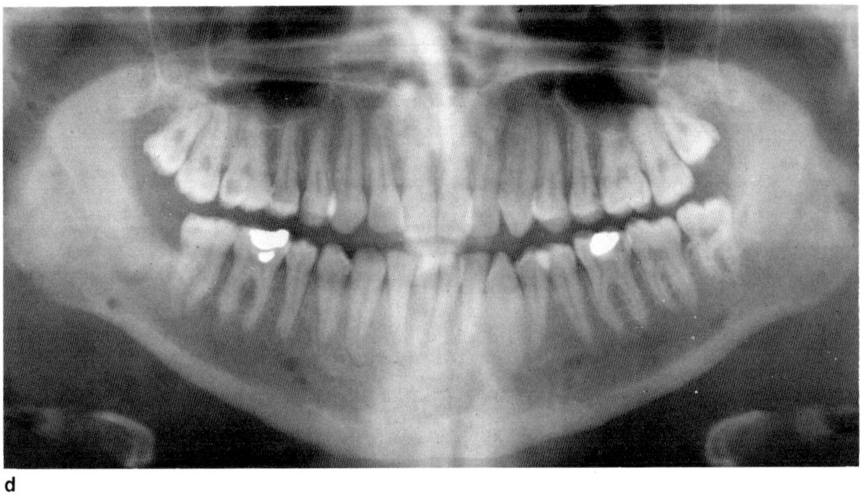

d

4.2.2.7.3 Prophylactic Use of External Fixation

Another problem is impacted teeth in the atrophic or edentulous mandible. In one such case (Fig. 99 a) external fixation was applied prophylactically to maintain continuity of the mandible while the tooth was extracted (Fig. 99 b).

Spontaneous fractures and deformations, which occur rarely in association with progressive facial hemiatrophy, fibrous dysplasia, eosinophilic granuloma, or cysts, cannot be optimally immobilized by conservative treatment or by internal fixation. External fixation offers an alternative in these cases.

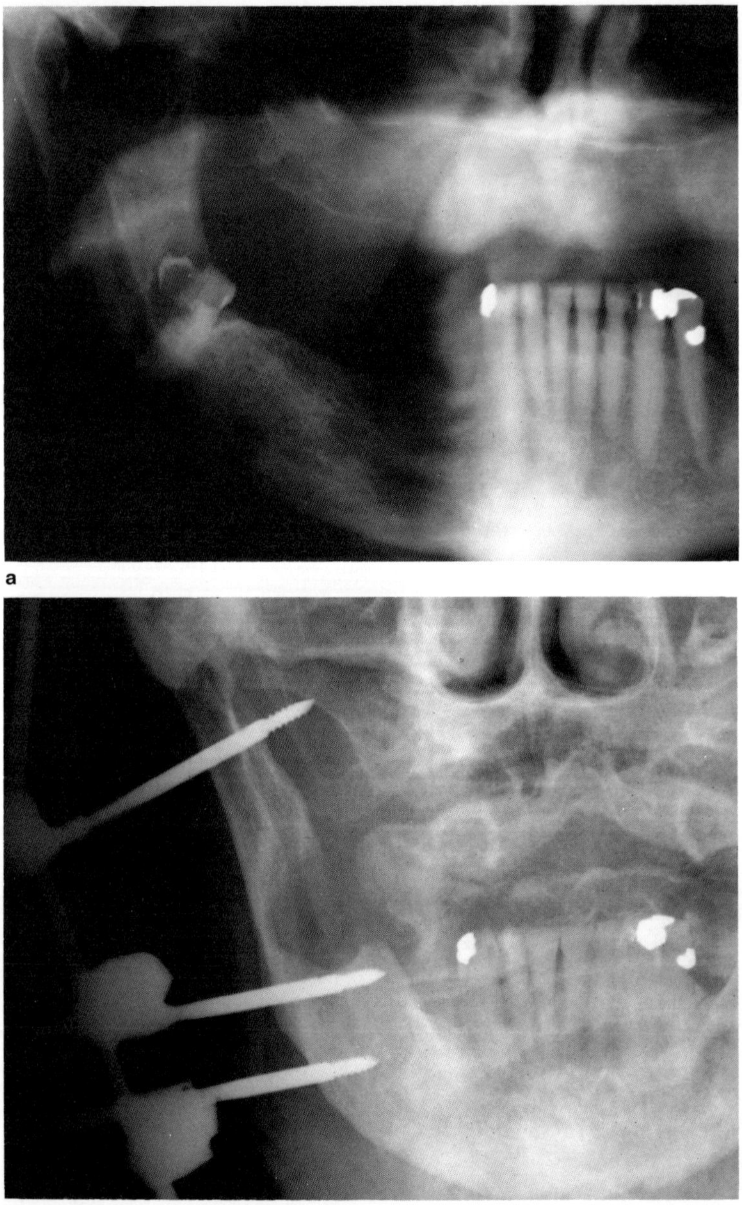

a

b

Fig. 99 **a** Typical high-risk situation for a fracture. **b** The impacted tooth was extracted under the protection of the external fixation device

5 ASIF Instrumentation

Functionally stable fixation is a challenging therapeutic goal. It requires an assortment of surgical instruments that are:

- tailored to the variety of fracture patterns that can occur;
- simple to handle and use;
- easily identified on the instrument table;
- standardized in their design and use.

With the help of Technical Committees comprised of surgeons, researchers, and manufacturers, the ASIF has been able to develop and test a line of surgical instruments of exceptionally high quality. Widely copied, the original ASIF instruments and implants are engraved with the ASIF trademark. Details on the design of the instruments and their arrangement into sets may be found in the monograph *AO/ASIF Instrumentation* by Sequin and Texhammar (1980) and *Functionally Stable Maxillofacial Internal Fixation*, a manual for operating room personnel, by Texhammar and Schmoker (1984).

5.1 Instrument Sets for Mandibular Surgery

The ASIF instruments and implants are supplied in modular sets that permit all maxillofacial bone operation to be performed with a relatively small number of basic instrument elements. The basic instruments for maxillofacial bone surgery consist of an instrument and implant set for internal fixations of the mandible (Fig. 100) as well as a set for sagittal split osteotomies (Fig. 101)[4].

The basic instrument sets are sufficient to deal with virtually any type of mandibular fracture. The sets should be checked before use to make certain that all the instruments are present and that the implant and screw sets are complete.

---

[4] A forther detailed information can be obtained from SYNTHES-MAXILLOFACIAL, P.O. BOX 1767 PAOLI, PA 19301-1222, USA or any other official distributor of AO/ASIF Instrumentation all over the World or ASIF-FOUNDATION, CH-3007 BERN, Balderstrasse 30, SWITZERLAND.

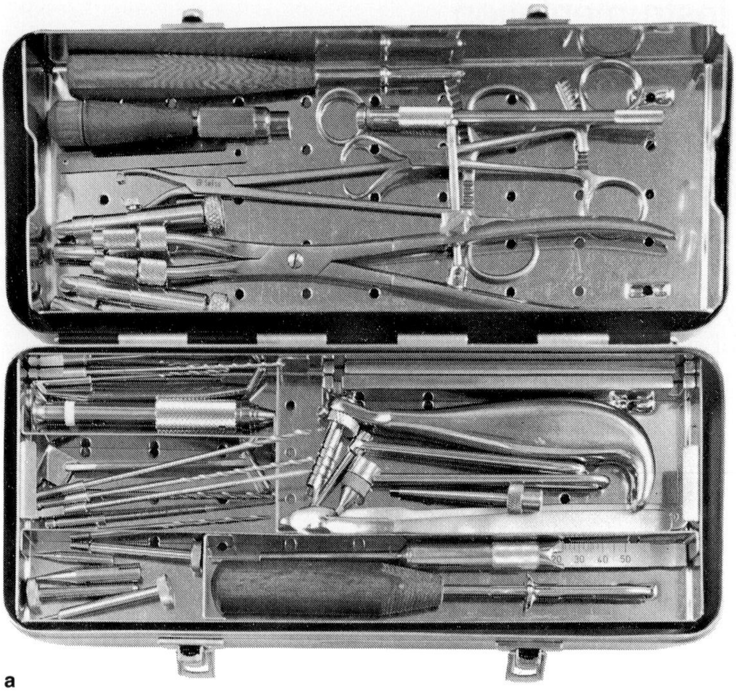

a

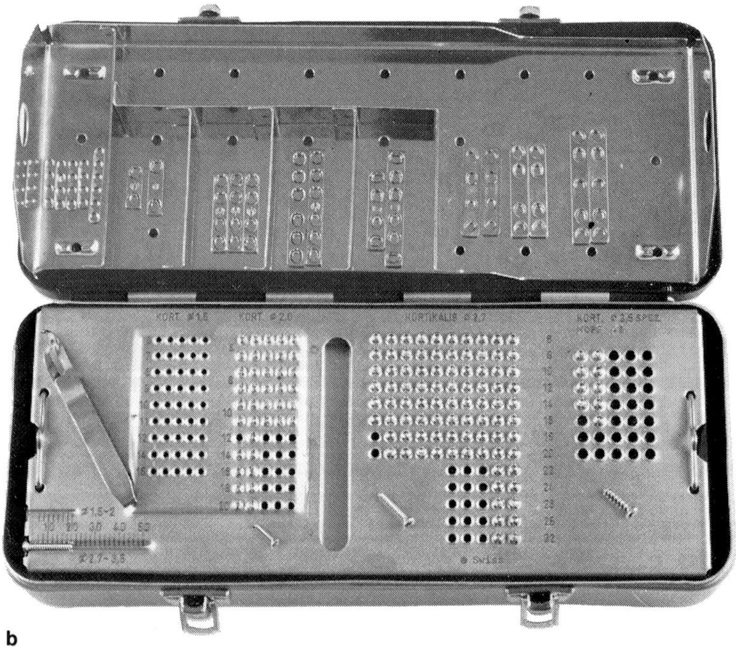

b

Fig. 100. a Instrument set for internal fixation of the mandible. **b** Implant set for internal fixation of the mandible

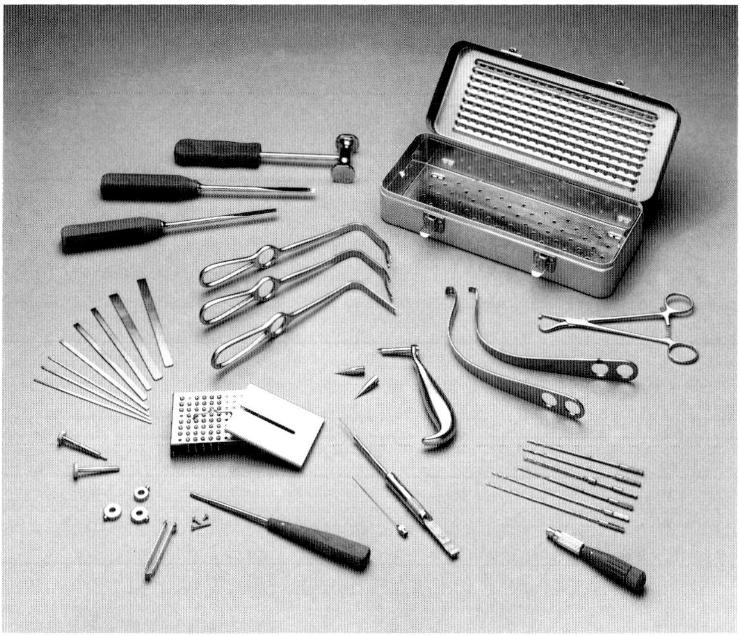

Fig. 101. Combined set for sagittal ramus osteotomy and percutaneous lag screw fixation. *Top left:* chisel and osteotome; *bottom left:* drill sleeves and screws; *center:* special retractors and transbuccal drill guide with handel; *bottom center:* depth gauge (extra-long); *right:* 2.7-mm and 2.0-mm drill bits (extra-long)

5.2 Materials

5.2.1 Materials for Mandibular Implants

The plates and screws are manufactured in accordance with national and international standards. ASIF implants are made from stainless steel or titanium. The stainless steel implants are composed of 18% chromium, 14% nickel, 3% molybdenum, 1.5% manganese and silicon, and less than 0.03% carbon and iron (AI American norm: AISI 316 L). In addition, special smelting processes are used that give the metal a crystalline structure of extremely high purity (Steinemann 1968). Thus, the stainless steel from which the ASIF implants are manufactured has the low-carbon quality of unsmelted steel, very high corrosion resistance, yet still meets prevailing national and international standards for surgical implant materials.

Pursuant to a 1986 resolution by the Technical Committee for Maxillofacial Surgery, all mandibular implants are also presently manufactured from titanium.

The titanium used for ASIF implants is a commercially pure grade metal reworked to yield the desired strength and ductility. The yellow-gold color is produced by an oxide coating applied during the special surface treatment process. Slight color changes are of no consequence and simply mean that the oxide layer has thickened as a result of sterilization, storage, or exposure to the biologic milieu.

Hence, the chemical composition and manufacturing processes ensure adequate corrosion resistance, good tissue compatibility, and optimum mechanical strength.

5.2.2 Materials for Instruments

The materials for surgical instruments must meet less stringest requirements in terms of corrosion resistance than the materials for implants. Material selection is based more on considerations of function, weight, durability, ability to retain a cutting edge, wear resistance, and ease of maintenance. The ASIF uses:

- chromium-nickel steel for instruments that do not need to meet special requirements, so that simplicity and economy of manufacture are the major concerns.
- stainless chromium hardened steel for cutting instruments such as drill bits, taps, and chisels.
- stainless heat-treatable chromium steel for forceps, periosteal elevators, etc.

The latter two groups are not completely rustproof and require good care to prevent corrosion. The rubber and plastic materials used for instrument handles, bearings, seals, and hoses can be sterilized by autoclaving at 140 °C.

5.3 Mandibular Instruments

5.3.1 Reduction and Compressing Instruments

1. The *reduction-compression forceps* (Fig. 102) is used without pressure rollers to distract the fracture surfaces for removal of entrapped material and to accurately appose the bone ends while applying a manual compression of 10–15 kg (forceps prestressing). The ends of the forceps branches (slotted tubes with a sliding collar) are fixed to the inferior border of the mandible via two 8-mm cortex screws (see Fig. 157). We use the 2-mm drill guide and drill sleeve (Fig. 103, see also Fig. 112) to insert the screws. If there is sufficient room, we recommending attaching the pressure rollers (Fig. 104) to obtain a uniform pressure distribution over the fracture site (pressure roller prestressing).
2. The *reduction forceps with extra-long points* is an atraumatic grasping forceps. With its points anchored in the cortex (Fig. 105), the forceps can be used to hold the reduced fracture together and apply compression.

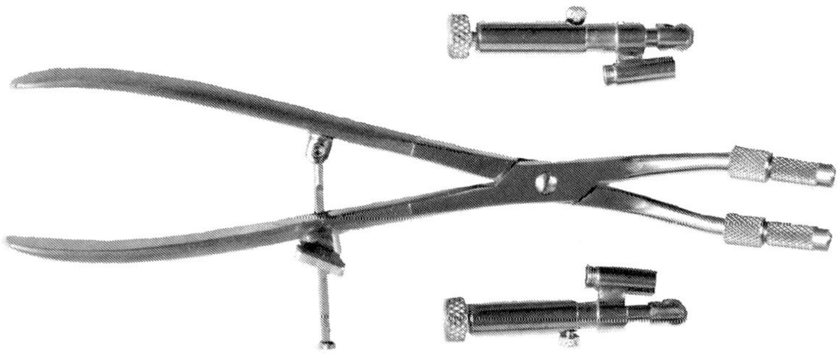

Fig. 102. Reduction-compression forceps with detachable pressure rollers

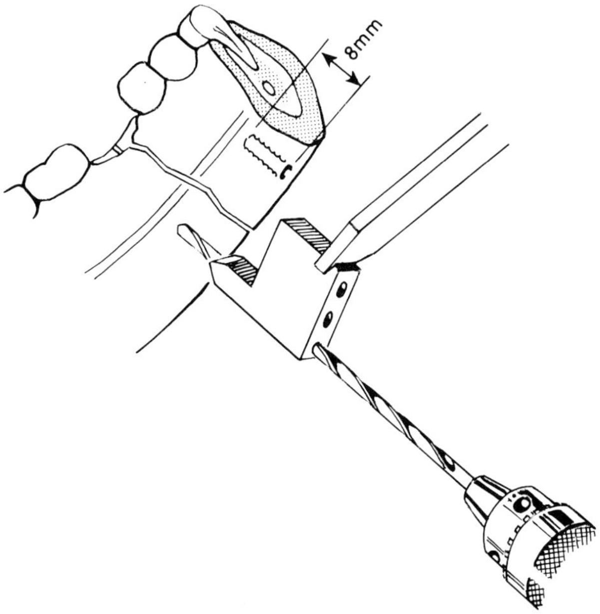

Fig. 103. The 2.0-mm drill guide, placed at the apex of the inferior border of the mandible, is used to drill the holes for inserting the anchoring screws for the reduction-compression forceps. Typical depth of the drill hole: 8 mm

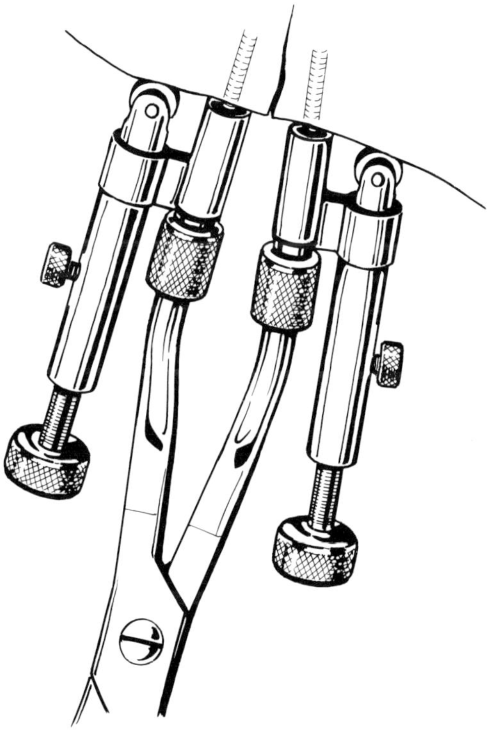

Fig. 104. Function of the pressure roller mechanism: convergence of the compressive forces on the alveolar side of the fracture

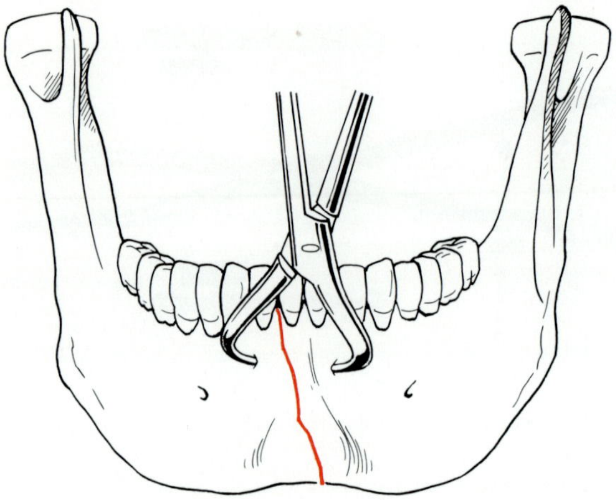

Fig. 105. Reduction forceps with extra-long points (may be used to prestress the tension side when anchored bilaterally in the cortex)

5.3.2 Instruments for Screw Insertion (see Figs. 106–113)

5.3.2.1 Instruments for Direct Screw Insertion (see Figs. 114–118)

Comments on the Use of the Eccentric Drill Guide (see Fig. 114)

1) The arrow must point toward the fracture (see Figs. 30 and 31).
2) The diameter of the drill guide is less than the diameter of the plate hole so that, when the plate is strongly contoured, the guide can be placed within the deformed plate hole. This also provides leeway for selecting the degree of eccentricity of the drill hole.
3) For *maximum* compression the end of the drill guide is placed *away from* the fracture in the plate hole (compressive displacement of 0.8 mm; see Fig. 29).
4) For *minimum* compression the end of the drill guide is placed *close to* the fracture in the plate hole (compressive displacement less than 0.8 mm).

Note: The hole should be drilled at maximum eccentricity in the oblique hole of the EDCP in a mandible of normal height. The hole should be drilled at minimum eccentricity in the edentulous *atrophic* mandible.

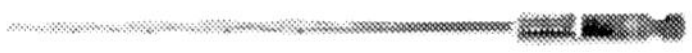

Fig. 106. Drill bit, 2.0 mm diam., for making the thread hole for the 2.7-mm cortex screw

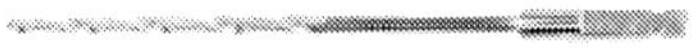

Fig. 107. Drill bit, 2.7 mm diam., for making the gliding hole for the 2.7-mm cortex screw when used as a lag screw

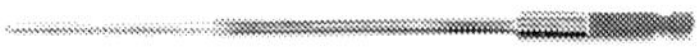

Fig. 108. Tap, 2.7 mm diam., for the 2.7-mm cortex screw, fits the quick coupling of the tap handle

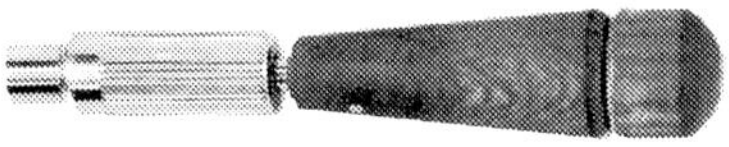

Fig. 109. Tap handle with quick coupling

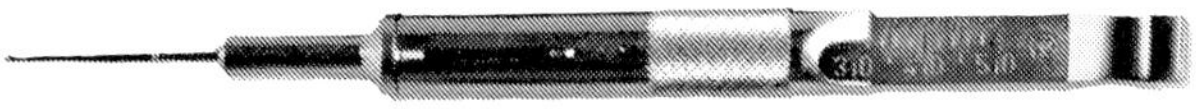

Fig. 110. Depth gauge for determining screw length

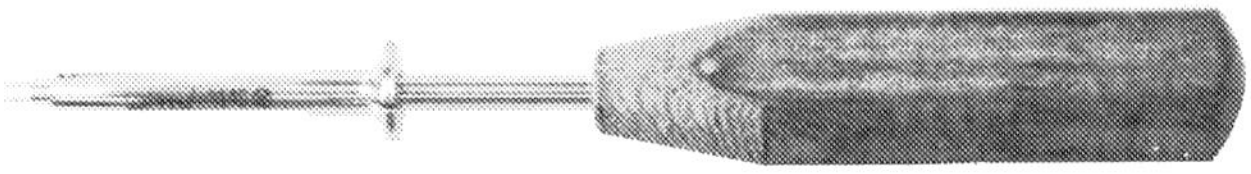

Fig. 111. Hexagonal screwdriver, width across flats 2.5 mm, for the 2.7-mm cortex screw

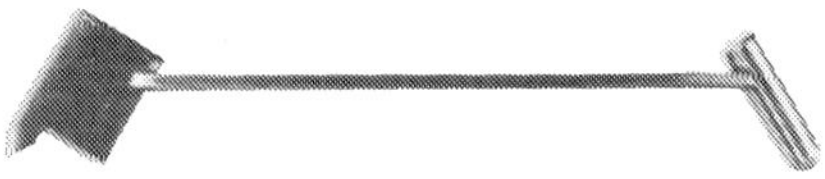

Fig. 112. Drill guide and drill sleeve, 2.0 mm diam., has serrated lower edge to prevent slipping of the drill bit

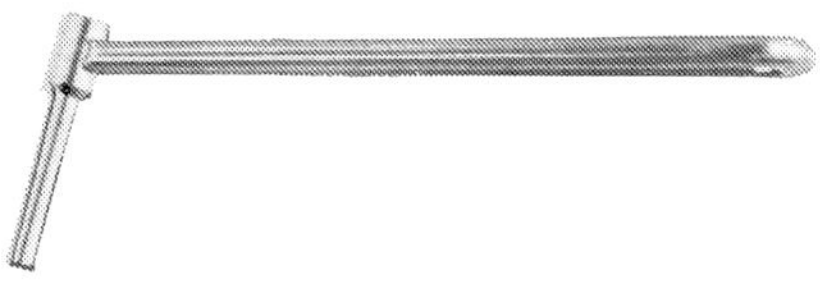

Fig. 113. Tap sleeve, 3.5 mm diam., protects soft tissues during use of the 2.7-mm tap

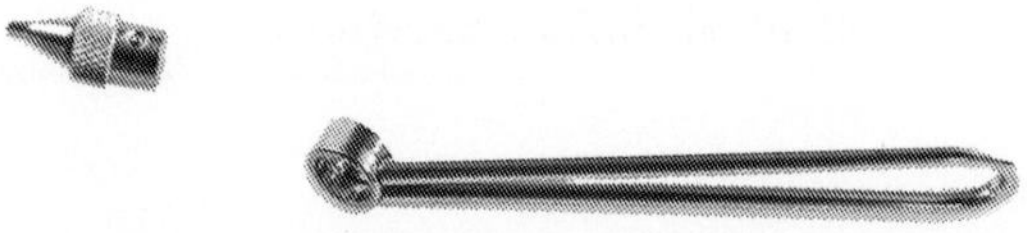

Fig. 114. DCP drill guide with handle, 2.0 mm diam., with two settings marked 0 and 0.8. The 0 setting centers the guide for drilling the 2.0-mm thread hole at the exact center of the DC hole, resulting in a *neutral* screw position. The 0.8 setting places the guide for the 2.0-mm thread hole off-center in the plate hole so that the screw effects compression (see Fig. 31)

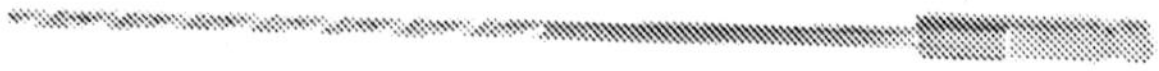

Fig. 115. Extra-long drill bit, 2.0 mm diam.

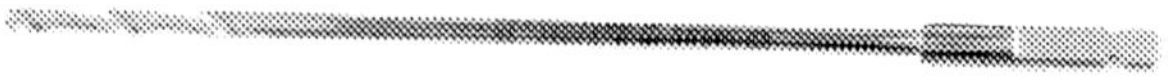

Fig. 116. Extra-long drill bit, 2.7 mm diam., for making the gliding hole for the 2.7-mm cortex screw when used as a lag screw

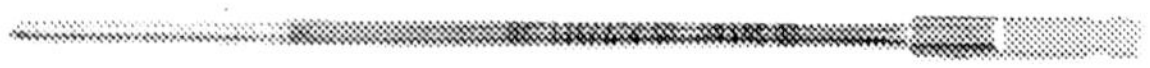

Fig. 117. Extra-long tap

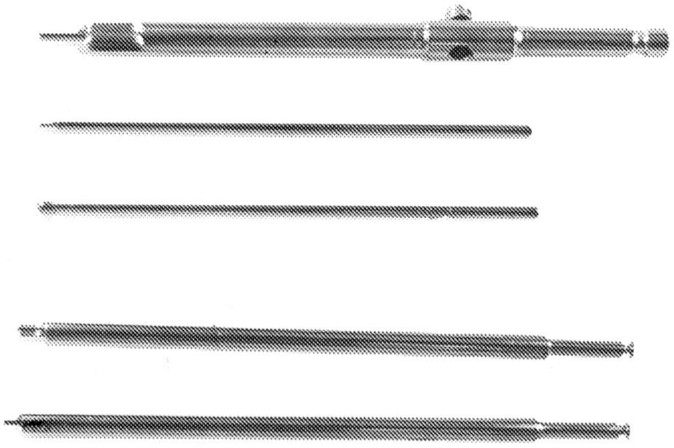

Fig. 118. Long countersink with interchangable centering sleeves for 2.7-mm and 2.0-mm screws, used to sink the screw head flush with the bone surface (see p. 118)

5.3.2.2 Instruments for Transbuccal Screw Insertion

See Figs. 119–123, also Figs. 111 and 380.

5.3.2.3 Small Air Drill with Quick Coupling (Fig. 124)

Advantages: Compressed air is a readily available power source and permits the construction of machincs that are autoclavable. Air-driven machines can be stopped quickly because of their low inertia. Speed is easily regulated, and the machines are easy to handle owing to their light weight.

The small air drill is used for drilling holes up to 5 mm in diameter, for tapping, and for the insertion and removal of screws.

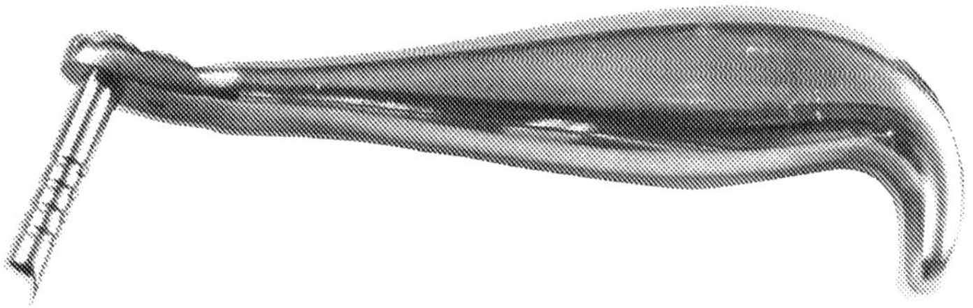

Fig. 119. Transbuccal trocar with tissue protector (see also Fig. 72)

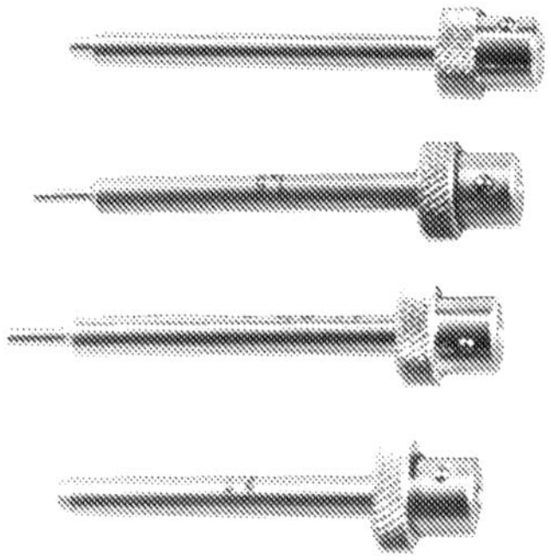

Fig. 120. Four inserts for the transbuccal trocar two for lag screw fixation in sagital split osteotomies (see Fig. 380) and two special long DCP drill sleeves, for the gliding hole and the threaded hole (see Fig. 145)

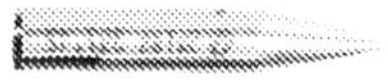

Fig. 121

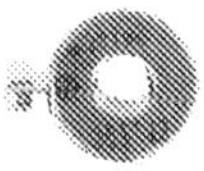

Fig. 122

Fig. 121. Removable trocar point

Fig. 122. Ring-shaped buccal retractor; mounted on the transbuccal trocar intraorally after removal of the trocar point (see p. 344)

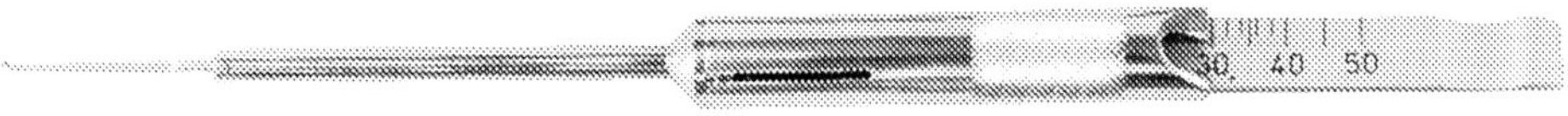

Fig. 123. Depth gauge, extra-long, for the 2.7-mm cortex screw (see Fig. 146)

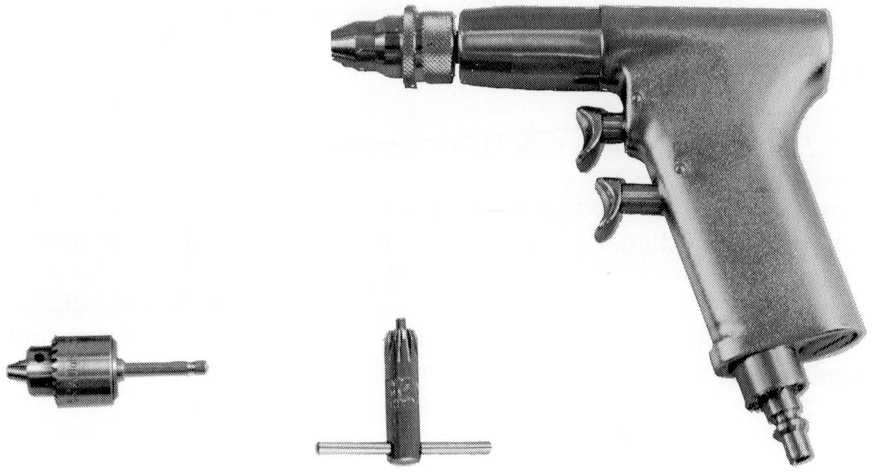

Fig. 124. Small air drill

Technical specifications: Single- or double-hose model, reversible, variable speed to approx. 600 rpm, quick coupling for compatible instruments, regulator pressure 6 bar (600 kPa), air comsumption approx. 250 liters/min, weight approx. 600 grams, autoclavable to 140 °C.

Functions: Drill speed is controlled with the lower trigger, operated by the middle finger. The upper trigger, operated by the index finger, is for reversing the drill during operation.

Quick coupling and instruments: Instruments are available with ends that fit the quick coupling of the small air drill.

Attaching the instruments: The sleeve of the coupling is pushed forward, the instrument shaft is inserted and rotated to find the keyway, then the shaft is fully inserted and the sleeve is released.

Removing the instruments: The sleeve of the coupling is pushed forward and the instrument is withdrawn. A small chuck with key for dental drills is also available.

Operation of the drill: Normally the drill is operated with the lower trigger, producing a clockwise rotation from the operator's view. Reverse operation may be helpful in some instances to remove the drill bit from bone.

Accessories: Small chuck with key for Kirschner wires. Pressure reducing valves, filters, and a drip oiler (with lubricating connector, if needed) may be required depending on the type of drill and air supply.

The pencil-shaped mini compressed air machine (Fig. 125) is also available for drilling, sawing, and the insertion of Kirschner wires.

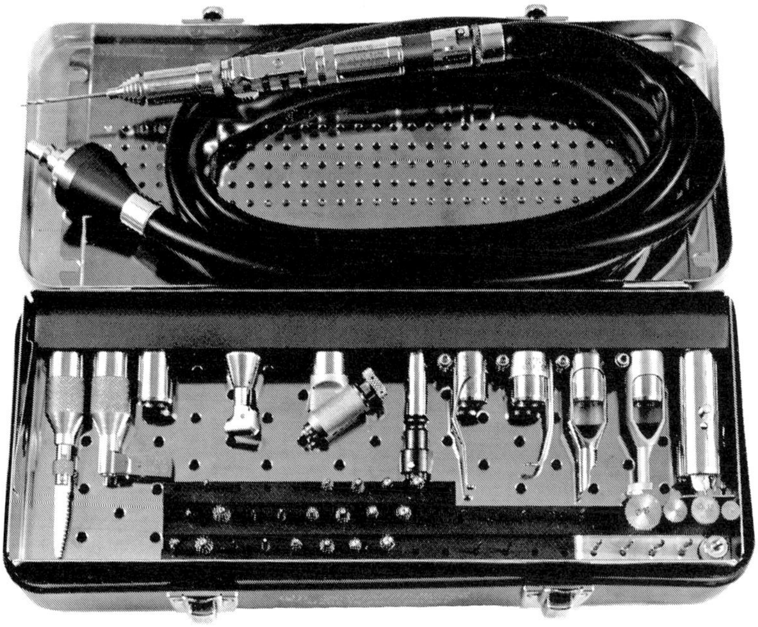

Fig. 125. Mini compressed air hand-piece, used for drilling, sawing, and K-wire insertion

5.3.2.4 Instruments for Bending and Twisting

We make a strict distinction between bending and twisting. The bending of a plate for adaptation to the bone is done exclusively with the appropriate bending pliers (Fig. 126a). The knob at the end of the pliers is turned to lock the plate between the jaws. The interchangable anvil (Fig. 126b) is specially designed for mandibular plates and makes it possible to bend the plate or bar without creating a sharp angulation (Fig. 126c). Plates should always be bent between the holes.

The contour of the mandible often makes it necessary to twist the plate with a separate bending iron (Fig. 127). There are two bending irons for this purpose (Fig. 128). The iron is applied to a specific site on the plate and used like a lever to apply torque.

Difficult contouring should be done with the aid of a separate, malleable template (Fig. 129) that is manually bent to the shape of the bone surface.

The three-dimensional bending of a reconstruction plate is done with two special pliers (Fig. 130a) that enable the plate to be bent edgewise or on the flat, twisted, and restraightened. Two special bending irons are available for additional adjustments (Fig. 130b).

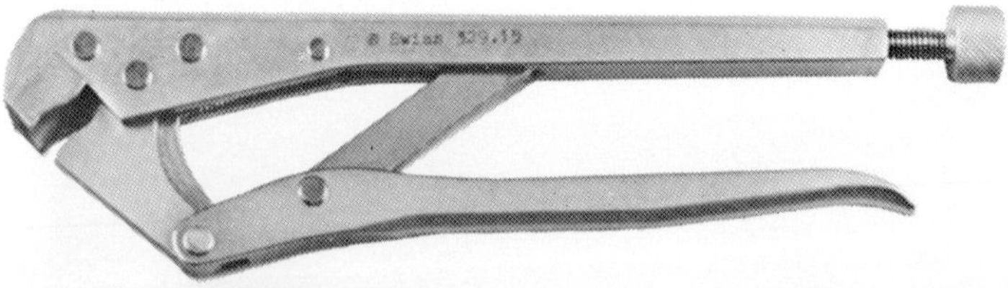

a

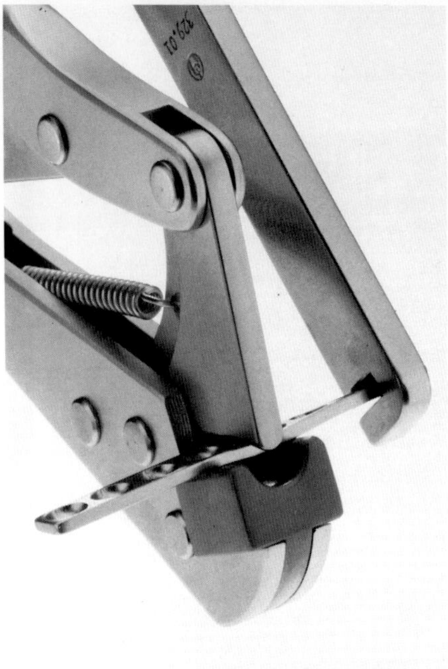

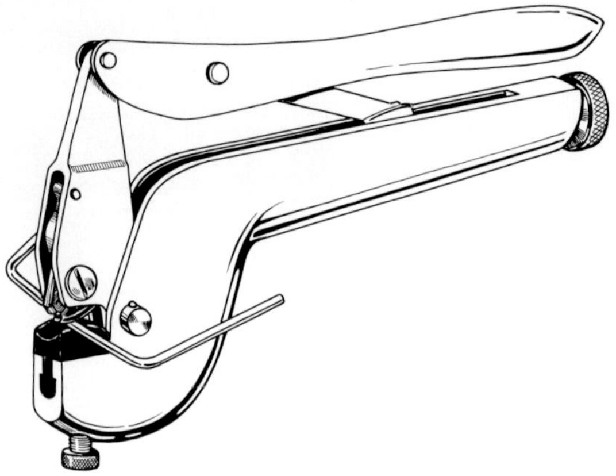

c

b

Fig. 126. **a** Plate bending pliers. **b** Bending an 8-hole plate with an appropriate anvil (interchangable). **c** Plate bending pliers with interchangable anvil for bending the connecting bar of the external fixation device (see Fig. 74)

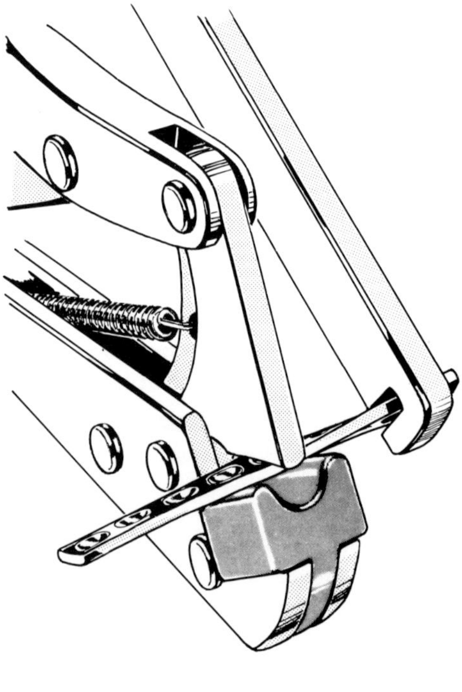

Fig. 127. The plate can be locked in the bending pliers while one end is twisted with the bending iron

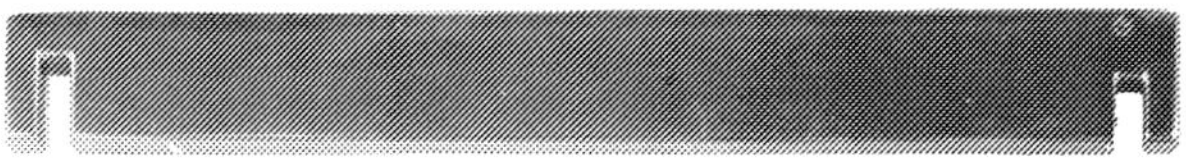

Fig. 128. Bending iron

Fig. 129. Malleable templates for contouring bone plates

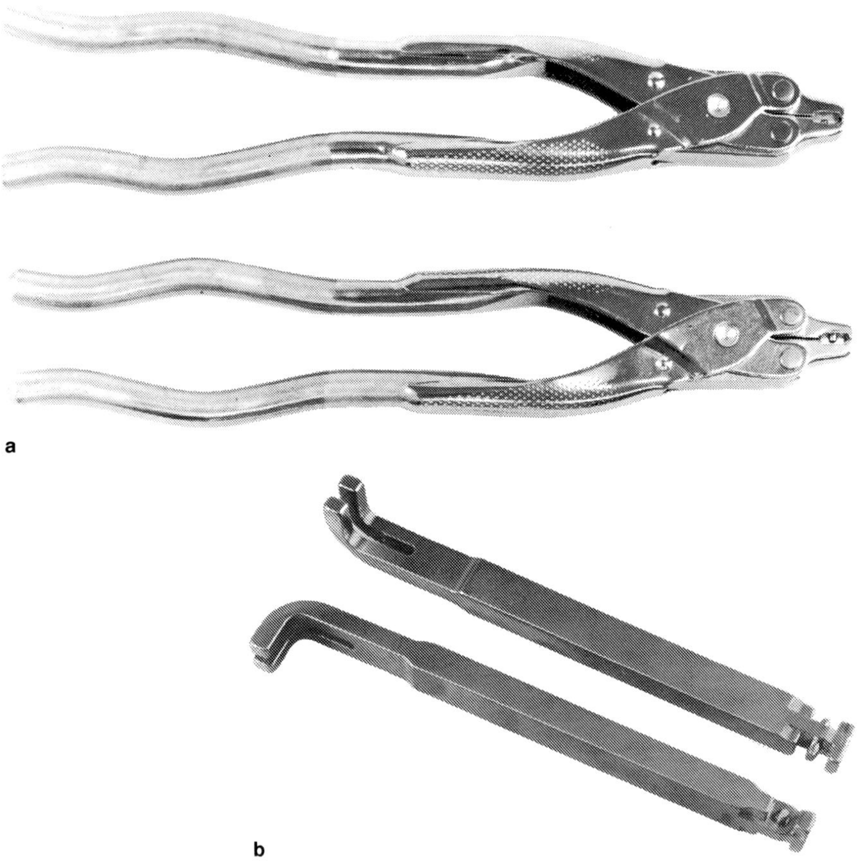

Fig. 130. **a** Special bending pliers for reconstruction plates. **b** Bending irons for reconstruction plates

5.4 Mandibular Implants

The temporary implants used for internal fixations of the mandible consist of plates, screws, and in some cases wires. The implant set for mandibular surgery, consisting of plates and screws, is supplied in an aluminum case. The assortment of implants is sufficient to deal with the most common fractures and is available in stainless steel or titanium.

5.4.1 Mandibular Plates

The plate serves to neutralize bending forces and so is designed primary to withstand tensile loading. Torsion and shear forces are absorbed either by the arrangement of the fixation system (e.g., a plate combined with a tension band, see pp. 21 and 59) or by the use of a stronger implant (reconstruction plate). This makes it possible to keep the size of the plate small, commensurate with the small anatomic dimensions of the mandibular region.

We make reference in internal fixation to the compression plate, neutralization plate, buttress plate, bridge plate, and reconstruction plate, depending on the function of the device. Two types of plate system are utilized in the mandible: the *linear* system and the *universal* system.

Plates of the linear system are straight and can be deformed in only two dimensions. Despite this limitation, they have a greater range of applications than plates with an angular or U-shaped cross-section.

The plates of the *universal* system are deformable in three dimensions and can be applied at any site. They are thicker than the linear plates, which makes them excellent for buttressing and bridging comminuted fractures and segmental defects.

Both plate systems possess satisfactory strength and elasticity. Their ductility (deformability at room temperature) enables them to be adapted to the bone by bending.

5.4.1.1 Linear System: DCP and EDCP (see Figs. 131–136)

The DCP (dynamic compression plate) offers the following advantages:

1) Axial (interfragmental) compression.
2) Angling of the plate screw. The screw can be angled through 25° axially and 7° transversely. Thus, if necesary, a screw can be placed very close to a fracture line without crossing it (Fig. 132a) or can be lagged across the fracture site to give added stability (Fig. 132b). A screw also may be angled transversely to spare important anatomic structures such as a nerve or dental root (Fig. 132c). This capability should be applied judiciously, for it is not the number of screws that determines stability *but the placement of the first two screws close to the fracture line. These screws, firmly anchored in both cortices, have the most important static compression function.*
3) Fixation of the plate to the bone without danger of distraction by using the DCP drill guide in the neutral position.

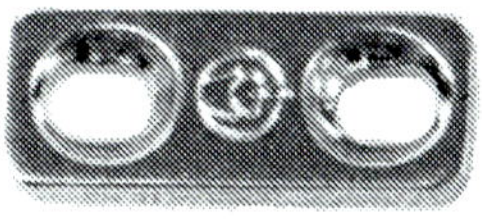

a

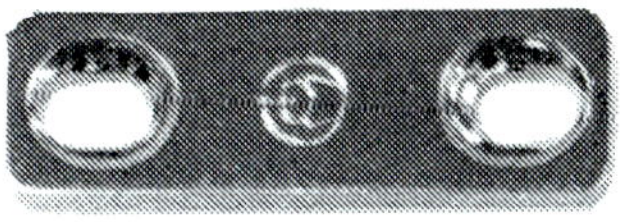

b

Fig. 131 a, b. The 2.7-mm DCP (dynamic compression plate for 2.7-mm screws). The 2-hole model, short or long, is used as a tension band plate on the mandibular angle. The 4- and 6-hole model is used as a stabilization or neutralization plate and may be supplemented by a tension band splint or tension band plate

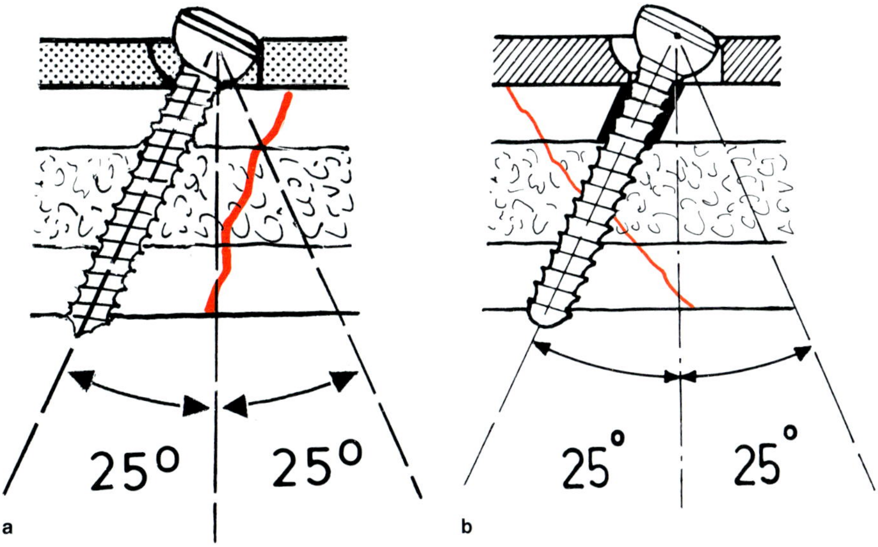

a b

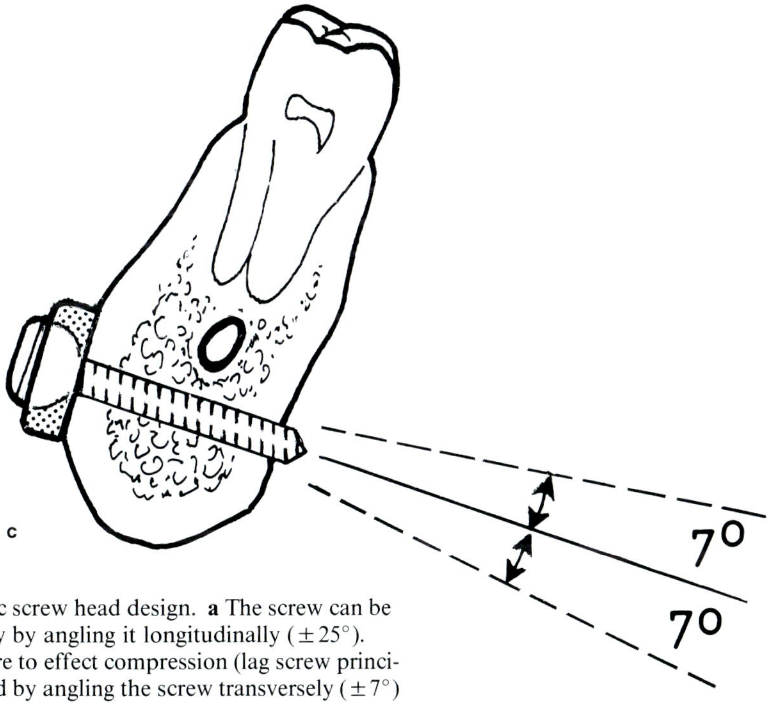

c

Fig. 132 a–c. Advantages of the hemispheric screw head design. **a** The screw can be placed close to the fracture where necessary by angling it longitudinally (±25°). **b** The screw can be angled across the fracture to effect compression (lag screw principle). **c** Anatomic structures can be preserved by angling the screw transversely (±7°)

4) Final coaptation of an imperfectly reduced fracture by utilizing the 0.8-mm compressive displacement of the plate. This is done by placing the second screw in the maximum "load" position using the yellow DCP drill guide (Fig. 133, see also Comments on p. 98).
5) Sequential compression of multiple fractures (Fig. 134).

The EDCP (eccentric dynamic compression plate, Figs. 135 and 136) produces a convergence of the compressive forces through a centric (axial) and eccentric arrangement of the plate holes (see p. 60).

Note: During attachment of the 75° EDCP, the sloped edge of the transverse hole (active edge) must be lowermost at the inferior border of the mandible (Fig. 136 b). *Only the 75° EDCP has been manufactured since 1987, because this angle provides optimal compression at the alveolar side of the fracture.*

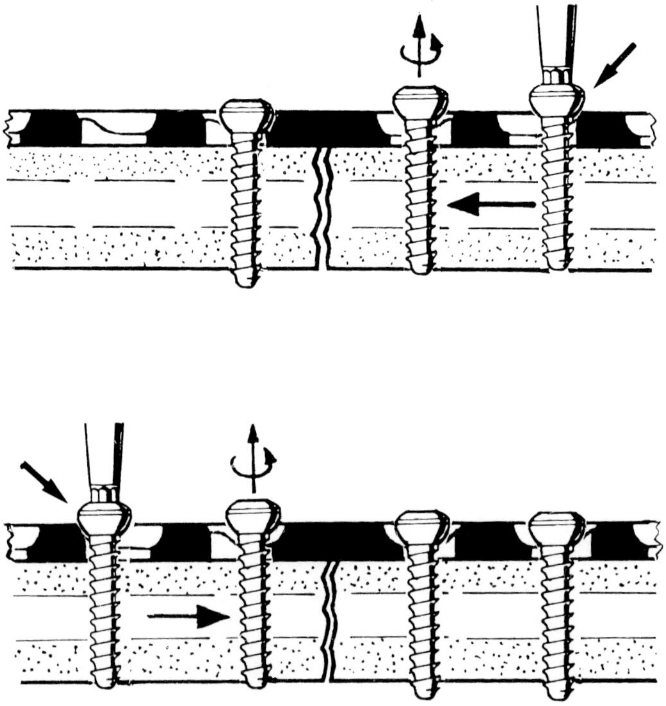

Fig. 133. Approximation of the fragments by utilizing the DC principle on both sides of the plate: The screw adjacent to the fracture is loosened, and the more distant screw is inserted eccentrically in the maximum "load" position

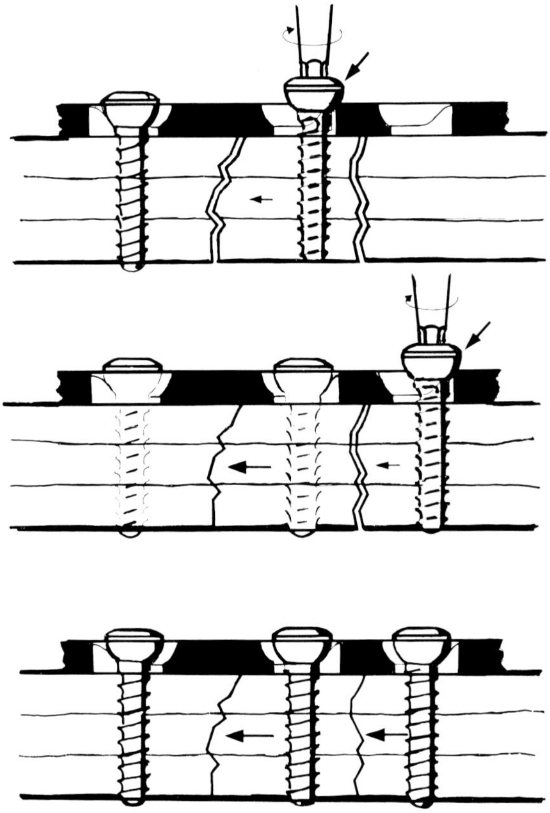

Fig. 134. Sequential compression of multiple fractures

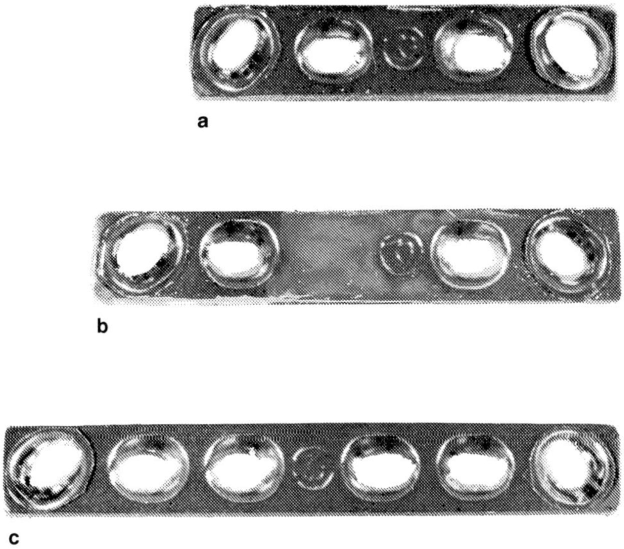

Fig. 135 a–c. Experimental version: EDCPs with 45° outer holes

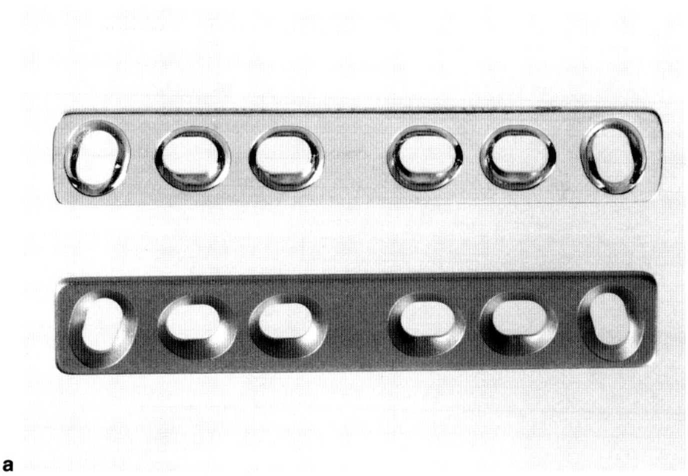

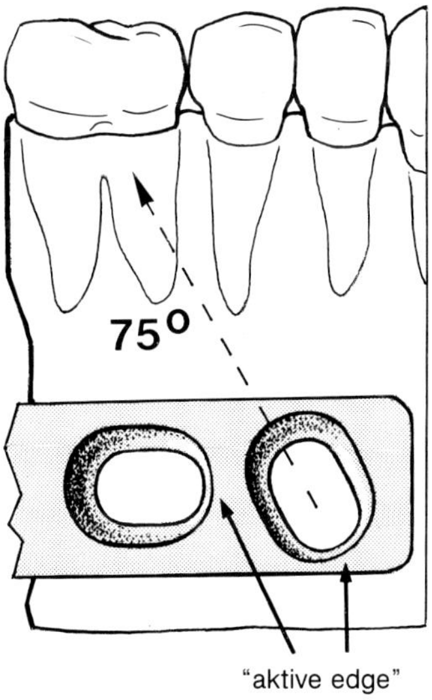

Fig. 136 a, b. Six-hole mandibular EDCP with 75° outer holes. The sloped edge of the tranverse hole can be seen on both sides of the plate. **b** The sloped edge of the plate hole is the "aktive" edge

5.4.1.2 Universal Plate System: Reconstruction Plate (Fig. 137)

As stated above, the universal *reconstruction plate* is used primarily for buttressing and bridging. These functions are dependent on two conditions:

1) functionally stable retention of the mandibular stumps or fragments in an anatomically correct position (see Fig. 346);
2) mechanical rest and, with an interposed bone graft, access for undisturbed revascularization.

A review of the literature from 1945 to 1978 (Schmoker 1986) demonstrates the wide range of devices that have been developed for the bridging of defects - 33 methods in 33 years - and underscores the problem of mandibular reconstruction.

Development of an ASIF reconstruction plate began in Basel in 1973. The current plate is the product of positive clinical experience (in Basel, Bern, Freiburg, Toronto, Buffalo, and Syracuse) and extensive experimental studies which Schmoker (1986) performed in 44 minipigs. The plate is 2.7 mm thick, 7.8 mm wide, has an arched cross-section, and is notched along its edges. The DC holes are spaced 8 mm apart and are designed to accept 2.7-mm cortex screws. The strength is optimal for bridging of comminuted areas in trauma. These plates are loaded for the limited period of time until the fracture has united.

The holes are bidirectional, i.e., they permit compression to be applied in either longitudinal direction. The notches, which increase the area available for vascular ingrowth into grafted bone, enable the plate to be bent edgewise and faciliate twisting. However, the plate may become weakened or deformed if bent more than 15° on edge, so it is best to use the standard preshaped plates (Fig. 137b) for fractures involving the apex of the mandibular angle. The plates can withstand considerable bending without losing their biotechnical properties. Even so, we strongly recommend that bending be performed with the plate bending pliers, and twisting with the bend-

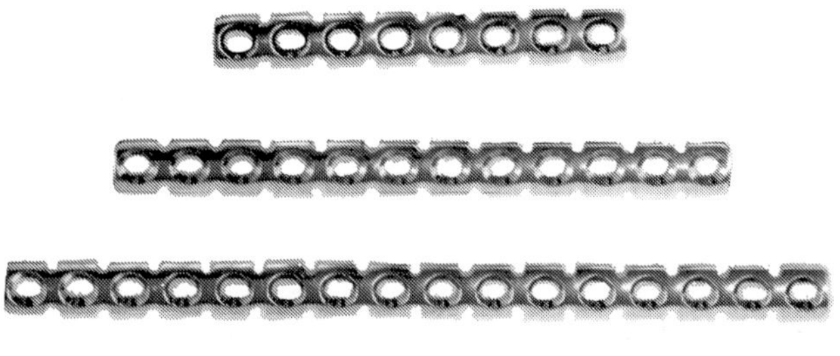

a

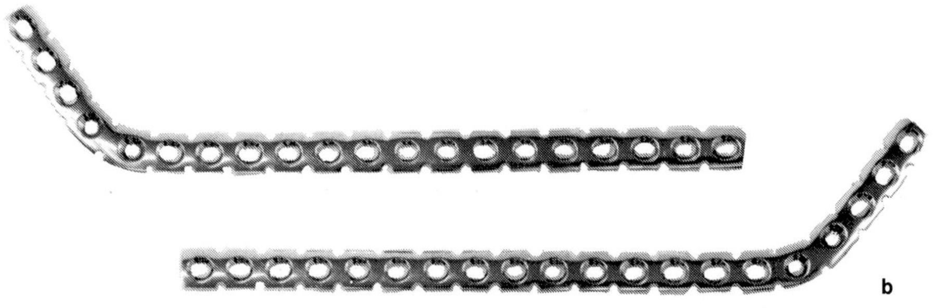

b

Fig. 137 a, b. Legend see page 111

Fig. 137 a–e. Universal plate system. **a** Straight reconstruction plates, narrow, 6–24 holes. **b** Angled reconstruction plates, left and right, 20–24 holes. **c** Mandibular reconstruction plate (body reconstruction), small: 26 holes, medium: 28 holes, large: 32 holes. **d** Angled reconstruction plates with condylar head, left and right, each available in three lengths. **e** Articular prosthesis (see Fig. 360)

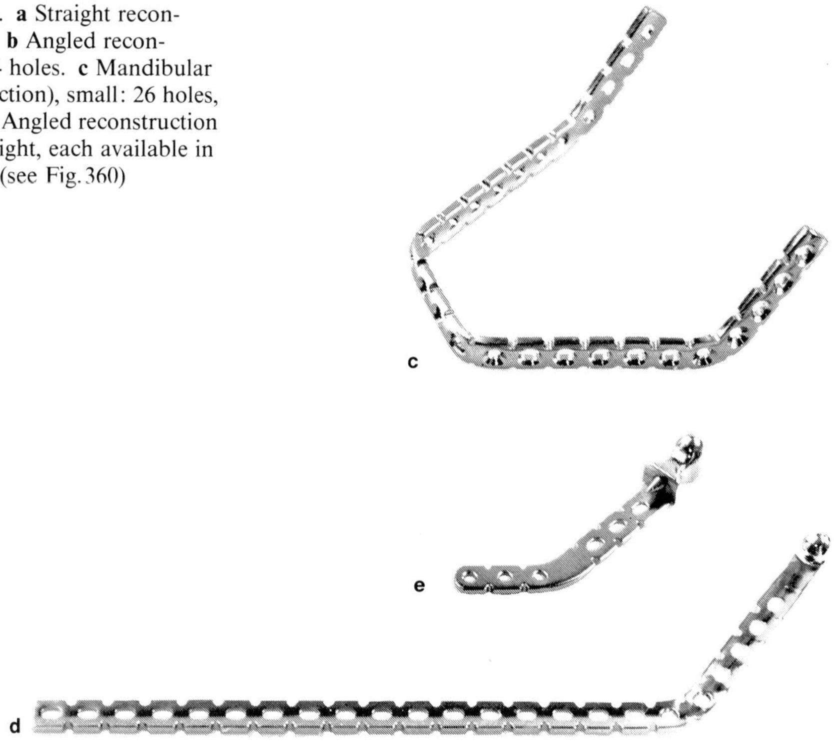

ing irons and/or the special pliers for mandibular reconstruction plates (Fig. 138 a, b). The plate should never be bent at a sharp angle, and all bending and twisting should occur at the notches between holes. Bending the plate back and forth will strain the metal, alter its surface, and predispose to corrosion and failure. Plates that have been repeatedly bent and twisted should be replaced. By the same token, implants should not be reused after removal.

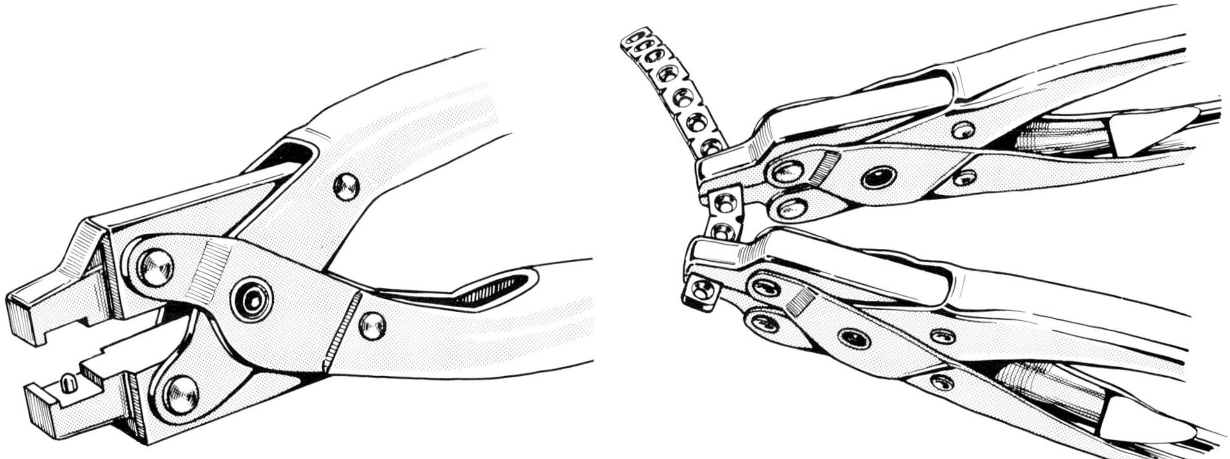

a b

Fig. 138. **a** The special bending pliers have box-shaped jaws with a central peg to hold the reconstruction plate securely for bending on edge and for twisting. **b** Use of two pliers for edgewise bending of the plate

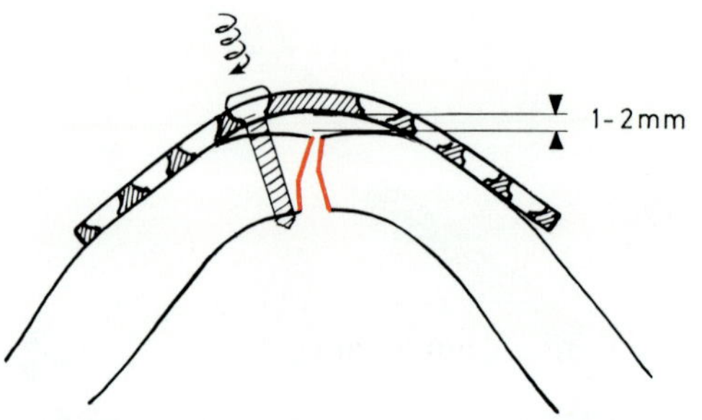

Fig. 139. Overbending the plate creates a "leaf spring" mechanism that improves interfragmental compression. Once the two central screws have brought the bone flush the plate, the remaining screws may be inserted (see also Fig. 18)

5.4.1.3 Principles of Plate Bending

Adaptation of the plate is an important part of a technically sound internal fixation. It consists of *contouring* and *overbending*. First the plate is adapted to the bony surface at the site where it is to be applied. This may be done with the aid of a template if desired. Then the plate is overbent. A bending pliers is used to give the plate a slightly arched shape so that a gap of 1-2 mm remains between the center of the plate and the fracture (Fig. 139). The slight discrepancy between the shapes of the plate and bone increases the interfragmental compression and improves its distribution, especially on the lingual side of the fracture (see Fig. 32a, b). This occurs when the first pair of screws are placed closely adjacent to the fracture line, and the remaining screws are inserted from the center of the plate outward. The basal outer surface of the mandible is flat to convex. The arched plate section is longer than the opposing segment of bone and therefore acts as a leaf spring when the screws are inserted in the neutral position. The remaining screws are not inserted until the two central screws have been tightened and the plate is flush with the bone.

The procedure for attaching the EDCP is somewhat different: the *central* screws are inserted first (longitudinal holes, eccentrically away from the fracture), and the *end* screws are inserted second (the 75° oblique holes eccentrically towards the inferior border). Finally the remaining screws are inserted outward from the center in a neutral position (see Fig. 57).

5.4.2 Mandibular Screws

The ASIF screw is the essential means for effecting interfragmental compression. It may be used individually as a *lag screw* or in conjunction with a plate as a *fixation screw*.

5.4.2.1 Cortex Screw

The 2.7-mm cortex screw is the standard *lag screw* and *fixation screw* for mandibular surgery. It is *fully threaded*. When used as a lag screw, it produces interfragmental compression obliquely or at right angles to its long axis by the classic lag screw mechanism. Used as a fixation screw, it represents one element of a system that, in conjunction with the DCP, produces both transverse compression and axial interfragmental compression. The magnitude of the transverse compression determines the quality of the plate fixation, which is proportional to the number of threads that grip the cortex. The screw passes freely through the plate hole, and its head presses the plate against the bone surface. Axial compression between the fragments results from the geometric interaction of the sphere and cylinder as modeled in the spherical gliding principle (see p. 41).

5.4.2.1.1 Thread

The thread of the cortex screw has the same diameter from the head to the tip (Fig. 140 a) so that even the last thread will gain a perfect hold. The wide, deep screw threads with a broad, flat pressure-bearing surface provide a secure hold over the whole length of the screw. This ideal design is fully utilized when the screw is inserted into a tapped hole. The debris formed by the tapping process collects in the flutes of the tap (Fig. 140 c) and is removed along with the cutting instrument. Removal of this material affords a definite advantage over the self-tapping screw: the drill hole needs to be only slightly larger than the core of the screw, so the full width of the threads can grip the bone (see Fig. 140 b).

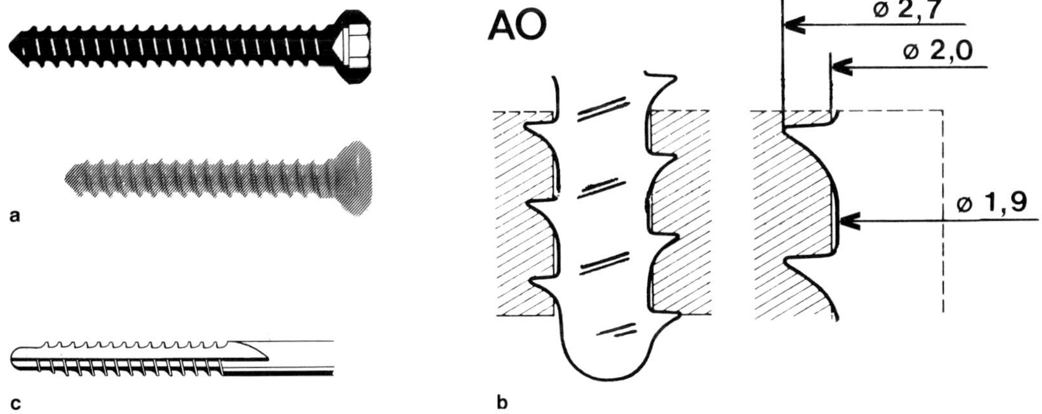

Fig. 140 a–c. Technical principle of the AO/ASIF screw. **a** The thread has a constant diameter from head to tip so that even the last thread will afford a perfect hold. **b** The thread has a sawtooth profile with flat load-bearing surfaces at right angles to the screw axis. It is not fluted like a self-tapping screw. **c** The flute in the tap is for collecting and removing bony debris

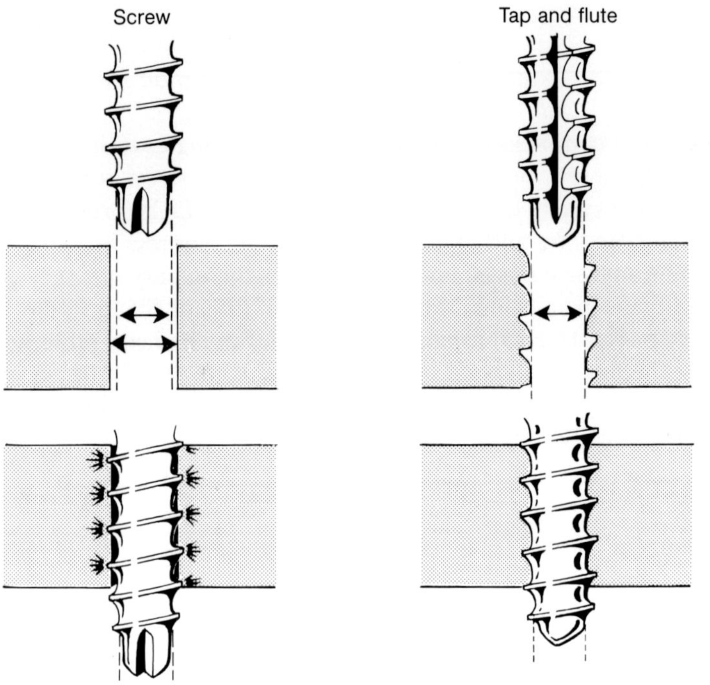

Fig. 141. Comparison of the Sherman and ASIF principles.
Left: The Sherman (self-tapping) principle yields a *less secure hold* because:
1) The drill hole must be larger than the core diameter of the screw (almost as large as the outer thread diameter).
2) Only the tips of the threads engage the bone.
3) Peak loads can easily tear the threads from the bone.
Right: The ASIF principle yields an *optimum hold* because:
1) The drill hole is approximately the same size as the core of the screw, because the thread is cut over the full length of the hole, and the debris collects in the flutes of the tap
2) The threads cut in the bone are deeper and wider
3) The right-angle surfaces of the threads can bear maximum pressure; and 4) the screw hold is not degraded by temporary removal and reinsertion (e.g., preliminary attachment of a reconstruction plate prior to a mandibular resection)

In the self-tapping screw, the rate that the flute fills with bone is proportional to the size of the hole; the smaller the hole, the more rapid the rate of filling. Consequently the drill hole must be relatively large. This means that only the tips of the narrow, V-shaped threads gain a purchase in the bone. Thus, the supposed advantage of a universal self-tapping screw is in fact a disadvantage (Fig. 141: comparison of a Sherman self-tapping screw with the ASIF screw driven into a tapped hole; see also Fig. 8a).

5.4.2.1.2 Spherical Head

The hemispheric screw head was developed as an adjunct to the dynamic compression plate (see p. 41). The hexagonal recess in the screw head enables the screw to be inserted and removed without applying axial pressure. This ensures optimum stress transfer and avoids damage to the recess, as long as the screwdriver is precisely coaxial with the screw.

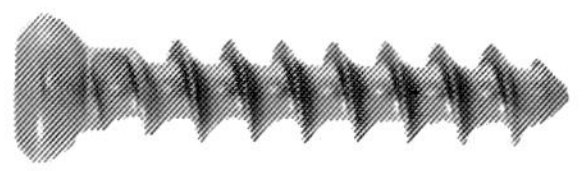

Fig. 142. The "emergency" screw can be inserted to replace a cortex screw that has stripped its precut thread

5.4.2.2 Emergency Screw

Faulty technique, such as drilling without a drill sleeve or power tapping in porous bone, can easily result in a defective threaded hole that does not afford good purchase for the cortex screw. This becomes apparent when the screw strips the hole during insertion. A possible solution in this situation is to replace the cortex screw with an "emergency screw" whose thread profile matches that of a 3.2-mm cancellous screw (deep thread with a high pitch, Fig. 142). The specially deepened thread will cut its way through the stripped hole and should gain a secure hold.

5.4.2.3 Technique of Screw Insertion

Every screw insertion consists of a specific sequence of individual actions such as drilling, length measurement, tapping, and insertion and tightening of the screw.

5.4.2.3.1 Drilling the Screw Hole

Lag screw fixation requires the use of two drill bits of different size, one for the gliding hole and the other for the thread hole. The diameter of the gliding hole matches the outer thread diameter of the screw (Fig. 143); the diameter of the thread hole matches the core diameter of the screw (Fig. 144).

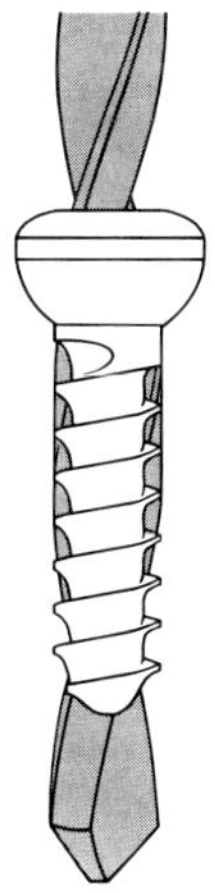

◁ **Fig. 143.** The gliding hole matches the thread diameter of the 2.7-mm screw

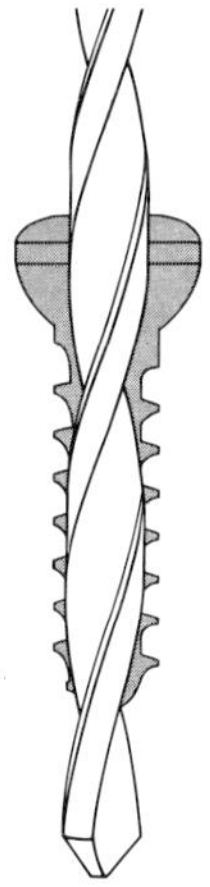

Fig. 144. The compression hole matches the core diameter of the screw (1.9 or 2.0 mm diam.). (From Brinker et al. 1984) ▷

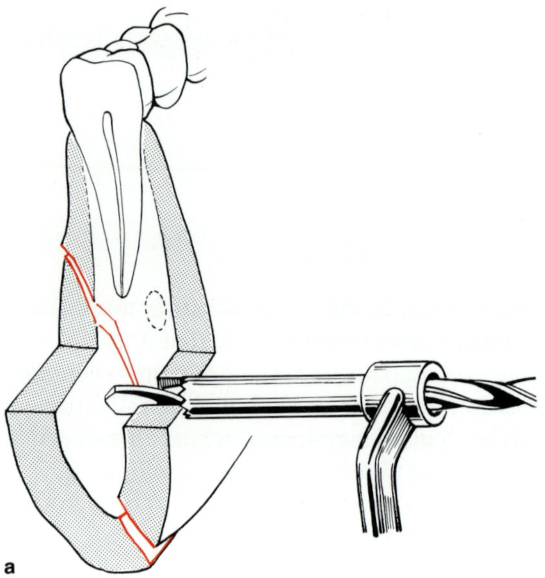

a

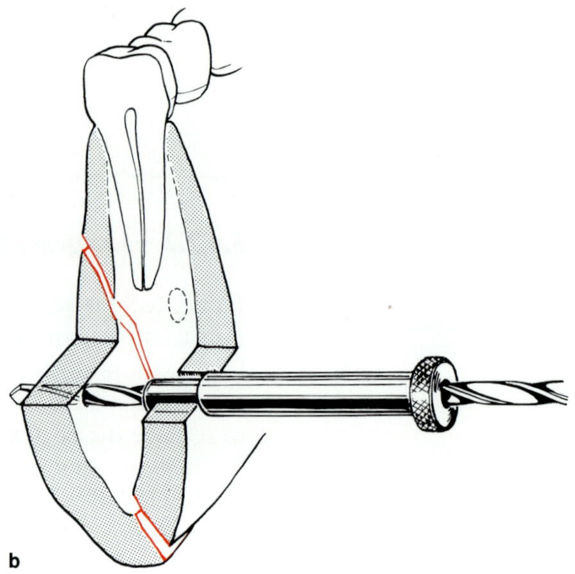

b

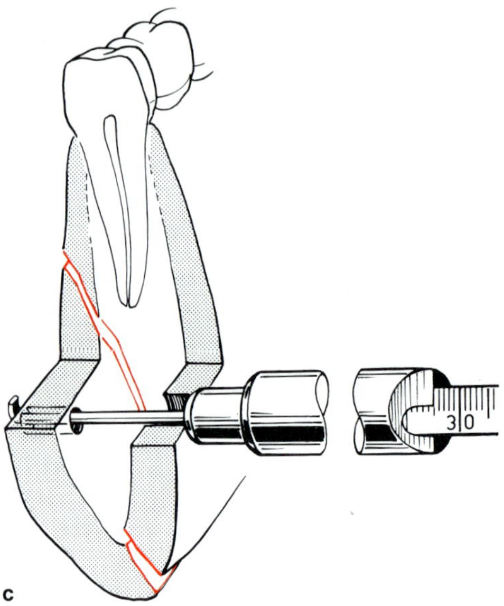

c

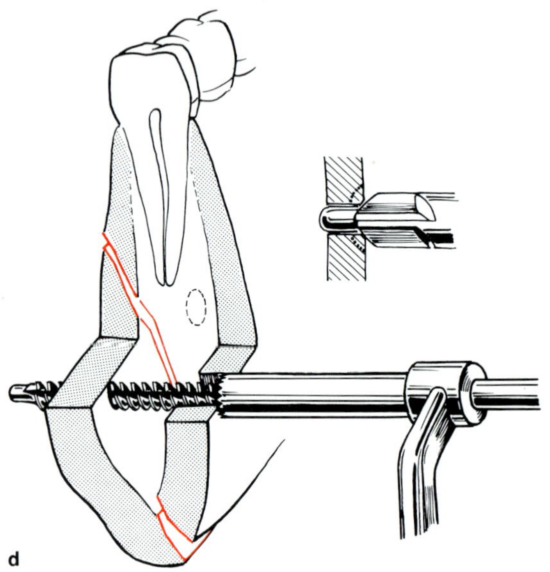

d

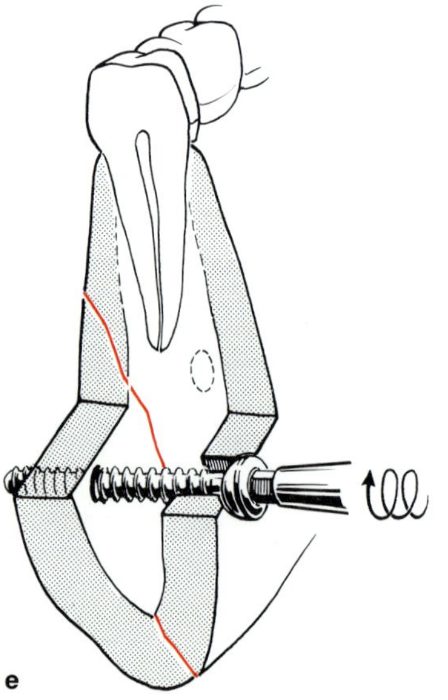

e

Fig. 145 a–e. Technique of lag screw fixation. **a** Drilling the gliding hole (2.7 mm). The tap sleeve, placed against the bone in orthogonal fashion, guides the 2.7-mm bit for drilling the gliding hole in the near cortex. **b** Drilling the compression hole (2.0 mm). The 2.0-mm drill sleeve is seated in the gliding hole for drilling a coaxial 2.0-mm hole in the far cortex. **c** Determination of the screw length. The depth gauge should be used before the hole is tapped. **d** Tapping the hole in the far cortex. The tap sleeve is used to help direct the tap through the predrilled hole. (In the atrophic or osteoporotic mandible, preliminary countersinking of the weakened cortex is advised.) **e** Insertion of the lag screw

Unless the drill sleeve is used systematically, there is a danger of:

- soft-tissue damage and widening of the drill channel by the unsteady shank of the drill bit,
- slippage of the tip of the drill bit on the opposite cortex.

The correct technique for inserting a lag screw is illustrated in Fig. 145 a–e. Some additional technical points should be noted:

1) As the drill bit nears its point of emergence from the far cortex, the drill speed is reduced to ensure that the bit does not fracture the cortex or perforate the soft tissues.
2) As the bit is withdrawn, normal forward operation of the drill should be continued to ensure removal of the drilling debris from the hole (reversing the drill will leave debris in the hole).
3) Never drill without irrigating with Ringer's solution!
4) Never use a drill bit whose flutes contain bony debris!
5) Never use a blunt bit!

Increasing the drilling pressure will not compensate for a blunt drill bit. It will only increase the danger of bone necrosis despite cooling irrigation, and the bowed shank of the bit will widen the drill channel.

5.4.2.3.2 Measuring the Screw Length

The length of the drill hole should be determined *before* the hole is tapped. The measurement should be performed with *one hand,* as this provides a better feel for the position of the depth gauge and avoids damage to the edge of the drill hole, especially on the opposite side. The screw length *includes* the height of the screw head. The definitive length is 2 scale marks more than indicated on the gauge to be sure that the screw threads fully engage the hole in the far cortex. This means that the tapered tip of the screw will project 1–2 mm from the bone (Fig. 146).

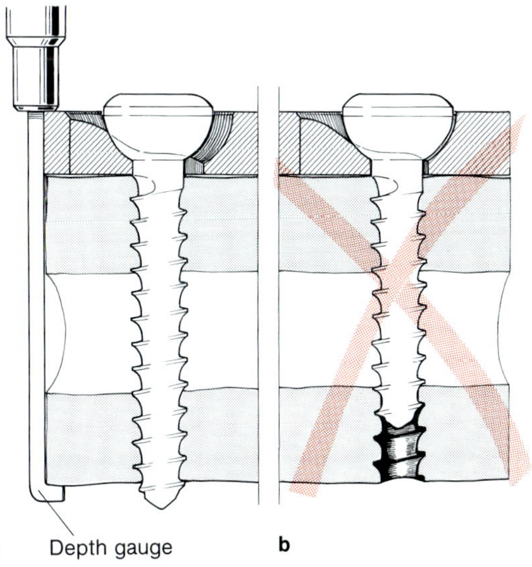

Fig. 146 a, b. The calibration of the depth gauge includes the height of the screw head. Two scale marks are added to the measured length

5.4.2.3.3 Countersinking the Lag Screw

The head of the lag screw should be partially countersunk so that it will not act like a wedge. An appropriate countersink is used for this purpose. Countersinking is mandatory for the single lag screw fixation of an angle fracture due to the necessarily acute angle of the screw insertion relative to the bone surface (see p. 50).

Slight countersinking is also recommended for the screw fixation of a sagittal split osteotomy, depending on the thickness of the cortex. Except for these indications, routine countersinking is not considered necessary because of the very high strength of the mandibular compact bone. It is extremely unlikely that the screw will split the bone when tightened unless severe atrophy or osteoporosis exists. In that case a washer can be used to create a more favorable pressure distribution.

5.4.2.3.4 Tapping (see Fig. 145 d)

The creation of a perfect intraosseous thread depends on how well the tap is aligned with the predrilled hole. A hole should never be tapped without using the appropriate tap sleeve to guide the tap accurately to its destination. For the same reason we prefer manual operation of the tap over tapping with a power drill. The tap is twisted slowly by hand in the clockwise direction. We always use the tap handle with quick coupling (see Fig. 109), as this makes it easier to direct the tap accurately. A palpable lessening of resistance indicates that the tip of the instrument has traversed the second cortex. The tip may slip on the far cortex unless a tap sleeve is used (Fig. 147).

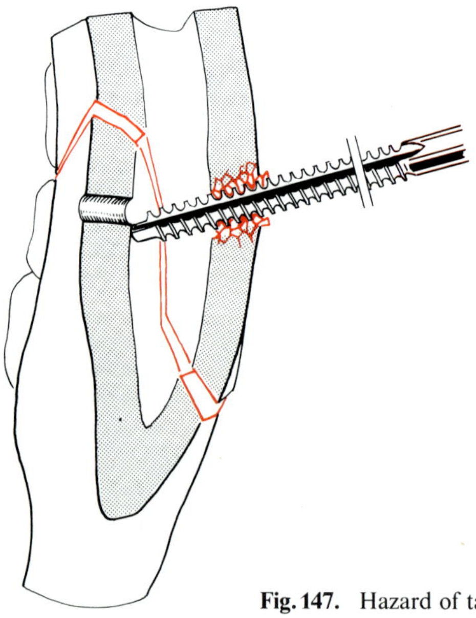

Fig. 147. Hazard of tapping *without* a tap sleeve

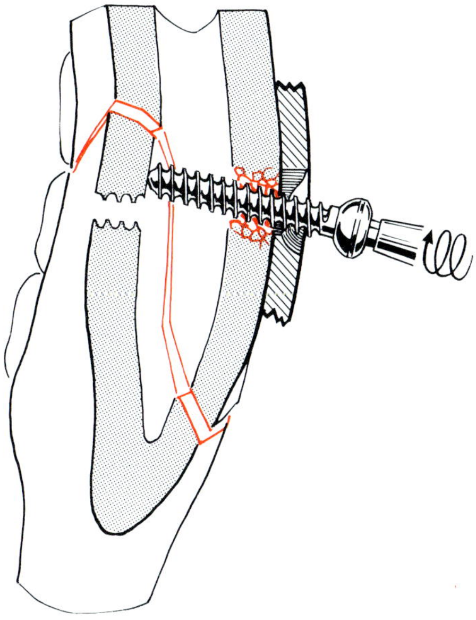

Fig. 148. "Forcing" the screw when resistance is felt can destroy the cortex. Instead, the screw should be withdrawn and its line of insertion checked

Failure to cut a proper thread may cause the screw to strip the hole when inserted. If the emergency screw is of no help in this situation, the screw hole must be left vacant. Because this mishap is not always preventable, we recommend strict observance of the *"three screw rule."* It is axiomatic that *the two screws adjacent to the fracture, solidly anchored in both cortices, are the key to stability.* This key relies upon a perfect thread (see also p. 108).

5.4.2.3.5 Inserting and Tightening the Screw

It is self-evident that the screw must be inserted carefully in the same direction in which the hole has been predrilled and tapped. A misdirected screw will damage the near cortex (Fig. 148), miss the opposite hole, and skid along the inner surface of the far cortex.

Most surgeons quickly learn how to tighten the screw until the proper compression is achieved, i.e., just to the point before the screw begins to strip its precut thread. However, it is remarkable how much force can be applied when tightening the screw if the thread has been properly cut.

5.4.3 Wire as a Fixation Material

Both rigid (Kirschner wire) and flexible wires (e.g., wire sutures) are utilized in orthopedic and trauma surgery. The wires are supplied in separate sterile packages because of the infrequency of their use. There is little occasion for the use of Kirschner wires in the mandible. Wire sutures and cerclage wires also are fixation materials of second choice in the lower jaw. They are most commonly used in the treatment of pediatric fractures (see p. 266).

Wires are occasionally used for graft fixation in cases where plating is not possible (see Fig. 335). When a plate is used to buttress a comminuted fracture, it is sometimes helpful to anchor an intermediate fragment to the reconstruction plate with a simple wire loop (Fig. 149).

Double wire loops offer a simple solution to the problem of the oblique fracture (e.g., beak fracture) in the edentulous, atrophic mandible (Fig. 150). It is important that the wires be applied under tension, and for this purpose the ASIF has adopted a well-known industrial method of wire tightening. After the wire is passed around the mandible, its end is brought through the eye of the wire, then through the oval hole of the tightener, and finally through the hole in the crank (Fig. 151).

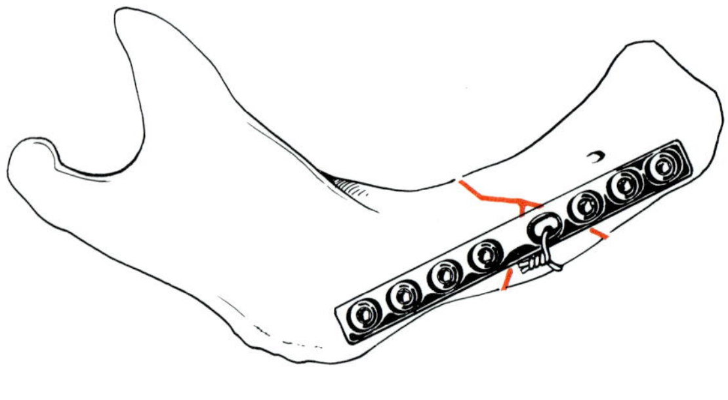

Fig. 149. Wire fixation of a fragment that cannot be fixed securely with a screw

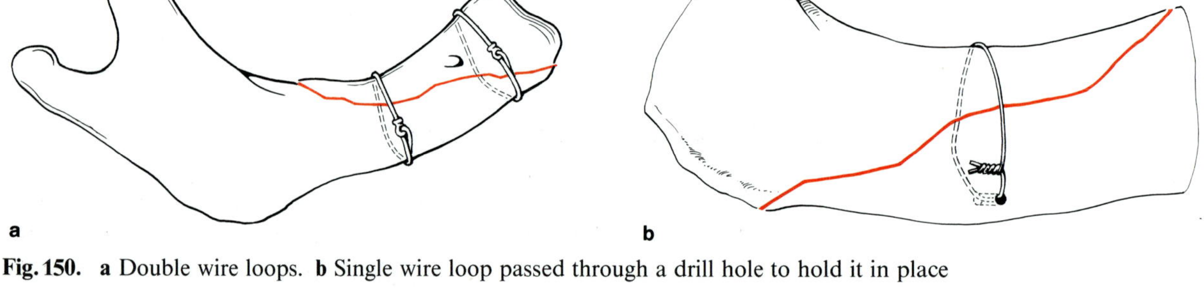

a **b**

Fig. 150. **a** Double wire loops. **b** Single wire loop passed through a drill hole to hold it in place

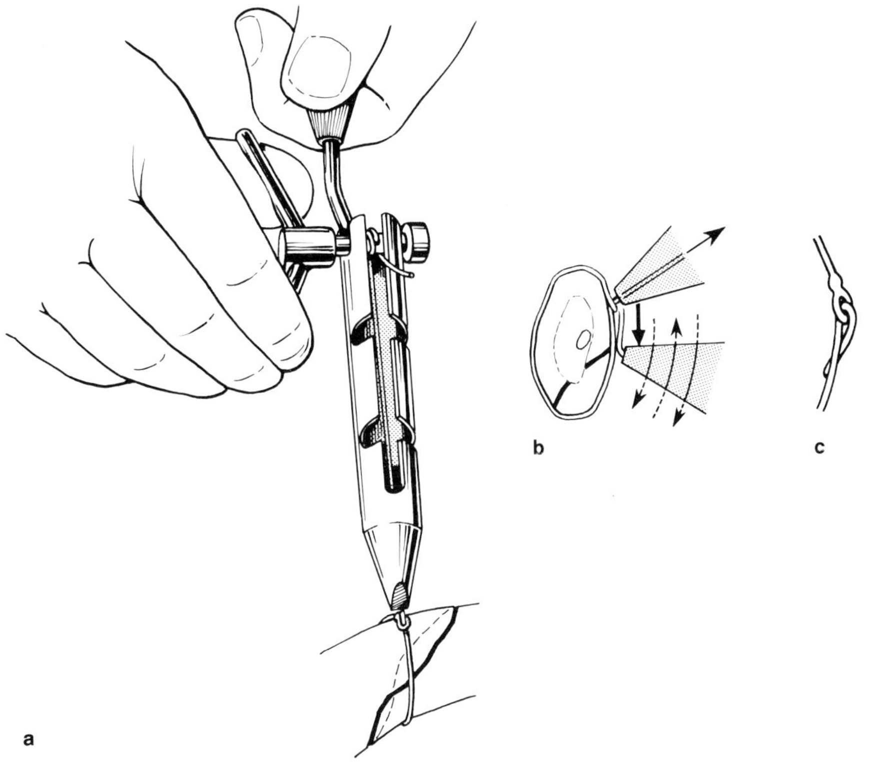

Fig. 151 a–c. Technique of wire tightening. **a** The wire is slowly tightened by turning the crank in the slot. **b** As soon as the wire begins to stretch, the free end is tipped through a 90° angle and released. **c** The wire is cut about 1 cm from the bend, and its free end is tucked under

5.5 Wire Acrylic Splint (Schuchardt Splint)

5.5.1 Functions: Reduction, Retention, Tension Band

The wire acrylic splint is used for reduction, retention, and especially as a tension band. For reduction one may use either a sectional splint or intermaxillary elastic if the splint has not yet been stiffened with acrylic.

5.5.2 Materials and Instrumentation

The splinting material (Fig. 152) consists of a prefabricated arch bar with cross-pins, ligating wire, and self-curing resin (Fig. 152). The arch bar itself is a semiround, soft-annealed Randolf or silver wire 2 mm in diameter. The length of the bar corresponds to the average length of the mandibular arch.

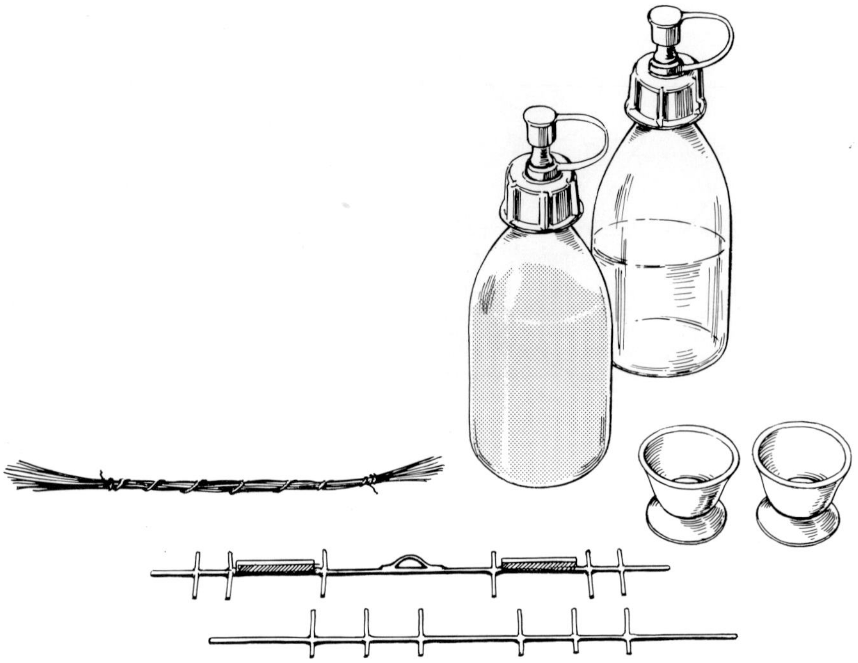

Fig. 152. Prefabricated arch bar with ligating wires and self-curing acrylic resin

Each bar carries 6 cross-pins 1.4 mm in diameter. For the treatment of maxillary fractures, the arch bar is fitted laterally with a pair of rectangular tubes to accommodate extraoral rods and with a central eyelet for attaching a sagittal traction device. For craniofacial suspension we use an arch bar with wire eyelets soldered to the sides of the appliance.

A steel wire 0.35 mm in diameter is best for ligating the arch bar to the teeth. Once the bar is in place, saddle extensions or bite rims with a palatal plate may be added if desired. Generally this is done freehand. We use Palavit self-curing acrylic resin.

5.5.3 Splinting Technique

First the "auxiliary" splint is wired to the nonfractured jaw. If both jaws are fractured, the maxilla is usually splinted first.

5.5.3.1 Placement of the Arch Bar

Before the arch bar is adapted to the teeth, the occlusal ends of the cross-pins are bent toward the occlusal surface at the level of the molars and incisors to form temporary clasps (Fig. 153 a). The bar is adapted freehand to

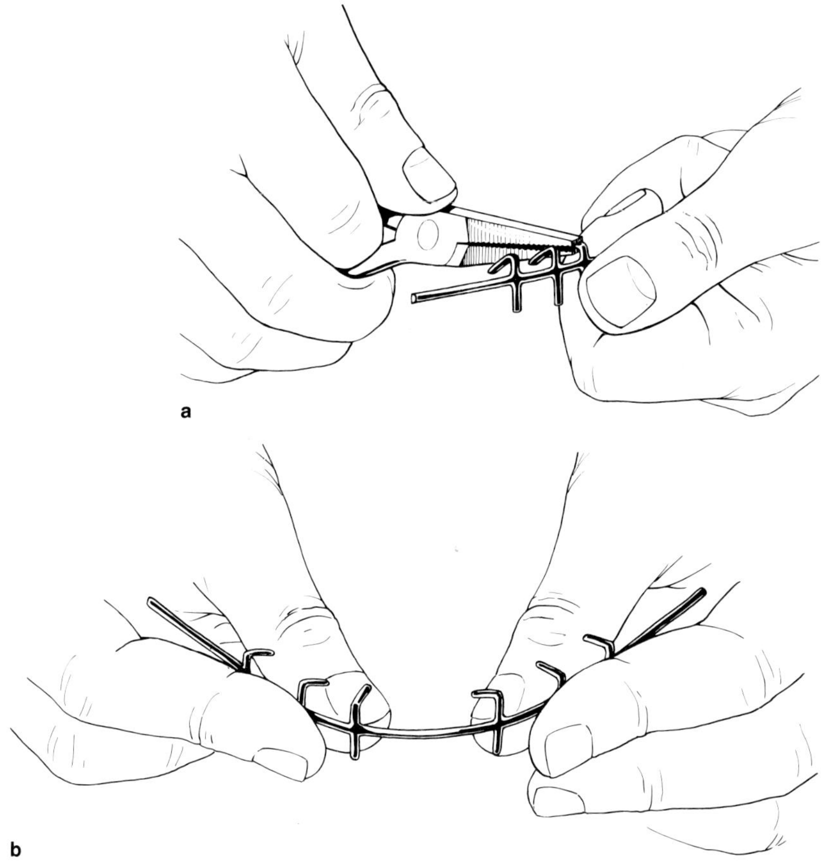

Fig. 153. **a** Bending the cross-pins (occlusal hooks). **b** Adaptation of the arch bar (see text)

the dental arch (Fig. 153 b). The bar should be positioned midway between the edges of the teeth and the gingival margins. The clasps will keep the bar from slipping during placement of the wires. The occlusal clasps are cut off after the wiring is completed and the resin has been applied.

5.5.3.2 Wiring the Arch Bar to the Teeth

We generally employ a *simple interproximal ligature* with one limb of the wire passed gingival to the arch bar and the other passed occlusal to the bar (Fig. 154 a).

First we ligate the arch bar to both premolars on either side. The fingertip places slight tension on the wire as its ends are twisted together. This makes it easier to tighten the wire sufficiently without overtightening and breaking it. When placing the ligature on the last molar, we grasp the free end of the wire distal to the tooth with a suitable instrument and hold it steady until it can be firmly apposed to the neck of the tooth below the bent end of the bar. The wires are shortened to a length of 5 mm (Fig. 154 b). We then use a flatnose pliers to give the wire ends a final twist and bend them back against the bar.

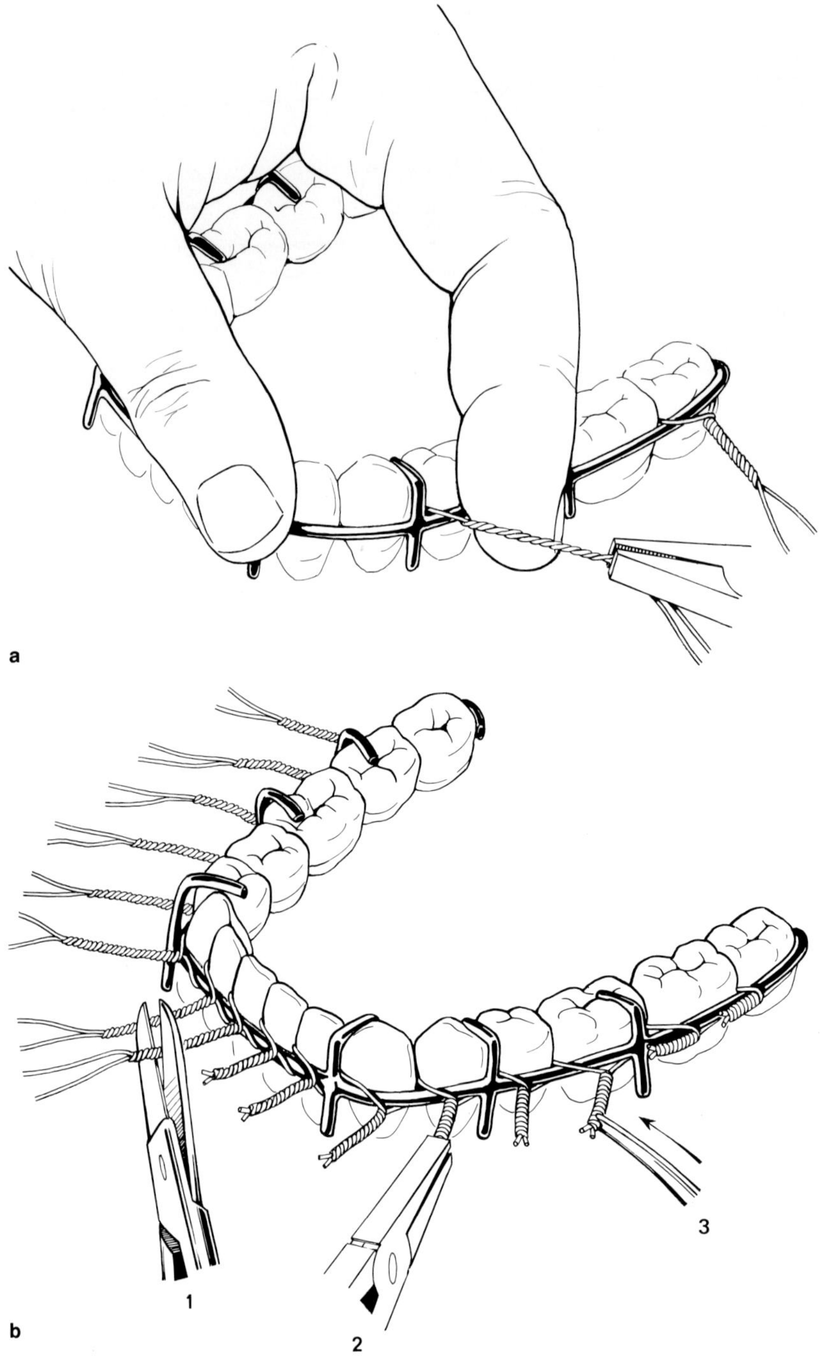

Fig. 154. **a** Wiring the arch bar to the teeth. **b** Shortening the wires

5.5.3.3 Stiffening the Arch Bar

Before the resin is applied, the oral cavity is throughly irrigated with saline solution. The liquid is removed with suction, and the dental arch and bar are dried with an air jet. The viscous resin is applied over the arch bar in sections (Fig. 155 a) and smoothed with a liquid monomer. Finally the occlusal hooks are cut off with wire cutters and smoothed with a grindwheel (Fig. 155 b).

The vestibular ends of the cross-pins will serve later as retention hooks for intermaxillary fixation while the internal fixation is carried out (Fig. 155 c).

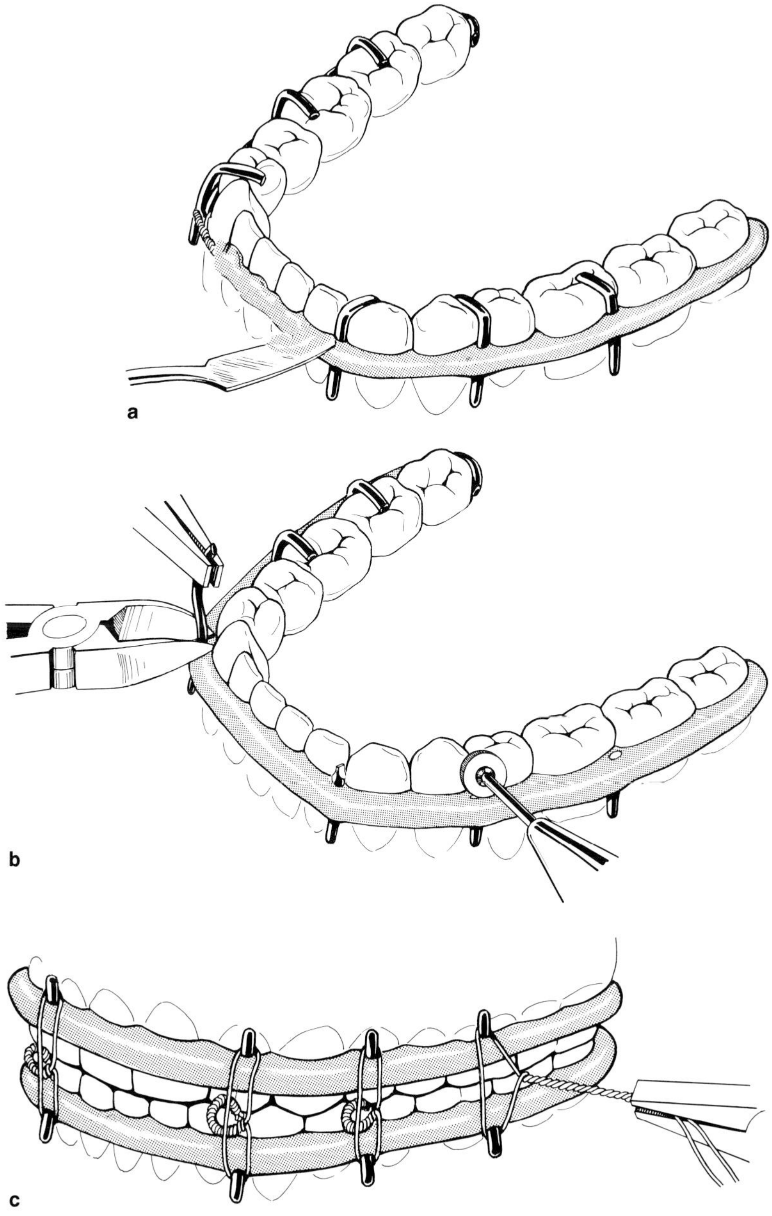

Fig. 155 a–c. Stiffening the arch bar, removal of the occlusal hooks, and intermaxillary fixation

6 Preoperative, Intraoperative, and Postoperative Guidelines

6.1 Organizational Requirements

There is no higher priority in bone surgery than asepsis. The strict maintenance of asepsis depends more on the training and discipline of the physicians, nurses, and orderlies than on any technical refinements. The quality of asepsis is measured by the infection rate, which should not exceed 2% in elective procedures and closed injuries, regardless of whether the procedure is done by the intraoral or extraoral route.

The focus of surgical endeavors in internal fixation is stabilization of the fracture. This requires a high degree of precision and carries a high technical cost. Accordingly, the operating room should have an adequate array of instruments that includes the specific sets for internal fixation and the tray with the general surgical instruments. The organizational advantages of a standardized instrument system and standard operating technique become apparent in this setting.

We have had very good results with the operating room setup illustrated in Fig. 156.

6.2 Priorities in the Care of Multiple Trauma Patients

Border (1984) conducted an informative study on the treatment of patients with multiple trauma. Half the patients were managed conservatively, while the other half were treated by immediate open reduction and internal fixation of their fractures. Both groups received the same intensive care and, where indicated, the same operative treatment of injuries to body cavities. The number of days on the respirator and the total duration of intensive care, including care for metabolic derangements, were significantly less in the patients who received immediate and definitive operative treatment than in the group receiving nonoperative care. An analysis of the data clearly indicates, and a similar study by Johnson et al. (1985) confirms, that a number of complications in multiply injured patients are caused not by the initial trauma but by modalities of conservative therapy. The author characterized these with the term "crucifixion position." One such modality is intermaxillary fixation for concomitant mandibular fractures. The study confirms the benefits of aggressive trauma care, which should include the early stabilization of all fractures.

As Graph 6 indicates, most multiple trauma patients with injuries of the facial skeleton receive definitive treatment for those injuries within one

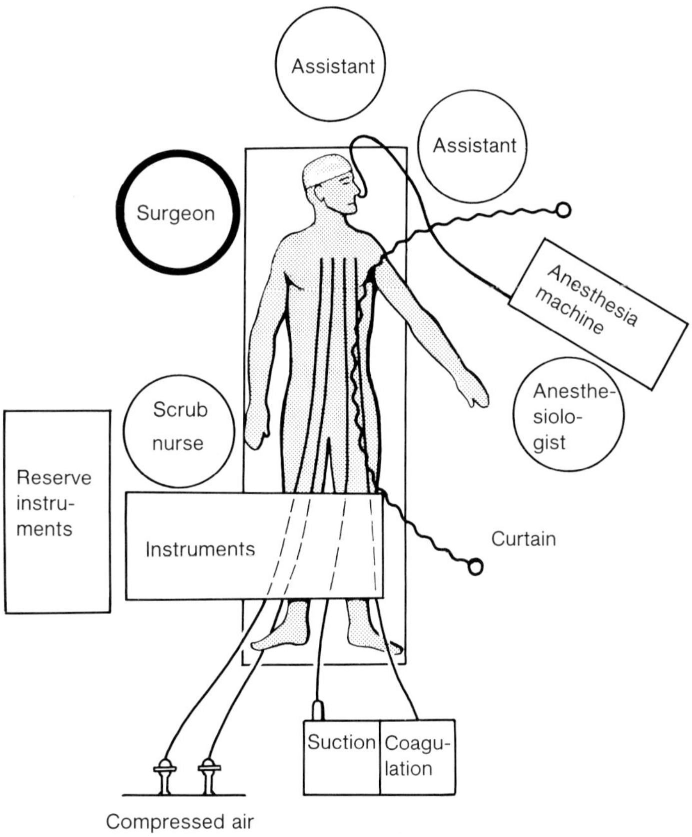

Fig. 156. Disposition of the operating team

week after they are admitted for care. Two conditions must exist in order for this early functional treatment to be provided:

1) an integrated treatment concept (see p. 160ff.).
2) uncompromising application of the principles of stable skeletal fixation.

The integration of all special services makes possible a comprehensive, *phased* approach to patient care (Wolff et al. 1978). We have found that, following resuscitation, it is rarely necessary to intervene acutely with a surgical procedure for the control of bleeding. In most cases aggressive, intensive medical care will enable definitive treatment of the jaw injury to be performed during or at the end of the "stabilization phase" (phase in which vital functions become stabilized). The timing of tracheostomy tube removal and of surgical treatment are determined in consultation with the neurosurgeon and the ICU physician. This coordinated approach has led to a significant reduction in late morbidity. Instances of hypertelorism, enophthalmos, and dish facc have become very rare among our patients and, if they occur at all, are the result of extraordinary circumstances or very severe trauma.

The question of priorities in polytrauma patients is an interdisciplinary decision made under the direction of the emergency physician in charge. The decision concerning primary or postprimary treatment depends on the threat to life posed by blood loss and on the degree of injury to cranial, thoracic, and abdominal organs. The prevention of posttraumatic respiratory problems continues to be a major concern until blood gas analyses show satisfactory values.

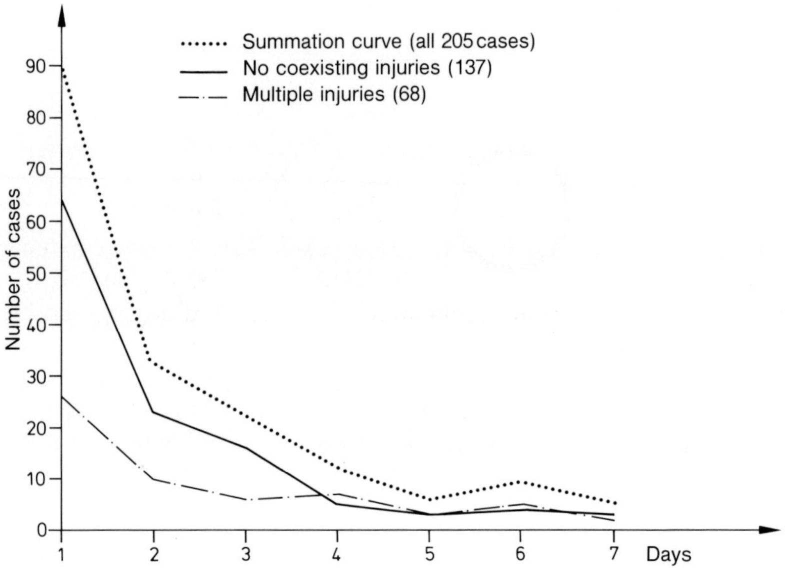

Graph. 6. Interval between the occurrence and internal fixation of 205 mandibular fractures treated in Basel from 1976 to 1982

Postprimary treatment, if required, consists of the operative control of life-threatening bleeding (e.g., from the maxillary artery) performed concurrently with other life-saving procedures on the head, chest, and abdomen.

In Basel we have found that the immediate and definitive treatment of long-bone fractures in polytrauma patients greatly facilitates intensive care. The same applies to the treatment of major mandibular injuries, which can be stabilized while a second team is operating on a fractured lower extremity (see p. 162).

6.3 Timing of Operation

The benefits of immediate or early fracture treatment in multiple trauma patients are well established (Allgöwer and Border 1983). If the fracture cannot be stabilized before the onset of swelling, it is common practice to defer treatment until swelling has subsided. But this rule does not have the same force in mandibular fractures as it does in fractures of the extremities. The mandibular fracture, whether open or closed, may be stabilized even two or more days after the traumatic episode, and even when there are signs of incipient or established infection. The main concern is the absolutely stable fixation of the fracture (see Indications for External Fixation, p. 69).

6.3.1 Plan of Operation

Preoperative planning is based on clinical and radiographic findings with emphasis upon the classification of the mandibular fracture, the "FLO" formula (fracture category, fracture site, and occlusal status), and the grade of severity of the injury (see p. 152ff.). With difficult Grade III and Grade IV fractures, it is best to intubate the patient before proceeding with the manual examination, as a thorough examination is most easily conducted under general anesthesia; sterile gloves should be worn at this time. With the results of the manual examination and selected radiographic views in hand, it will be possible to formulate a plan of operative treatment and discuss it with the operating team. Personnel should be clearly apprised as to the instruments and instrument sets that will be needed for the retention of occlusion, bone grafting, possible dental extractions, and the definitive stabilization of the fracture.

6.3.2 Preparation of the Operative Field

Some preparations are aimed at the prevention of further infection. If the patient is taken directly from the emergency room to the operating suite, wound dressings should not be disturbed until anesthesia has been induced and the dressings can be removed under sterile conditions.

The same precautions are applied to the splinting of open fractures. Extensive shaving is not only unnecessary but potentially harmful. Facial hair removal, if required, should be limited to the immediate area of the incision. Even in elective procedures shaving should be done at the time of the definitive skin prep, just prior to surgery, rather than on the day before the operation.

Cleansing should follow the "inside-to-outside" principle and should be done in the preparation room where anesthesia is induced. Cleansing is best achieved with a spray or jet lavage, with Ringer's solution and hydrogen serving as the primary media. Of course, antiseptic sprays such as Betadine or hexachlorophene also may be used. Embedded foreign particles should be removed from wounds by scrubbing with a stiff brush.

The head is dorsiflexed before sterile drapes are applied. Topographic landmarks or reference lines will aid the surgeon in making the correct incision (see p. 170).

6.4 Postoperative Care

It is our practice to leave sutured wounds uncovered. Twice daily the wound is cleansed with an antiseptic solution following copious irrigation of the oral cavity with a saline spray. The nursing staff is instructed to enforce oral hygiene measures after every meal, stressing the importance of tooth brushing rather than simple rinsing. The lips should be smeared with bepanthene ointment or Vaseline, especially if intraoral splints are present.

Cold, moist compresses are applied continually to promote swelling reduction and relaxation of the soft tissues.

Vacuum drainage bottles are changed twice daily. The drain should be suctioned at this time to keep it clear and functioning. The drain is removed after two to three days if less than 5 cm^3 of seroma fluid is collected.

Follow-up radiographs should be taken no later than one day before the patient is to be discharged.

The length of hospitalization for a mandibular fracture alone is four to seven days. The patient is fed a soft diet during that time.

6.5 Atraumatic Operating Technique

6.5.1 Handling of the Soft Tissues

The target organ of internal fixation is the bone. Its exposure requires a meticulous dissection and anatomically exact division of the soft tissues. This is necessary to ensure uncomplicated healing, an acceptable scar, and the preservation of essential nervous structures.

6.5.1.1 Value of the Scalpel Technique

The progress of healing depends to a large extent on the handling of the soft tissues. Atraumatic soft-tissue handling requires a mastery of the scalpel technique. With this technique thin tissue layers can be successively divided *without pressure,* and severed blood vessels will present cleanly on the wound surface where they can be coagulated with a fine splinter forceps. Bleeding vessels are coagulated at once so that they will not obscure the field. Hemostatic clamps should be kept out of the field if at all possible. The division of tissue with a scissors inflicts considerably greater tissue and cellular injury than cutting with the sharp blade. Any surgical act that increases the volume of necrotic tissue will tend to aggravate edema and inflammation.

The interchangeable blade, splinter forceps, and small wound retractors (instead of surgical forceps) are the instruments that need to be mastered in order for successful atraumatic handling of the soft tissues to be accomplished.

6.5.2 Prevention of Infection

The wound bed is irrigated approximately every 15 min with isotonic Ringer's solution to protect the tissues from drying and infection. Blood and tissue fluid should be removed by suction whenever possible; swabs are rarely used.

Hematoma formation and posttraumatic infection are most effectively prevented by meticulous hemostasis and by the consistent use of vacuum drainage following closure of the wound.

6.5.3 Handling of the Bone

Bone is a bradytrophic tissue, and its mechanisms of compensating for a sudden disturbance of blood flow take time to become operative. Recognition of this fact dictates the manner in which the bone must be handled.

Preservation of maximum blood supply during fracture exposure requires:

- sharp division of the periosteum;
- elevating rather than scraping the periosteum from the bone (smoothly elevated, uninjured periosteal surfaces are a sign of atraumatic technique);
- limiting exposure to the basal part of the fracture (the alveolar part has already been reduced and retained by the intermaxillary fixation);
- respecting the intact lingual surface of the bone;
- avoiding excessive periosteal stripping by planning the details of the fixation in advance and determining the number of plate holes that will have to be occupied by screws.

Neglect in these areas can spoil an initially stable fixation due to circulatory deficits and loss of bone strength, resulting in gradual loosening of the implant. The cause of this complication, known as "secondary instability," can be difficult to pinpoint in a given case, although the studies of Hörster (1985) offer a plausible explanation (see p. 141 ff.). The reduction-compression forceps (Fig. 157) is an excellent aid to preserving the osseous blood supply. This instrument makes it possible to limit the exposure to the dimensions of the bone plate and makes it unnecessary to strip periosteum from the lingual aspect of the jaw. The self-centering bone forceps (see

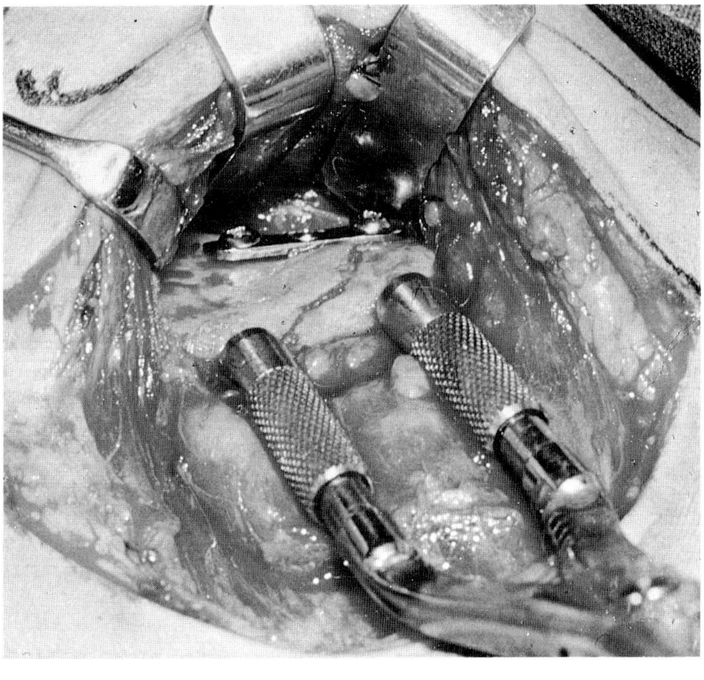

Fig. 157. Reduction-compression forceps attached with screws to the lower border of the mandible. This instrument simplifies the reduction, allows manipulation of the fragments in a narrow field, can distract the fragments for removal of interposed material, and produces axial precompression

Fig. 105) and single-prong hook are also useful aids in difficult reductions. In special cases the disturbance of blood flow is minimized by using two separate approaches (see Fig. 263 a).

6.6 Antibiotic Prophylaxis (General)

At all times the oral cavity is colonized by facultative pathogens that are capable of inciting a purulent infection, especially since *Staphylococcus aureus* predominates over coexisting organisms like *Actinomyces, Streptococcus (viridans),* and *Candida.* Closed fractures that are treated intraorally are at significant risk of infection from endogenous bacterial flora. The danger becomes acute when host resistance is weakened as a result of age, diabetes, leukopenia, or drug addiction. It is unclear just how frequently "opportunistic infections" develop in fractures that are treated by the intraoral surgical route. However, prophylactic antibiotics are clearly indicated in cases where it is apparent prior to surgery that systemic resistance or local defenses are compromised. Jaques investigated the value of prophylactic antibiotics in elective maxillofacial procedures at our center in 1976 and concluded that preventive chemotherapy was not routinely justified. For some years the ASIF has rejected routine antibiotic prophylaxis in fracture treatment due to the danger of promoting resistant strains. This policy is based upon the low infection rate of 2% that is associated with such procedures.

The concept of antibiotic prophylaxis has changed considerably since the studies of Burke (1963). At one time the prophylaxis was taken to mean the intra- and/or postoperative use of antibiotics. But Burke's animal studies showed that an antibiotic can prevent infection only if an active concentration of the drug is already present in the blood and tissues immediately before the incision is made. To achieve the necessary "minimal inhibitory concentration," high initial and maintenance doses of the antibiotic must be given *before* the operation as well as *during* the operation, depending on its duration. We routinely follow this protocol for internal fixations that are judged to be difficult or presumably of long duration (more than 2 h), in cases where there are teeth in the fracture line that require extraction, and in other circumstances that pose an exorbitant risk of endogenous infection (e.g., apical or marginal foci in close proximity to the fracture line).

Our protocol at the present time is to initiate cephalosporins parenterally at the time of induction. A dose of 2 g is administered initially and is repeated every 2 h for 2 days.

Other, more specialized aspects of antibiotic prophylaxis are discussed on p. 245.

6.7 Interaction Between the Implant and Tissue[5]

Both *biomechanical* and *biochemical* interactions can occur between the implant and tissue in internal fixations. Often no distinction is drawn between these aspects in the interpretation of physiologic reactions, yet this is important in terms of identifying the cause of the reactions and finding a possible remedy.

6.7.1 Mechanical Interactions

a) Pressure from the implant or relative motion between the implant and soft tissues can produce irritation. Occasionally this is seen when the integument is very thin.

b) When relative motion between the implant and bone reaches a critical level, it incites bone resorption, which in turn loosens the hold of screws and progressively weakens the stability of the fixation (Perren et al. 1972).

   Primary instability of the fixation with delayed union or secondary instability with associated bone resorption or infection is a frequent cause of cyclic, alternating loads acting upon the implant ("load cycling"). If the duration of the loading is prolonged and the stresses are of sufficient magnitude, the implant may eventually succomb to fatigue fracture (see p. 299).

c) Relative motion between implant components such as plate holes and screw heads (fretting) can cause mechanical wear at the sites of contact. The wear debris impregnates the tissue and in some circumstances can cause physiologic reactions. Studies have demonstrated the extremely fine particulate debris that can result from the fretting of titanium implants.

Stainless steel implants are subject to frictional corrosion as well as mechanical wear at sites of contact. Generally, frictional corrosion is so minimal that it can be detected only with a scanning electron microscope. Fretting and fretting corrosion typically occur at sites of plate-screw contact in the area of comminuted fractures, in individually fixed bone fragments, and at the ends of plates, i.e., areas where radiographs show signs suggestive of relative motion (Pohler 1983).

---

[5] I am grateful to Prof. G. Pohler, Ph. D., for her contributions on this point, which is always a source of lively discussion at ASIF courses.

6.7.2 Chemical-Physiologic Interactions

There are various mechanisms by which metal can enter tissues from implants.

a) Friction or frictional corrosion can lead to the release of greater amounts of metal than the mechanisms described in b) and c).
The fine titanium wear debris reacts at once with ambient oxygen to form a stable compound, titanium oxide (TiO_2). The oxide particles are chemically inert and are either phagocytized or deposited at extracellular sites.
The wear debris from steel may passivate and become deposited about the implant. The degradation of corrosion products is a fairly selective process. Nickel is usually not found in the tissue around implants, indicating that it goes into solution; this is consistent with the solubility of its corrosion products. Chromium impregnates the tissue around the implant, apparently as a stable chromium oxide, while iron is partially dissolved and removed and partially deposited at intra- and extracellular sites in nearby tissues.
Histologic investigations of excised tissue that has been in contact with clinical implants and biocompatibility experiments indicate that the wear products and corrosion products of stainless steel and titanium normally remain in the tissue without causing irritation. However, it has been noted that tissue in contact with titanium implants may contain a greater number of blood vessels and a larger population of fibrocytes than tissue in contact with stainless steel implants.
Local reactions in the form of erythema and swelling are occasionally seen over stainless steel implants that are shown to be free of infection. Often these changes relate to instability and regress when the instability is corrected. They do not interfere with bone healing and disappear completely after the implant is removed. These observations are particularly common in internal fixations of the distal tibia, where the soft-tissue envelope is thin, the bone elastic, and the circulation often poor. Redness and swelling have not been seen in the mandible following internal fixations with ASIF appliances.

b) Stainless steel and titanium derive their high corrosion resistance from a protective surface film that forms spontaneously. This "passive layer" is only a few atoms thick and regenerates very quickly when mechanically disrupted. That is why the surfaces of the implants remain generally free of corrosion. (The passive layer on stainless steel may not regenerate quickly enough when constant friction is present, resulting in local frictional corrosion.)
Through electrochemical processes, the surfaces of implants can become a source of very minute quantities of metal ions. A migration of ions occurs when the implant is introduced into the body and forms a passive layer that is in equilibrium with the milieu; it also occurs when the implant is functioning within the body and the passive layer is being maintained. The amounts of metal released are negligibly small compared, say, with the quantities ingested daily with the food, and they can hardly be detected in tissues even with modern analytic techniques.

c) Rarely, a patient may have a generalized allergy to particular metals. The nickel allergy is the best known example. One solution is to substitute other metals as allergens in a patient who is sensitive to a given metal. Contact with the offending metal is sufficient to precipitate an allergic response; corrosion need not occur. So far allergies to titanium are unknown, and in the few patients to date who have demonstrated allergies to steel implants, symptoms have disappeared promptly when the steel was replaced by titanium. Titanium implants have also proven effective in cases judged to be at risk for infection, e.g., cases where there is compounding into the oral cavity or there is suspected devitalization of the bone.

6.7.3 Observations in Mandibular Implants

Implants for maxillofacial application are exposed to significantly smaller mechanical loads than weight-bearing implants in the lower extremity. This explains why fractures of ASIF plates are unknown in maxillofacial trauma surgery. In the past 20 years the Straumann AG Institute has reported several instances of fatigue fracture in long reconstruction plates. All the devices were used to bridge mandibular defects without a bony buttress (usually across the midline), and all had been in place for longer than five years.

The frictional corrosion between screw heads and plate holes mentioned in the previous section is minimal in the maxillofacial implants. Again, this is due to the relatively small forces that are active in the maxillofacial region and also to the relatively rapid rate of healing in that region, which tends to shorten the period of instability. Mandibular resection plates that have been in situ for up to six years show little or no evidence of corrosion at contact sites or anywhere else on the implant surface. Figure 158a shows the frictional corrosion that occurred in the hole of a stainless steel reconstruction plate that had been in place for six years following a mandibular resection. The electron micrograph shows the junction between areas of flat frictional corrosion, wear channels, and the unaltered plate surface. The histologic section (Fig. 158b) demonstrates corrosion products from the stainless steel as phagocytized granules in the connective tissue cells. Figure 158c shows the area of contact between a titanium screw head and a titanium mandibular reconstruction plate, demonstrating sites of wear and particulate wear debris.

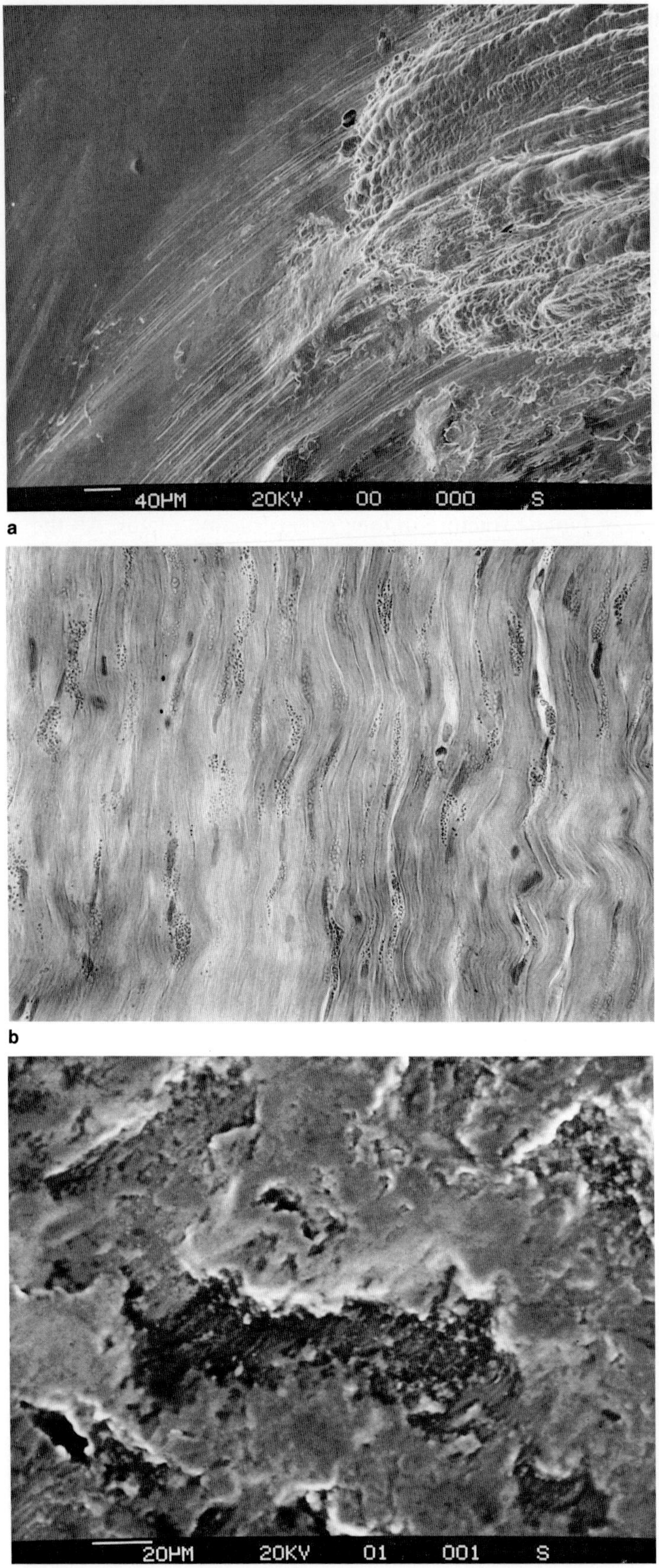

Fig. 158. **a** Hole of a stainless steel reconstruction plate that had bridged a mandibular defect for six years. Micrograph shows the junction between sites of frictional corrosion, wear tracks, and undamaged plate surface. **b** Histologic section through the connective tissue layer that had formed adjacent to a stainless steel plate. Fine particles of corrosion products have been phagocytized by the connective tissue cells. **c** Area of contact between a screw head and a titanium mandibular reconstruction plate showing wear sites and particulate wear debris

6.7.4 Implant Removal

It is the belief of the ASIF that implants should be removed once they have accomplished their purpose. There is no sound medical or biologic rationale for leaving a large foreign object inside the body once healing is complete. Obvious exceptions to this rule are patients in whom further surgery would pose an unacceptable risk (e.g., the elderly) or cases where the implant occupies a critical position or exercises a permanent function (e.g., bridging a mandibulectomy defect).

If implant removal is prohibited on legal grounds because of a perceived risk, as is presently the case in some countries, the patient should be instructed to notify his doctor at once if he experiences any symptoms referrable to the implant. Local irritation, complaints, and hypersensitivity to cold are always indications for implant removal.

It should be noted in this context that titanium implants are apt to cause the fewest problems when left in the body. The lower elastic modulus of titanium gives these implants a greater flexibility which approximates that of bone. Also, the tissue compatibility of titanium is superior to that of stainless steel (see Graph 3). These facts are generally known and cause us to be skeptical of firms which claim that the quality of their material is such that the implants may remain in place indefinitely, falsely implying that their implants possess a feature which those of other manufacturers do not.

6.7.5 Timing of Implant Removal

It has been shown that a plate applied under primary tension loses some of its tension during the course of bone healing. The associated decline of interfragmental pressure increases the physiologic stresses on the bone, and these have a stimulating effect on remodeling. Approximately one year of remodeling is needed for the mandibular bone to attain a completely homogeneous structure. After that point the fixation material may be removed.

6.7.6 Technique of Implant Removal

The number of screws used in the fixation will dictate the choice of surgical approach and anesthesia. For a lag screw fixation or plate fixation employing no more than six screws, the implants are retrieved through a combined intra/extraoral approach using a transbuccal screwdriver (Fig. 159). The procedure, which requires the vestibular exposure of the fixation site *in its entirety,* may be performed on an outpatient basis using either local or general anesthesia.

If more than six screws were used in the fixation, the external scar is incised for its full length or excised if it is hyperplastic. The plate is then exposed and removed through the reopened incision in the usual manner. Ordinarily the patient is hospitalized overnight for this procedure, which requires general anesthesia. Suction drainage should be maintained for 24 h after these minor procedures, since the risk of infection is equivalent to that in the original operation.

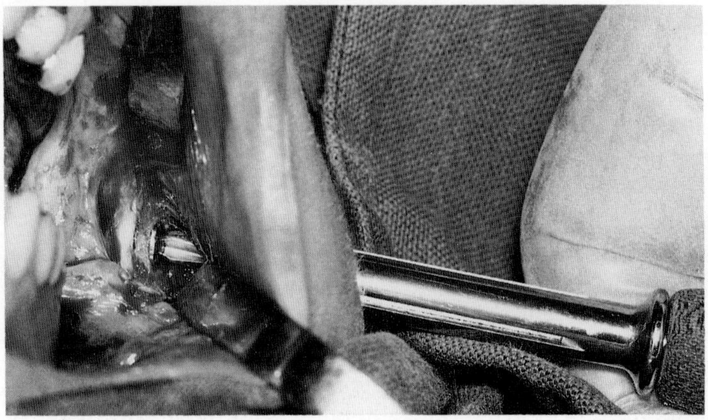

Fig. 159. The implant has been exposed intraorally, and the screw is removed with a transbuccal screwdriver introduced through an extraoral stab incision

6.8 Complications

6.8.1 Posttraumatic Bone Infection

Posttraumatic fracture-line osteomyelitis (Wassmund 1935) calls the efficacy of conservative fracture treatment seriously into question, for even without operative treatment the rate of infection is relatively high. The mandible, when fractured, is predisposed to infection by resident microorganisms. The quantity of bacteria and the types of species present are important factors in this regard. The oral cavity contains up to 10^9 organisms/ml saliva. Anaerobes predominate by a ratio of 30:1 (Knothe and Dette 1984). When the facultative pathogens leave their biotope and gain access to the normally mucosa-covered mandible, and if the systemic host resistance is weakened or local defenses impaired by motion at the fracture site, opportunistic bone infection is inevitable.

Would not an infection of this type contraindicate internal fixation? We can answer this question by describing a typical case which illustrates the benefits of postprimary internal fixation in a patient with a clinically manifest fracture-line infection. The patient was referred emergently at one week postinjury with a perimandibular abscess in an untreated fracture of the left mandibular angle (Fig. 160a).

Initially the abscess was incised and drainage established under antibiotic coverage. The molar in the line of fracture was extracted (Fig. 160b), and the mandible was immobilized. The acute inflammation resolved with two weeks' irrigation, at which time postprimary internal fixation of the fracture was performed. The present case involved an oblique-surface fracture that could be optimally stabilized with a very small amount of internal fixation material. The granulation tissue was removed by curettage, and the fracture surfaces were compressed with three lag screws (Fig. 160c, d). The fracture united without complications (Fig. 160e).

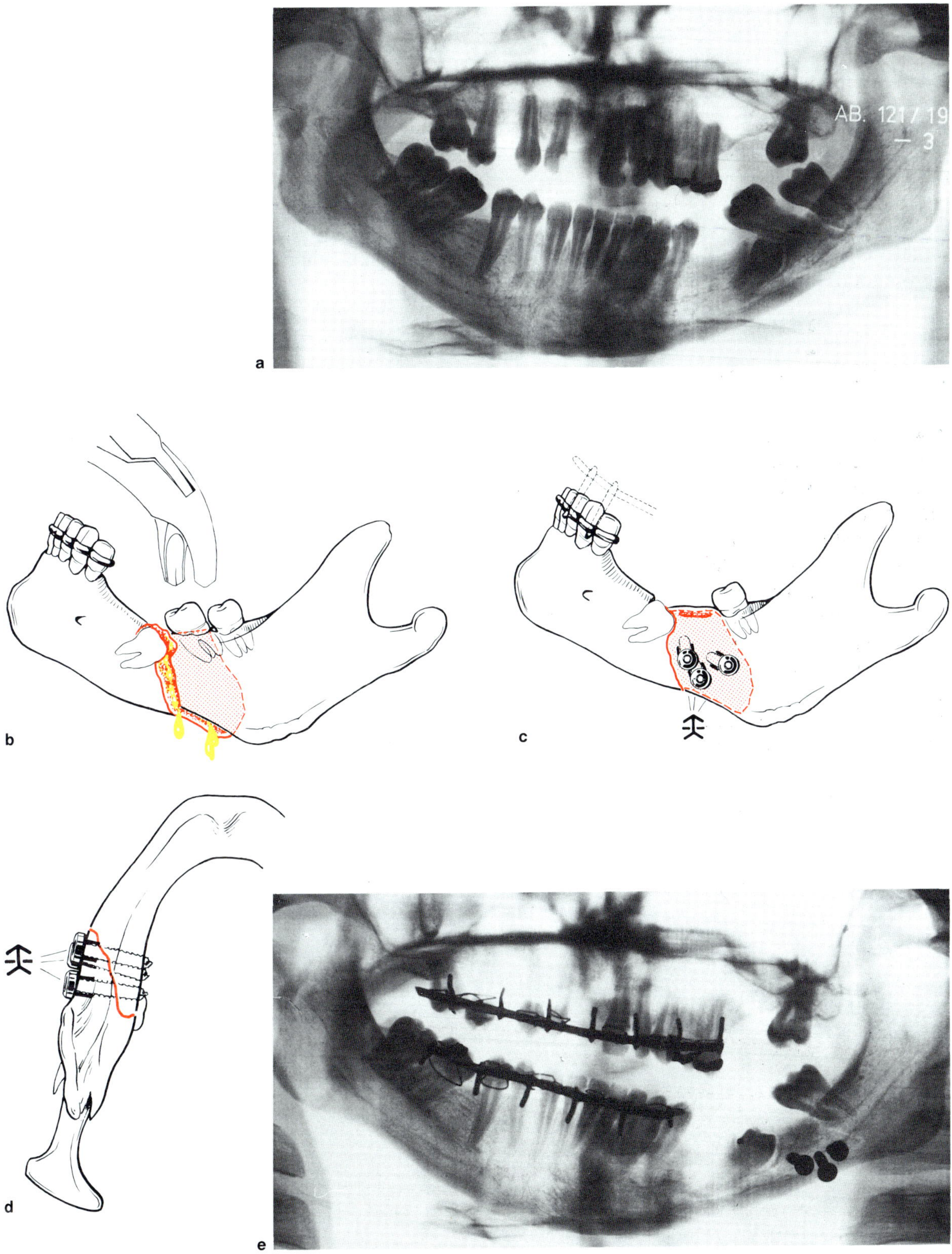

Fig. 160. **a** Infected, untreated oblique-surface fracture in the area of an impacted molar. **b** Infection is treated by incision, drainage, extraction of the tooth in the fracture line, and intermaxillary immobilization. **c, d** Postprimary fixation with lag crews. **e** Status after resolution of the infection. The intermaxillary fixation was removed to allow early mobilization

6.8.2 Postoperative Hematoma

The perifracture hematoma, which provides an excellent culture medium for bacteria, is most often a complication of nonoperative therapy. Postoperative hematomas are uncommon following meticulous hemostasis and vacuum drainage of the operative wound. If a hematoma develops, it can usually be managed by needle aspiration.

The situation is different when a frank postoperative hemorrhage exists that is producing marked skin tension. In this case the wound should be widely reopened, the hematoma evacuated by suction and irrigation, and the wound reclosed primarily.

6.8.3 Postoperative Pain and Inflammatory Edema

A well stabilized mandibular fracture should cause little or no pain by 24 h postoperatively. Pain after that time is related to edematous or infectious swelling of the soft tissues. Posttraumatic edema will subside appreciably in the initial days after surgery, assuming there has been early fracture treatment with atraumatic handling of the soft tissues. Increasing edema and pain may be attributed, then, to delayed treatment or traumatic exposure of the fracture site. These cases (and only these cases) warrant drug therapy for the control of swelling and pain and the use of moist compresses to relax the skin and alleviate pain.

Inflammatory edema is difficult to diagnose in the initial days after surgery. Close monitoring is needed for the early recognition of classic inflammatory signs. Usually these signs are accompanied by a low-grade fever and an elevated white count.

Broad-spectrum antibiotics should be administered for 3–4 days while the jaws are immobilized by intermaxillary fixation. This regimen will restore stability and blood flow to the cortical bone and create the best prospect for spontaneous resolution of the infection with no recurrence when the intermaxillary fixation is removed.

6.8.4 Postoperative Osteitis

6.8.4.1 Definition and Pathogenesis

Osteitis is an osteomyelitis that is localized or confined to the area of the fracture. The panosteitic form involving the periosteum, bone marrow, and cortex differs from the classic mandibular osteomyelitis in that it lacks the invasive component of marrow cellulitis and thus does not show the typical progression from a primary acute to secondary chronic stage. It is extremely common for the clinical picture of postoperative osteitis to begin with a paragenetic soft tissue abscess, which frequently is caused by a devitalized tooth or a tooth in the line of fracture. The actual osteitic process, however, is caused by the infection of necrotic areas of the cortex. The "infected necrosis" is the "component of the (primarily) chronic course," as Hörster (1985) noted in his morphologic studies of 100 posttraumatic bone infections. The infected necrosis has its onset in the immediate postoperative period and *results from the removal of periosteum during the internal fixation.* The injury to superficial nutrient vessels and vessels within the Haversian system very quickly incites resorptive changes involving the secondary osteons. If the intracortical blood flow is sufficiently impaired, sequestration may occur. Granulations form among the sequestra, and these also absorb and rarefy the bone ends until no more material is available for resorption. "Delayed union" is a variant of this process. It would be naive to assume that the mandible is exceptional in this regard. Given the discovery that the infected cortical necrosis is the principal agent of this rarefying inflammation, it is reasonable to attempt to reduce infection by practicing an operative technique that does not traumatize the periosteum and soft tissues unnecessarily.

Of course, the pathogenesis of infection also depends on the severity of the fracture and may be *exogenous* and/or *endogenous* in nature. It is not unusual to find anaerobic and aerobic organisms together in the same bacteriologic assay.

Several synergistic mechanisms play a role in the pathogenesis of postoperative osteitis:

1) traumatogenic and iatrogenic compromise of the superficial blood flow to the bone;
2) traumatogenic circulatory deficits at the bone ends;
3) infection by exogenous and endogenous organisms (contamination, hospitalism, resident flora);
4) devitalized bone fragments;
5) the general tendency of a bone plate and screws to promote devascularization and hinder revascularization, or the presence of unstable fixation material;
6) fracture instability.

6.8.4.2 Early Infection

Early infection (see Statistics, p. 245) is diagnosed when an abscess or infiltrate is noted in the initial weeks following operative fracture treatment (Fig. 161 a). If the heat, redness, and tenderness are refractory to conservative measures, *early reexposure* is indicated. Its purpose is to:

- eliminate factors interfering with extracortical blood flow to the soft tissues, and
- restabilize the fracture if necessary.

Reexposure involves reopening the original wound, taking samples for bacteriology, evacuating the potentially infected hematoma, and removing necrotic tissues. The wound is copiously irrigated with warm Ringer's solution so that the extent of the blood flow deficit can be assessed more clearly. The stability of the internal fixation should be carefully checked. If obviously stable, the implant is left in place, as was done in the case in Fig. 161 a. This case involved a fracture through the alveolus of the displaced third molar (Fig. 161 b), which was stabilized with a four-hole EDCP (Fig. 161 c). The fixation would have been revised with a six-hole reconstruction plate, but reexposure showed no evidence of instability, so there was no reason to revise the fixation. The suction drain was removed and a rubber tube inserted through which the site was irrigated once or twice daily. The infection cleared within two weeks (Fig. 161 d), and undisturbed consolidation ensued. Figure 161 e shows the status after removal of the screws and plate.

If the implant is found to be unstable, *it should be removed,* as illustrated by the case of a double fracture (Fig. 162 a) that had been poorly stabilized on the right side. After an uneventful three weeks, a swelling of fairly abrupt onset developed on the right side of the jaw and showed all the characteristic signs of a perimandibular abscess in the angle region (Fig. 162 b). The incision was reopened, and the area was drained. Inspection of the plate revealed four loose screws, which were removed together

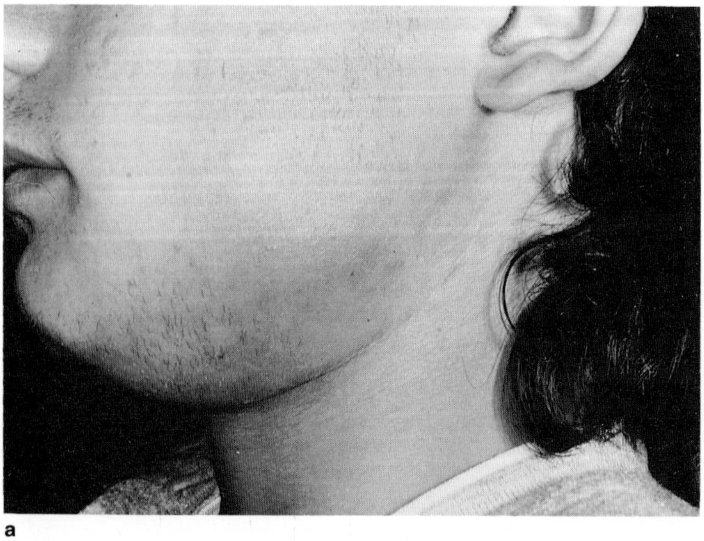

a

Fig. 161. **a** Classic signs of inflammation in an early infection. **b** Angle fracture through the alveolus of the third molar. **c** Fracture is stabilized with a four-hole EDCP. **d** Infection resolved after two weeks' inpatient treatment. **e** Status after removal of the plate and screws

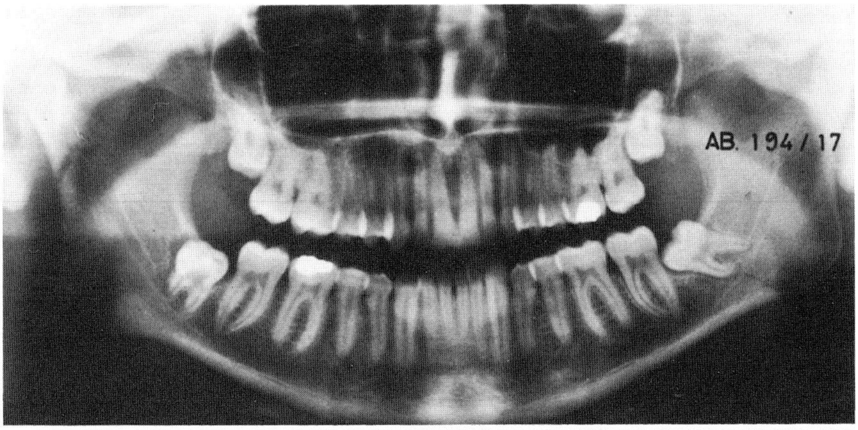

b

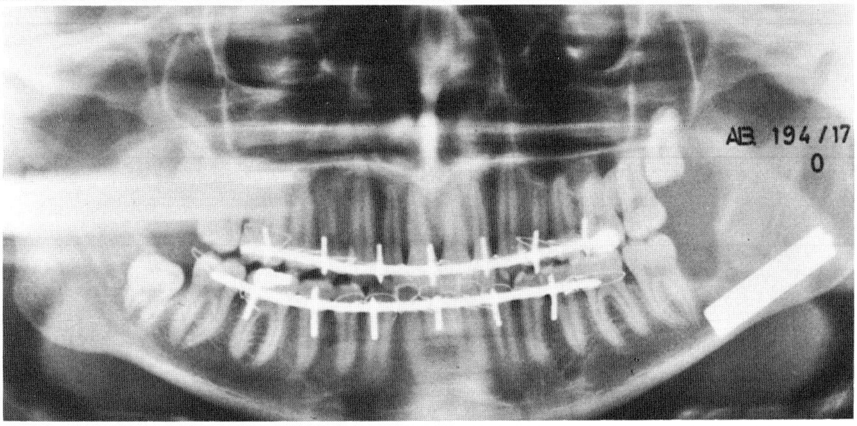

c

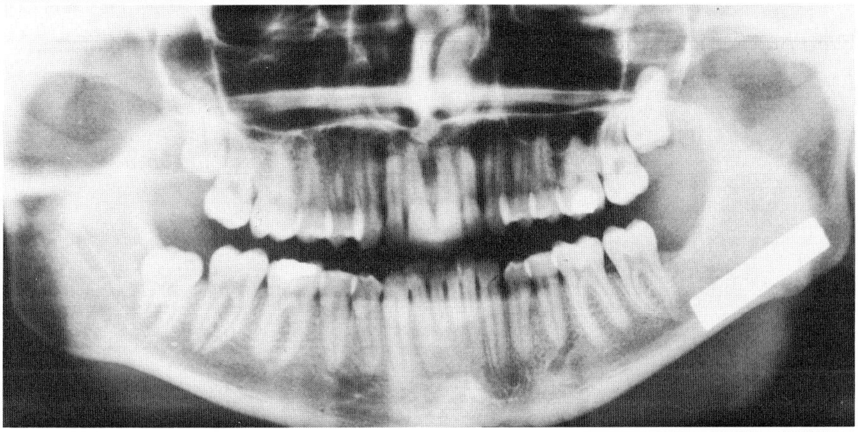

d

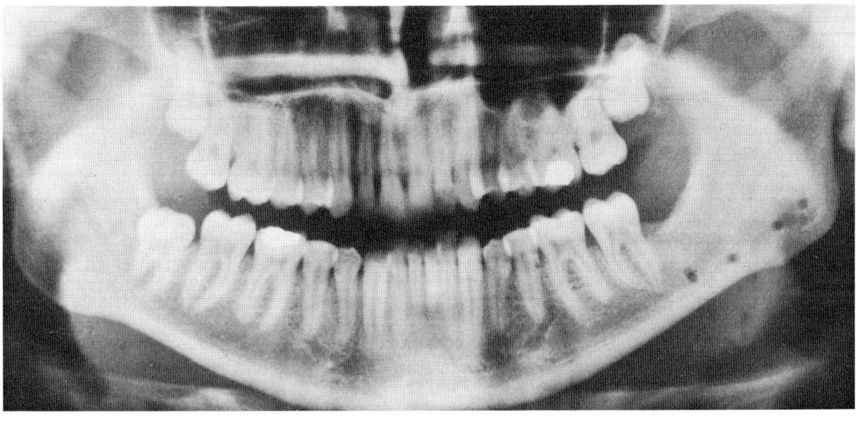

e

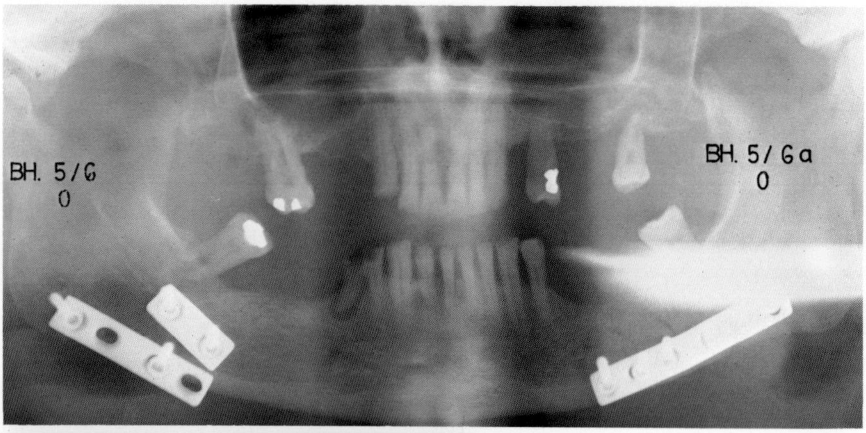

a

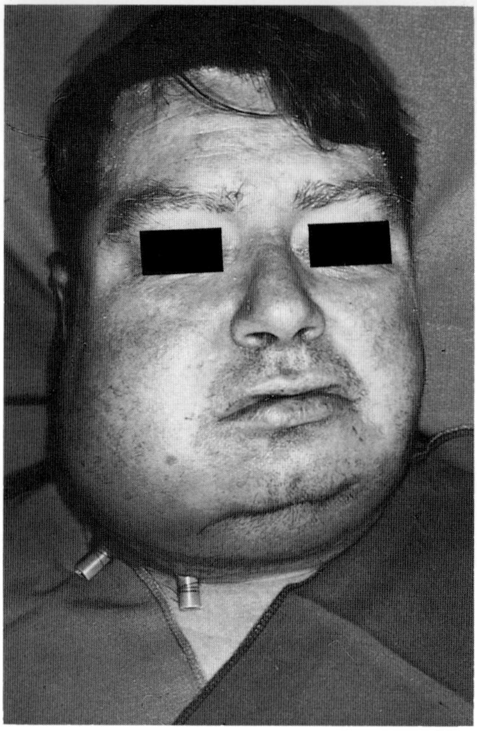

b

Fig. 162. **a** Faulty plate-and-tension-band fixation of a central angle fracture. Two errors can be seen: The distal screw of the tension band crosses the fracture line, and the attachment of the stabilization plate violates the three screw rule. **b** The primary instability led to infection of the fracture line with a perimandibular abscess. **c** Status after four weeks' irrigation therapy: The infection has resolved, and there is evidence of a nonunion. **d** The fixation was revised with a seven-hole reconstruction plate. **e** One year later the nounion is solid

with the plate. A small amount of fibrous callus was present at the fracture site, but the basal part contained multiple sequestra surrounded by infected granulation tissue. This situation called for a period of *intermaxillary fixation* rather than immediate revision. Antiseptic irrigations (e.g., with chloramine or Betadine) are more reliable than local antibiotic therapy and usually make it possible to undertake revisionary fixation within 3–4 weeks. In the present case a seven-hole reconstruction plate was applied to prevent the development of an established nonunion (Fig. 162c, d), while at the same time the implants were removed from the healed left side. The radiograph at one year (Fig. 162e) confirmed consolidation of the nonunion despite infection of the revisionary plate.

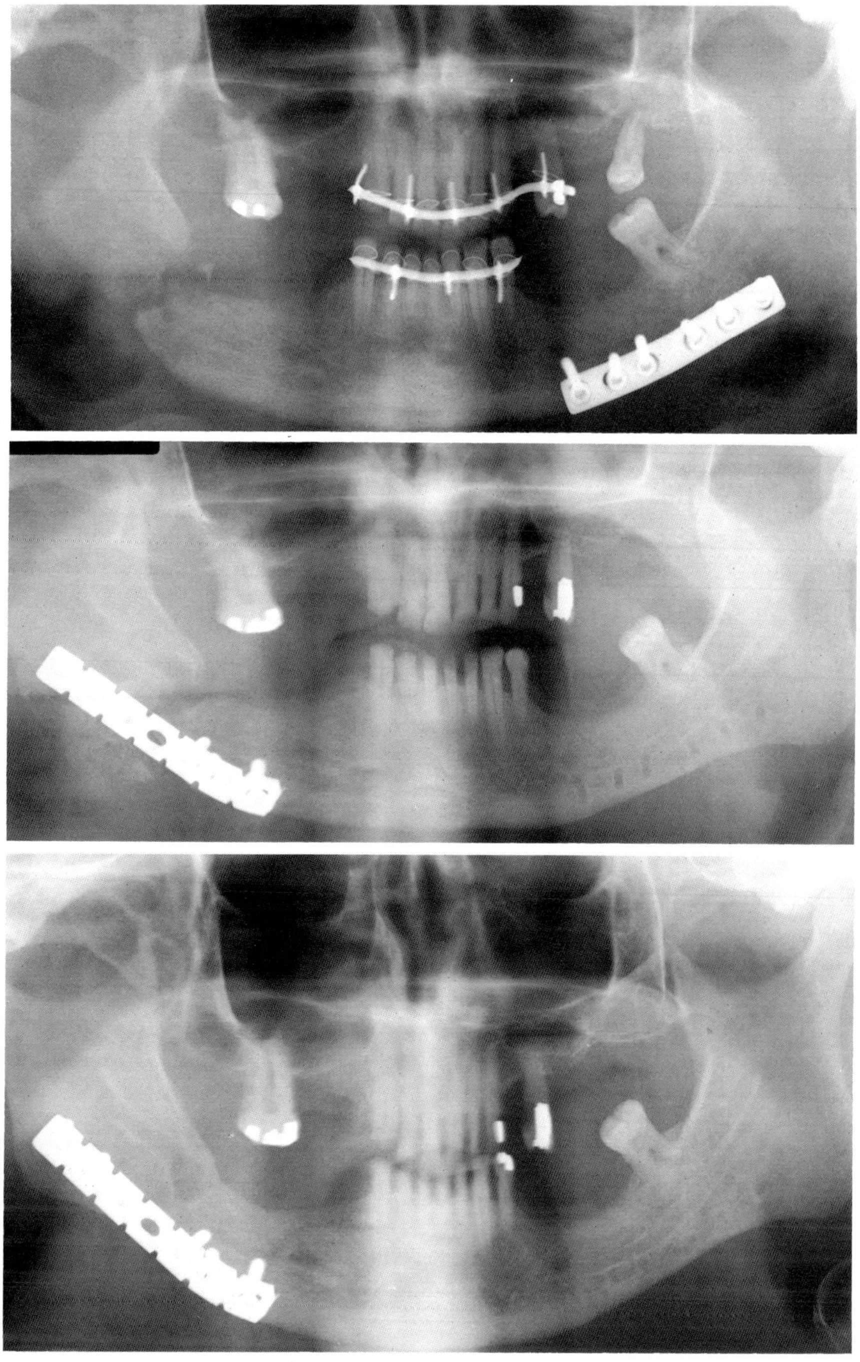

c d e

Fig. 162 c–e

Occasionally the plate may be left in situ if the replacement of one or two loose cortex screws by *emergency screws* (see p. 115) is sufficient to restore stability.

The decision concerning a *consecutive* revision of the fixation is more difficult. With a single fracture, the old screw holes often pose an obstacle to replacing the original plate with a longer one. In such cases we recommend removing the implant and applying intermaxillary fixation as the most reliable way to bring the infection quickly under control.

In comminuted fractures, however, there is no valid alternative to replacing the unstable plate with a *reconstruction plate* that has at least *two additional holes* on each side of the fracture. Grossly devitalized fragments are removed when the plate is applied.

6.8.4.3 Late Infection

Late infection is characterized by an inflammation-free interval of more than one month after operation.

Given the susceptibility of the stabilized fracture to infection, the patient should be informed prior to discharge about the fracture type, the type of internal fixation, and basic aspects of follow-up care and implant removal. As the weekly and then monthly outpatient follow-up visits become less frequent, competent self monitoring by the patient assumes greater importance.

Radiographs are of central importance in follow-up, even if they do not yield the same quality of information on fracture union in the mandible as they do in fractures of the long bones.

In a technically and anatomically perfect internal fixation of the mandible, a periosseous callus will not be visible on radiographs. Nevertheless, it is essential that follow-up films be taken at 6, 12, and 18 months to document the progress of healing.

Disturbances of fracture healing do not become apparent until the seventh or eighth postoperative week. The fracture line becomes unsharp but appears very prominent and widened as a result of osteolysis (Fig. 163a). These changes are usually accompanied by erythema, tenderness to pressure, and incipient fistula (Fig. 163b), which prompt the decision to reexplore the fracture. In the case presented, reexposure disclosed interfragmental callus and granulation tissue with small sequestra, especially in the basal part of the fracture, that had to be removed. The loosened plate also was removed (Fig. 163c, d). Even without fixation of any kind, the inflammation resolved quickly after removal of the implant, and the fracture went on to union. Figure 163e shows the status at two years.

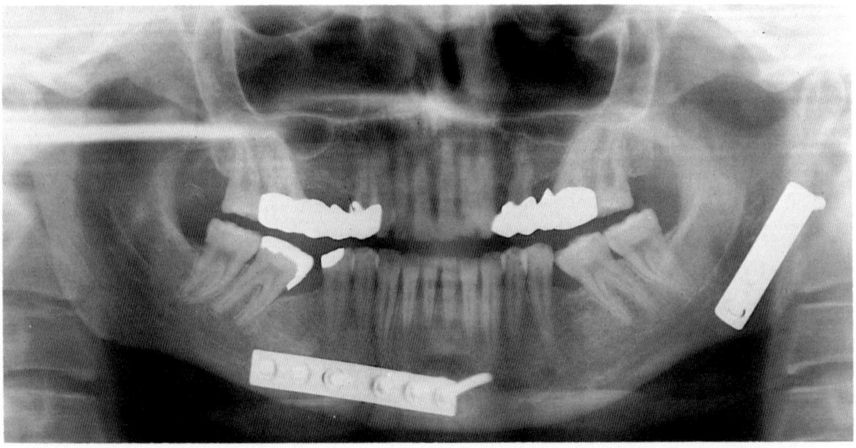

a **Fig. 163a.** Legend see page 147

Fig. 163 **a** Osteolytic widening of the canine fracture line in the inferior border of the mandible, opposite the center of the plate. **b** The scar shows inflammatory changes with erythema and a granulating fistula. **c** Reoperation disclosed fibrous callus and granulation tissue in the fracture line with demarcation of a sequestrum at the border. **d** Radiograph immediately after plate removal shows a widened fracture line extending to the apex of the canine tooth and osteolytic lucency in the area of the central screw holes. **e** Status after implant removal

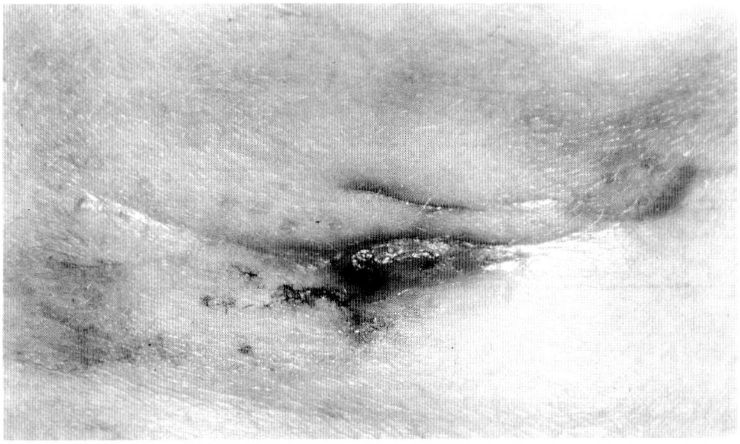
b

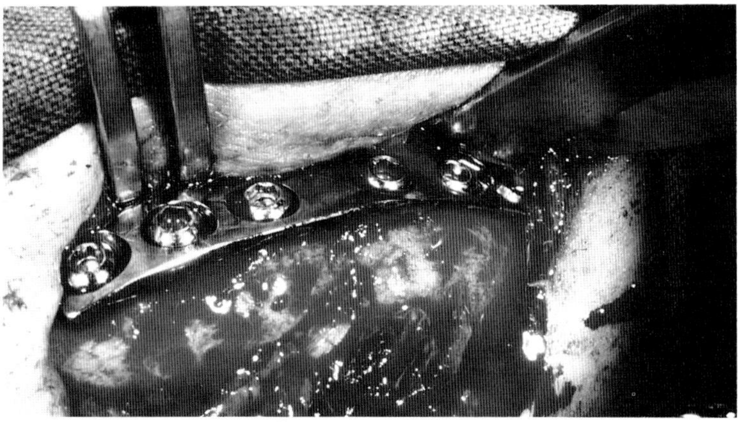
c

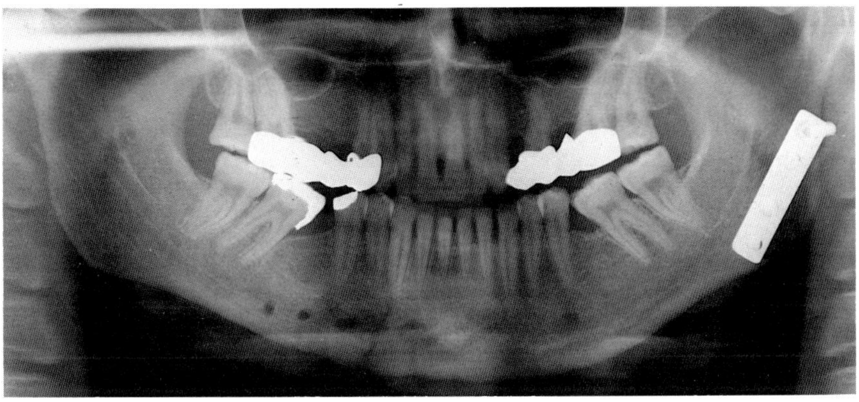
d

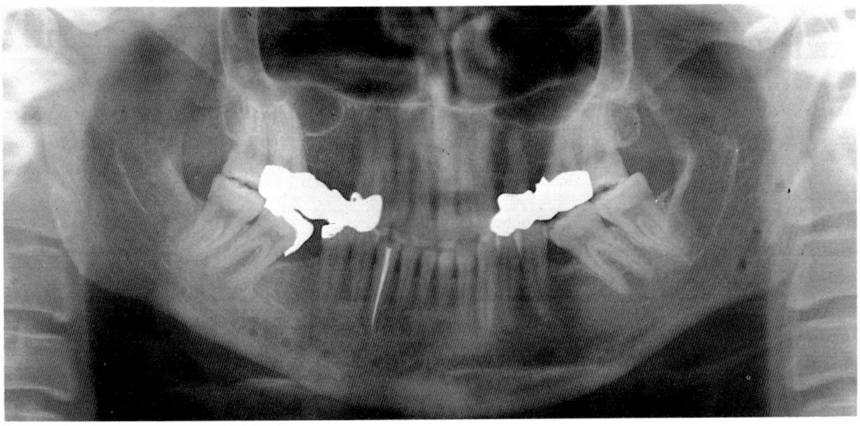
e

Occasionally radiographs will demonstrate poor fracture healing in the absence of a clinically manifest infection. If the internal fixation was performed three or more months earlier, a *delayed union* is said to be present (see p. 272). Cases of this type warrant close follow-up, and a soft diet should be consumed for the first 2–3 weeks. Generally the delayed union will consolidate without intermaxillary fixation.

Delayed union, because of its rarity, is considered a less significant late complication than osteitis (see also Figs. 2b and 3a, pp. 7 and 8). A strict protocol is followed in the management of late osteitic infection:

- removal of diseased bone into healthy tissue;
- removal of all sequestra;
- accurate excision of infected soft tissues, including the fistula;
- removal of the unstable internal fixation material and revision of the fixation (this is combined with bone grafting in the presence of a segmental defect or infected nonunion);
- continuous surface debridement by twice-daily irrigation through the drain.

6.8.4.4 Summary of Therapeutic Principles

The following treatment principles apply to the reexposure of an internal fixation complicated by osteitis:

I. Continuous debridement with drainage and irrigation until the infection resolves.
II. Assessment of stability.
III. Measures relating to stability.
   1. If immobility is confirmed: leave the implant in place.
   2. If mobility is noted, any of three situations may exist:
      a) Individual loose screws: replace with emergency screws.
      b) Deficient internal fixation and early infection:
         - Implant removal and intermaxillary fixation: *or*
         - Implant removal and primary revision of the fixation (with a grossly intact cortex);
         - Implant removal and secondary revision of the fixation (weeks later after clearing of infection).
      c) Deficient internal fixation and late or refractory infection:
         Phase 1: implant removal and intermaxillary fixation
         Phase 2: secondary revision of the fixation (e.g., with extensive areas of resorption or segmental defects or infected nonunion), generally combined with bone grafting.

Part II

Internal Fixation of Fresh Fractures

3.6 Contraindications to Internal Fixation and Exceptions

Internal fixation would not be indicated for single, minimally displaced fractures in cases where the avoidance of a surgical scar is a significant concern. These injuries are best treated nonoperatively.

In exceptional cases, anterior fractures of this kind may be treated through an intraoral approach. This can be accomplished with the transbuccal instrumentation of the ASIF (see p. 101). Most of these cases involve outpatients *who should be given considerable latitude in selecting the mode of treatment that is most acceptable.*

Other *exceptions* are incomplete fractures and undisplaced fractures associated with cysts or the attempted extraction of impacted teeth. In such cases internal fixation constitutes an adjunct to surgical treatment of the primary lesion.

3.7 Absolute Indications

Ongoing quality control studies (Eschmann 1974; von Euw 1982; Philps 1987) demonstrate the great therapeutic value of functionally stable internal fixation of the mandible. Consequently, the omission of internal fixation in a given case may do the patient harm. From this standpoint multiple fractures, comminuted fractures, and fractures with a bone defect constitute absolute indications for operative fixation. Displaced fractures that are closed extraorally are often included in this category, which means that all grades of severity except for group I (see Classification, p. 159) are an indication for internal fixation.

3.8 Condylar Neck Fractures: Their Significance as an Indirect Indication for Internal Fixation

A fracture through the neck of the mandibular condyle is not a favorable indication for internal fixation. In these cases it is not the internal fixation itself that is problematic, but the surgical approach. In theory, the slender neck of the mandible and the condylar head could be fixed as accurately and stably as fractures of the metacarpals and phalanges by using the small fragment instrument set, but the problem of access appears to be insoluble. The position of the temporomandibular joint under the skull base and the course of the facial nerve pose such serious obstacles that conservative therapy is traditionally preferred, especially when one considers the positive results of early functional treatment.

Temprorary extirpation and replantation of the condylar process to facilitate the application of fixation material is biologically and forensically unsound. Our idea of stabilizing the condylar process with a long lag screw inserted through the lower border of the mandibular angle (Spiessl and Schroll 1972) also has proved impractical. Petzel (1980) improved the technique and tested it clinically in 17 patients, but it has not come into routine use. Thus, the purely functional treatment of the condylar neck fracture continues to have value. Its success rests upon early mobilization. The urgency of this mobilization provides an *indication for the functionally stable in-*

ternal fixation of concomitant fractures of the mandible, even when they are single or undisplaced.

In principle there is only one *contraindication:* fractures in children. Pediatric fractures require a strictly conservative approach. Interosseous wire sutures or miniplates may be used in conjunction with intermaxillary fixation to approximate markedly displaced fragments (see p. 266).

4 Surgical Approaches

4.1 Inadequacy of Unilateral Fracture Treatment

Maximum success in fracture surgery depends on the *correct selection of the approach*. The basic rule is to select the most *direct* approach possible.

Despite the plausibility of this requirement, there is considerable ambivalence concerning the choice of operative approach. The tendency to perform internal fixations exclusively through an intraoral appraoch is motivated by the desire to avoid a visible scar and preserve the marginal mandibular branch of the facial nerve.

There is an equally good rationale for an exclusive extraoral approach, in that effective basal reduction of the fraction would appear to obviate the need for a dental splint and thus facilitate treatment. In reality, neither the intraoral nor extraoral approach is sufficient in and of itself to yield an optimum result.

As far as the scar is concerned, it must be considered that functionally stable internal fixation is indicated chiefly for difficult fractures which justify scar formation because of their severity. In one survey, 90% of 166 patients questioned did not consider their scar to be objectionable (Eschmann 1974; von Euw 1982).

As for nerve injury, 21 of 108 patients in one follow-up series reported sensory disturbances after their surgery. However, 17 of these patients had a preexisting neuropathy, so only 4 of the nerve deficits were referrable to the internal fixation (Eschmann 1974). In a later follow-up of 112 cases, 32 patients experienced sensory deficits in the area of the mandibular nerve (von Euw 1982), 6 of which were referrable to the internal fixation.

With regard to weakness of the mouth angle caused by traumatization of the marginal branch of the facial nerve, both authors found a total of only one case in their follow-up series. This may be a statistical accident. It is reasonable to assume that in centers which train postgraduates, the incidence of mouth angle weakness following internal fixation is approximately 3%–4%. When a systematic technique is followed in exposing the fracture (see p. 175 ff.), the avoidance of nerve injury should not pose a serious problem. This is evidenced by the fact that every resident practicing in our emergency department performs internal fixations autonomously. A staff physician lends support only in exceptionally difficult cases.

Other problems are associated with the exclusive intraoral approach, namely restricted access and contamination.

It is clear that meticulous, atraumatic handling of the bone and soft tissues is extremely difficult within the narrow confines of the oral cavity, especially when dealing with a displaced, postcanine fracture. Extensive stripping of periosteum will be necessary in the vestibular area in order to gain sufficient exposure.

When the bone is denuded to this extent, there is a high risk of cortical necrosis with subsequent osteitis. Hörster (1985) has demonstrated this in his histologic studies of 100 cases managed by bone plating. He thus confirms what has been presumed in operative fracture treatment for decades: that instability and *devitalized cortex* are the major causes of infection in internal fixations.

Although these studies pertain to internal fixations of limb fractures, there is no reason to believe that extensive periosteal stripping of the mandible would have a less devastating effect on osseous blood flow. The arborizing pattern of the intraosseous vessels cannot guarantee preservation of cortical flow in such cases due to the potential in some fractures for concomitant injury to the inferior alveolar artery. An even more severe consequence of the intraoral approach is bacterial contamination, which is unavoidable when the fracture is opened within the oral cavity.

As for the exclusive extraoral approach, the articulation and deformation problems that can result from neglected or inadequate occlusal reduction and retention are illustrated by the open fracture in Fig. 175a. The alveolar part of this fracture was reduced with only a partial splint placed on the mandibular teeth adjacent to the fracture (Fig. 175b), and a few wire ligatures were used to retain the occlusion. When the compression plate was applied through an extraoral incision, the intermaxillary wires became loose. The removal of small marginal fragments left a cortical defect on the lingual aspect of the fracture. The defect, combined with the loose intermaxillary fixation, was sufficient to cause the fragments to displace on the oral side when forceps compression was applied. The occlusal disturbance caused by this displacement was not appreciated by the operator. Only on completion of the procedure was it apparent from the open bite that the occlusion had been inadequately retained (Fig. 175c, d).

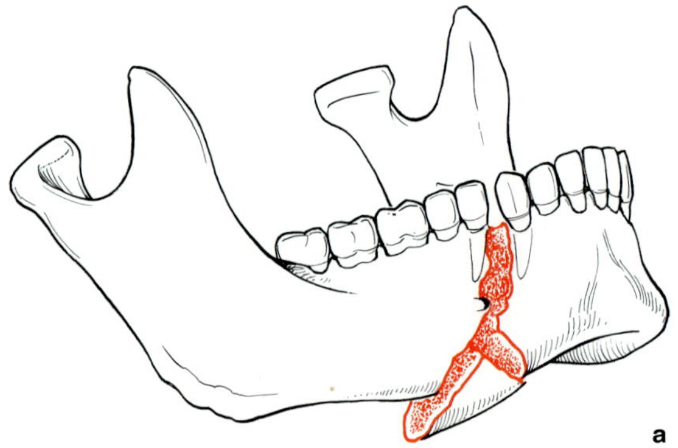

a

Fig. 175. **a** Drawing of a postinjury radiograph. The basal fragment and the width of the fracture gap suggest the difficulty that will be had in effecting and maintaining an open reduction. **b** The use of a too-short partial splint on the mandibular teeth and the absence of a maxillary splint resulted in unstable retention of the occlusion. **c, d** An open bite resulted from peroperative redisplacement. **e** A ten-hole reconstruction plate prevents relative displacement of the main fragments. **f** Status after the revision: The occlusion is restored. The intermaxillary wires were removed postoperatively

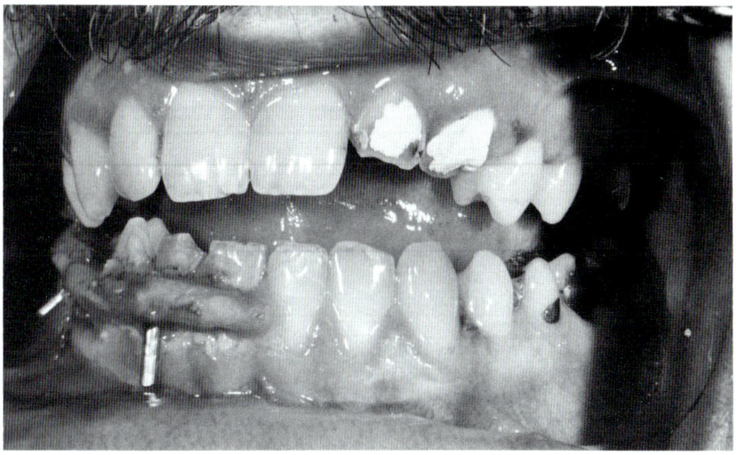

b

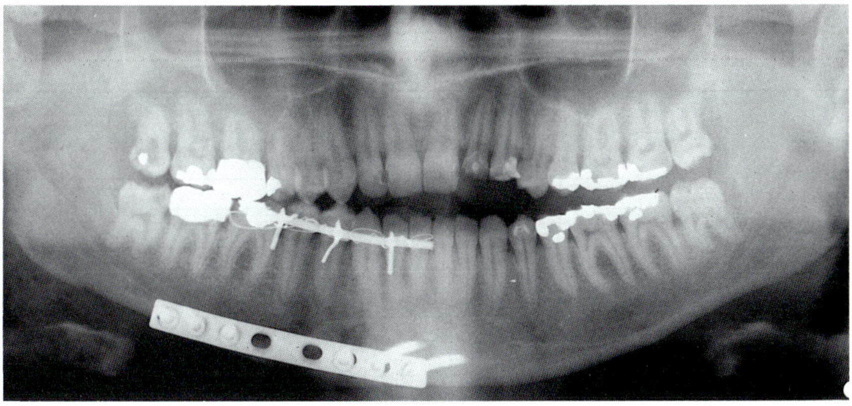

c

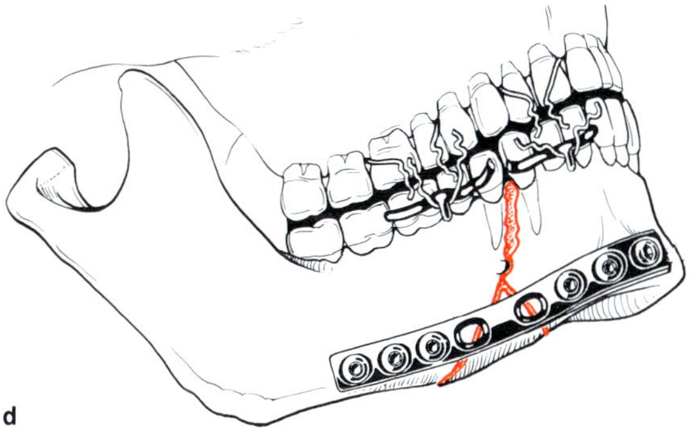

d

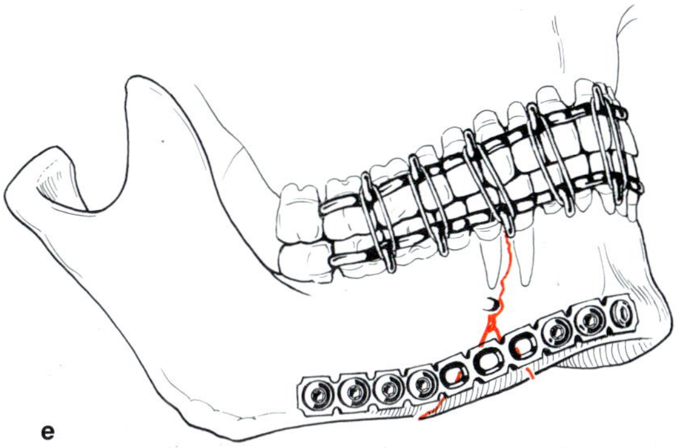

e

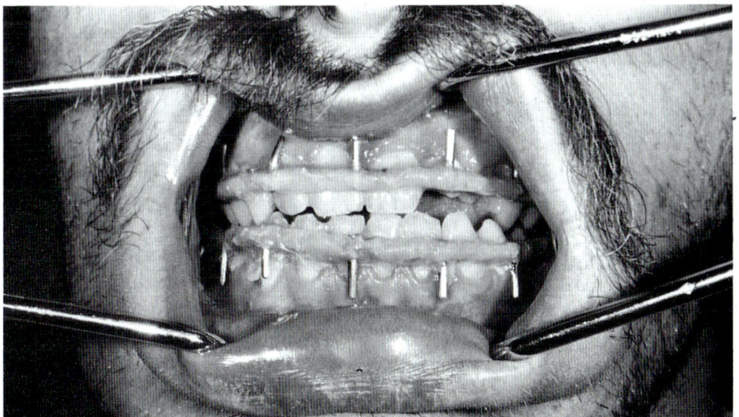

f

One week later the fixation was revised. This time the occlusion was retained with full-length maxillary and mandibular splints and intermaxillary fixation. A ten-hole reconstruction plate, attached with neutral screws, prevented relative displacement of the main fragments (Fig. 175 e). Normal postoperative occlusion (Fig. 175 f) confirmed correct alveolar and basal reduction of the fracture.

The postoperative occlusion provides a useful index of the quality of the internal fixation. Subjectively, even the most minute change in the relation of the dental arches will be perceived as disturbing by the patient. Arnold (1985) studied a group of 49 patients with full or good dentition to determine whether exact reestablishment of the occlusion was routinely possible following definitive reduction and stable fixation of the fragments. The follow-up results were compared with the prevalence data for various other forms of malocclusion present in the uninjured population (results of epidemiologic studies). It was found that the fully dentate patients of the study group had markedly fewer occlusion problems compared with the other groups and experienced fewer subjective and clinical dysfunctions.

4.2 Principle of Combined Fracture Treatment

The mandible is an essential component of the upper visceral tract. The alveolar process and teeth are placed within the oral cavity, while the basal part of the mandible is extraoral (Fig. 176 a). It forms the skeletal foundation for the external wall of the visceral tract, which in this region lacks a perivisceral space so that the inner lining and body wall form an enclosing soft-tissue envelope. The vertical ramus of the mandible and the temporomandibular joint are extravisceral in location.

This anatomic arrangement underlies the necessity of the combined (bilateral) approach, i. e., treating the intraoral part of the fracture (alveolar process and teeth) through the oral cavity while treating the extraoral, basal part of the fracture in its soft-tissue envelope through a direct approach from outside the mouth. The standard formula for bilateral fracture treatment may be stated as follows (Fig. 176 b, c):

Intraoral: occlusal reduction and peroperative retention of the occlusion.
Extraoral: open basal reduction and internal fixation.

This formula is based on the experience that

- the exclusive intraoral approach does not permit effective control of the basal reduction,
- the exclusive extraoral approach does not permit effective control of the occlusal reduction.

If the principle of the combined approach is followed without compromise, good results will be achieved with a high degree of consistency. We know this from our experience with more than 800 internal fixations that we have performed to date.

Given the great variability of fracture patterns in the mandible, the rule of the combined approach is not absolute, and there are exceptions to it

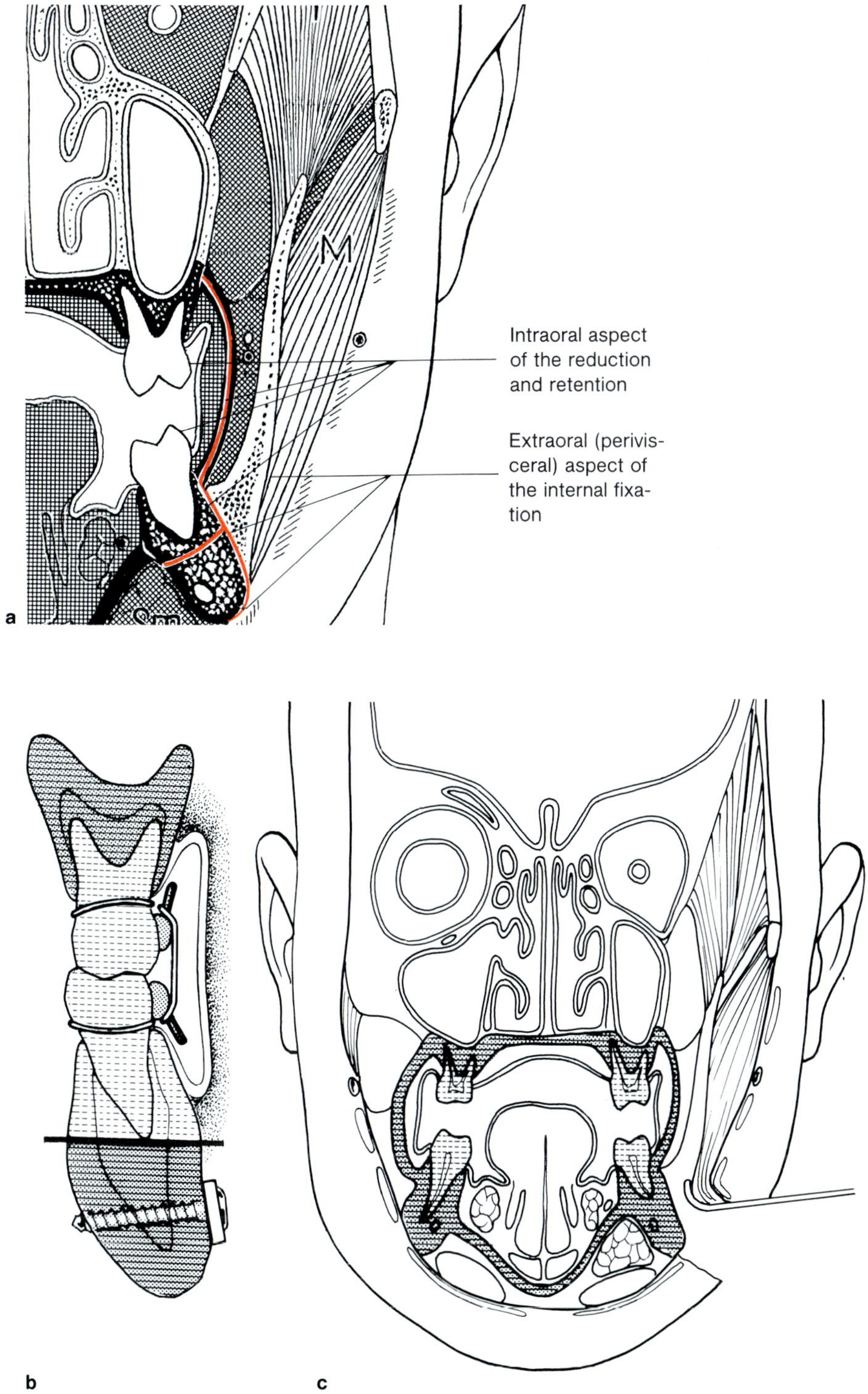

Fig. 176. **a** Coronal section of the facial skeleton at the level of the molars. The osseomuscular oral cavity consists of teeth and the alveolar processes *intraorally* and the mandibular base *extraorally*. (From Spiessl and von Hochstetter 1982). Formula for bilateral fracture treatment:

b Intraoral: occlusal reduction and peroperative retention of the occlusion.

c Extraoral: open basal reduction and internal fixation

(e.g., precanine fractures). However, the rule applies fully to segmental and comminuted fractures and to markedly displaced postcanine, angular, and supra-angular fractures, which cannot be satisfactorily managed by the unilateral application of ASIF principles.

The combined approach is entirely consistent with the principle of asepsis and is necessary for satisfying other essential conditions such as preservation of the blood supply and the appropriate selection and application of the plate.

4.3 Anatomic Landmarks for the Extraoral Approaches

The major landmarks for surgical approaches to the base and ramus of the mandible are the suprahyoid region and carotid triangle. In accordance with surgical requirements, the suprahyoid region is subdivided into a submental and submandibular region. The angle and ramus of the mandible are approached through the inlet of the carotid triangle.

4.4 Position of the Head

With the shoulder supported on a cushion, the head is dorsally extended and turned toward the opposite side. This increases the distance between the mandible and the hyoid bone and makes important topographic landmarks easier to recognize: the mental tubercle, the mandibular angle, the mastoid, the cervical crease at the hyoid bone, and the anterior border of the sternocleidomastoid muscle (Fig. 177). Swelling associated with hematoma and edema can make some of the landmarks difficult to identify, but the inferior border of the mandible is always palpable.

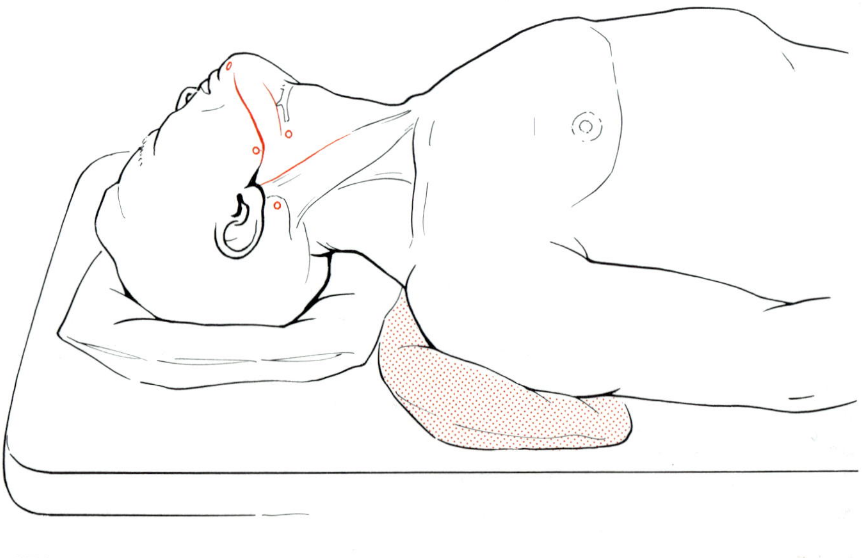

Fig. 177. Position of the head for operation

If there is concomitant injury to the cervical fascia, the hematoma will spread between the platysma and skin. In this case it will be harder to distinguish the blood-imbibed layers (platysma, overlying fascia, intervening nerve branches) when the incision is made. This underscores the importance of following a systematic exposure technique, which will allow the operator to maintain orientation even under difficult conditions.

4.5 Classification of Approaches

We distinguish the *subangular, submandibular,* and *submental* approaches in accordance with the potential sites of mandibular fractures (see Fig. 173). The angle and ramus are exposed through the subangular approach. The submandibular and submental approaches give access to the body of the mandible, consisting of the molar, premolar, and incisor portions.

4.6 Purpose of a Systematic Technique of Fracture Exposure

The major purpose of a systematic exposure technique is to avoid these complications:

1) weakness or paralysis of the mimetic muscles of the lower lip;
2) exacerbation of edema and pain, infection due to excessive traumatization of the soft tissues;
3) objectionable scar.

Surgical experience teaches that natural gliding surfaces and tissue planes provide routes of access that inflict minimal damage on nerves and blood vessels. The local magnitude of an operation is not necessarily a measure of traumatization. A "small" incision may divide more important structures and cause greater damage to the circulation (especially the terminal) than a more extensive approach that is made along natural tissue planes and avoids the transection of nerves and vessels. Accordingly, it has been found that exposing the mandibular border by the *subfascial route* yields superior results in terms of sparing the marginal branch of the facial nerve and the vascular supply.

It is not always possible to avoid the formation of a hyperplastic scar, which depends upon racial, hormonal, and age-related factors. Experience has shown that most patients consider the scar a necessary consequence of their surgery and place greater emphasis on an early restoration of masticatory function. The ability to open the mouth immediately after surgery gives the patient hope for a rapid and uncomplicated recovery. The scar does not have the impact on the patient's personal and social life that might be expected from a psychological standpoint. Rarely, a patient with a hyperplastic scar will desire revision by a plastic surgical procedure. In any case the operator treating the mandibular injury should always plan and conduct the *elective incision* in accordance with the principles of plastic surgery.

4.7 Directions and the Incision

The strategies for scar placement differ for closed and open fractures.

4.7.1 Closed Fractures

The incision for *closed fractures* is made either in the submental crease (submental sulcus) or in the natural cervical crease (hyoid sulcus). The latter is not directed toward the mandibular angle but runs roughly parallel to it, terminating as a point below the lobule of the ear. It is the standard incision for the subangular approach (Fig. 178). If the severity of the fracture requires extension of the incision, this may be done along the natural cervical crease despite its divergent course from the mandibular border.

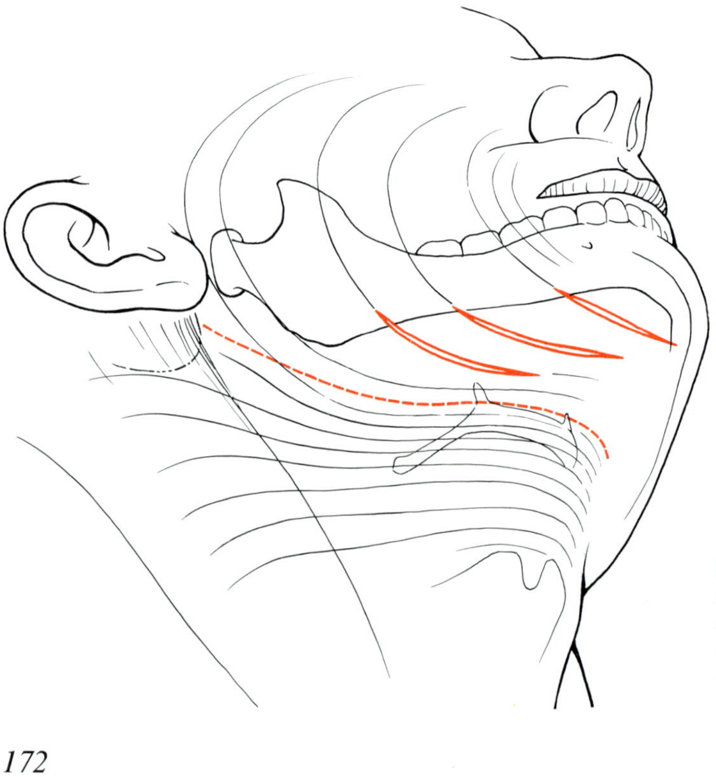

Fig. 178. Lines of election for scars correlated with fracture sites, following these principles:
- incision at right angles to the platysma fibers,
- respect for topography,
- utilization of natural skin crease (broken red line)

With a single fracture, there is a tendency to employ a short incision. If the incision is placed in the cervical crease (sulcus incision) at the level of the hyoid bone, the wound margin will have to be stretched excessively in the direction of the mandible. This additional trauma is compounded by the difficulty of performing the internal fixation through a small approach. Thus, the sulcus incision is not appropriate if a very limited exposure is desired.

The incision of choice in such cases is a paramandibular incision that closely follows the tension lines of the skin. These "lines of election for scars" (McGregor 1980), develop in the neck at right angles to the pull of the platysma. As the skin loses its elasticity with advancing age and subcutaneous fat is lost, the force of gravity causes thinned areas and creases to appear parallel to the hyoid sulcus.

4.7.2 Open Fractures

Open fractures of the mandible are associated with internal, external, or perforating injuries of the soft tissues (see Classification). The external soft-tissue damage is significant in terms of scar placement. It should be determined how and to what degree the principles of scar placement can be applied. Any of four options may be selected according to the extent and severity of the soft-tissue wound:

1) Expose the fracture through the existing wound.
2) Incorporate the wound into the incision (Fig. 179).
3) Make the incision separate from the wound, leaving a well perfused skin bridge between them (Fig. 180).
4) Incorporate the wound into the incision and add a small, separate incision for anchoring the plate outside the wound (Fig. 181).

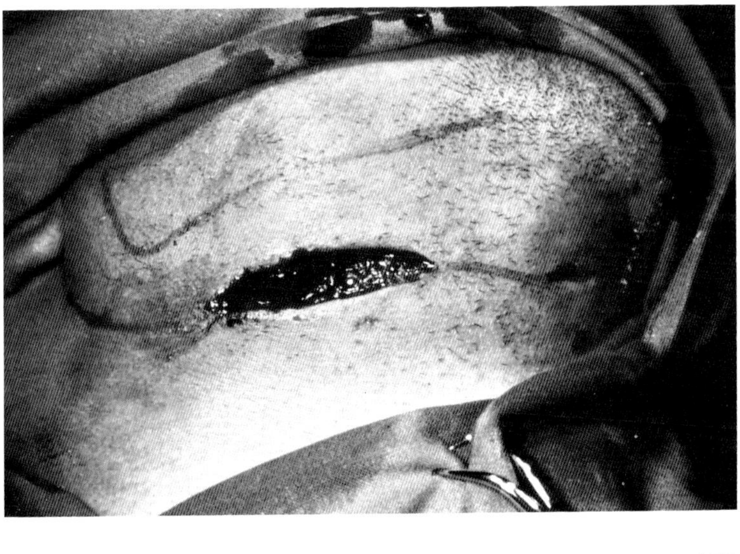

Fig. 179. Incision incorporating the traumatic wound

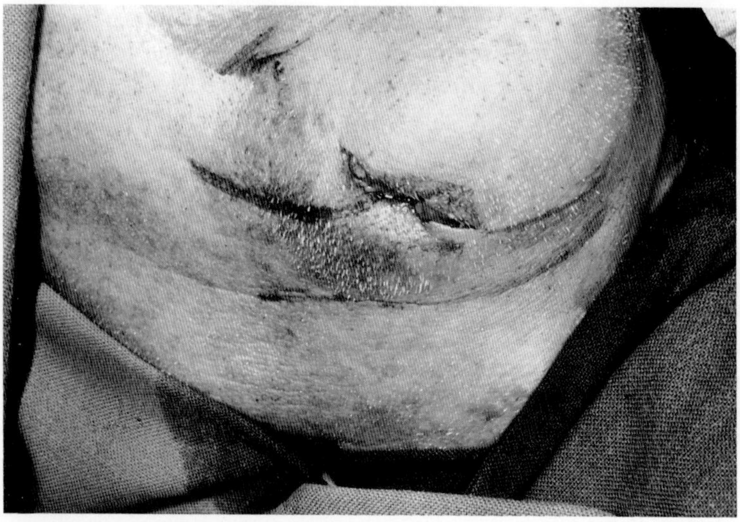

Fig. 180. Incision on the natural cervical crease, separate from the traumatic wound. (The paramandibular extension would produce a hyperplastic scar in a conspicuous site running across skin tension lines)

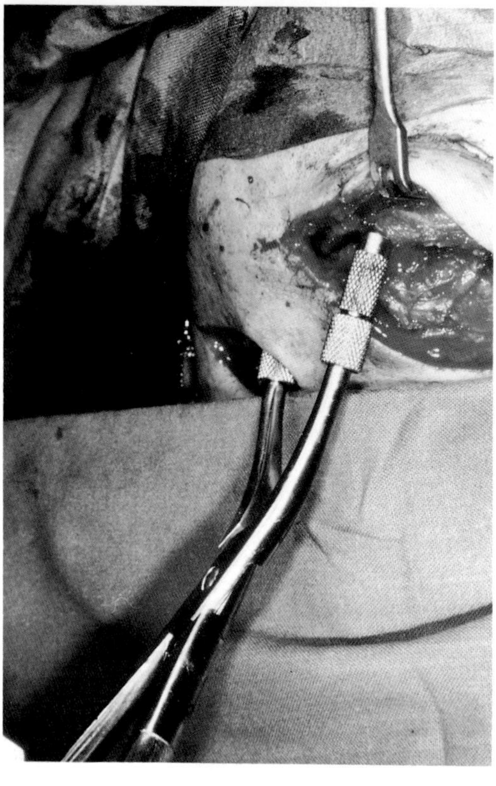

Fig. 181. Small, distally placed auxiliary incision to reduce the length of the scar

Regarding option 1), the size and position of the wound usually correlate so favorable with the fracture that an additional incision is unnecessary.

Option 2), where an incision is made that incorporates the wound, is occasionally used. The wound is extended in the direction of skin tension lines or the nearest cervical crease.

Option 3), a separate incision, is indicated when the wound is located 3–4 fingerwidths from the fracture. In exceptional cases a Z-shaped incision may be used if the soft-tissue injury is sufficiently close to the fracture. Otherwise this principle is reserved for secondary scar corrections. Generally it is unwise to extend a wound more than is absolutely necessary due to the infection risk and cosmetic result.

Option 4), where a second incision is made in addition to extending the wound, is very rarely employed.

4.8 Angle of the Incision

Scar formation depends upon the angle of the incision as well as its direction. Only an incision perpendicular to the skin surface will permit the wound margins to be reapproximated in an accurate, layer-to-layer fashion. The great mobility of the cervical skin, especially in older patients, can cause the incision to deviate inadvertently from the vertical direction. The oblique divided skin is susceptible to marginal necrosis, intracutaneous hematoma formation, and overlapping of the wound edges.

4.9 Surgical Anatomy of the Approaches

A knowledge of the special anatomy of the approaches is essential for a swift, sure, and nontraumatizing exposure of the fracture site that preserves functionally important substrates.

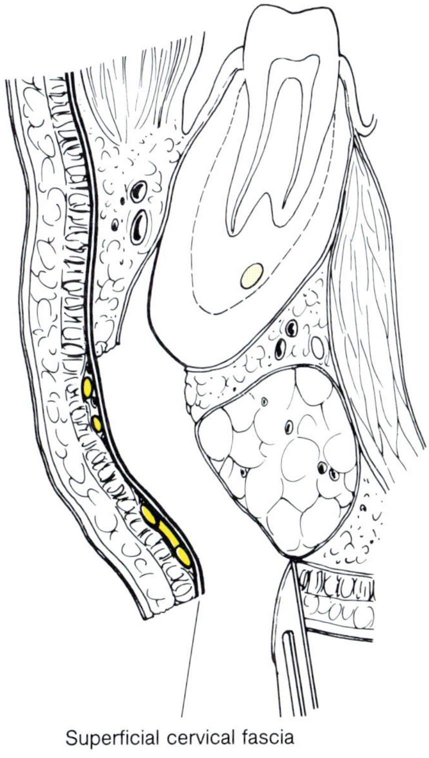

Fig. 182. The subfascial plane of approach to the fracture is bounded by the gland capsule and the loose tissue filling the space between the gland and the inferior mandibular border. The suprafascial layer contains the marginal branch of the facial nerve and the superficial ansa cervicalis, which form well-defined marginal and inframarginal nerve pathways (innervation zones)

Extraoral exposure of the mandible follows the fascial planes (Fig. 182). The nerve branches that are to be spared course superficial to the fascia in their own fibrous tissue layer. The path along the undersurface of the fascia leads directly to the bone, without risk of injury to an important nerve. This anatomic circumstance must be considered in all the approaches, along with the fact that the operative area is confined to the fascial layers above the level of the hyoid bone.

The area of interest encompasses three cervical triangles: the submandibular (digastric) trigone, the carotid trigone, and the submental trigone.

4.9.1 Submandibular Approach

The approach most commonly used is through the middle triangle, the digastric trigone. A double fascial layer stretches over this trigone between the mandible and hyoid bone: an inner layer covering the glandular bed and an outer muscular fascia applied to the undersurface of the platysma. Both, the fascia *and* platysma, should be regarded as a single unit 1) because of the nerve branches coursing between the fascial layers and 2) because the unit forms a guide plane for performing the paramandibular incision (see p. 178) and the submandibular incision in the hyoid sulcus.

Two zones of innervation occur between the fascia and platysma (Figs. 182 and 183): the marginal zone, which runs close and parallel to the mandibular border (marginal mandibular branch of the facial nerve), and the inframarginal zone, placed at the slightly more caudal level and containing nerve branches that run roughly parallel and at right angles (ansa) to the hyoid bone. The platysma itself if supplied by the cervical branch of the facial nerve and usually receives a collateral supply from the cutaneous nerve of the neck via the superficial ansa cervicalis. Both the cervical branch and the ansa must be spared to avoid postoperative mouth angle weakness. Thus, the incision through the platysma and fascia should be placed close to the hyoid bone. The hyoid bone is not always easy to palpate, for often it is covered over by the submaxillary gland. In this case the inferior border of the gland provides the landmark for orientation. Either of two surgical approaches may be taken through the platysma and fascia: the sulcus incision (classic submandibular incision) and the paramandibular incision.

4.9.1.1 Sulcus Incision: Incision in the Natural Cervical Crease (Hyoid Sulcus)

The cervical crease is located two fingerwidths from the angle of the mandible and three fingerwidths from its anterior border (mental tubercle). The increasing distance of the crease from the fracture site anteriorly must be compensated by increasing the length of the incision. Therefore this approach is best suited for multiple and comminuted fractures that require the application of a longer plate. The incision extends from the anterior border of the sternocleidomastoid muscle almost to the cervical midline. It lies precisely in the hyoid sulcus and thus is parallel to the hyoid bone.

The incision is carried vertically through four layers which are divided separately: the skin and subcutaneous fat, the platysma, a thin layer of loose connective tissue over the superficial cervical fascia, and finally the

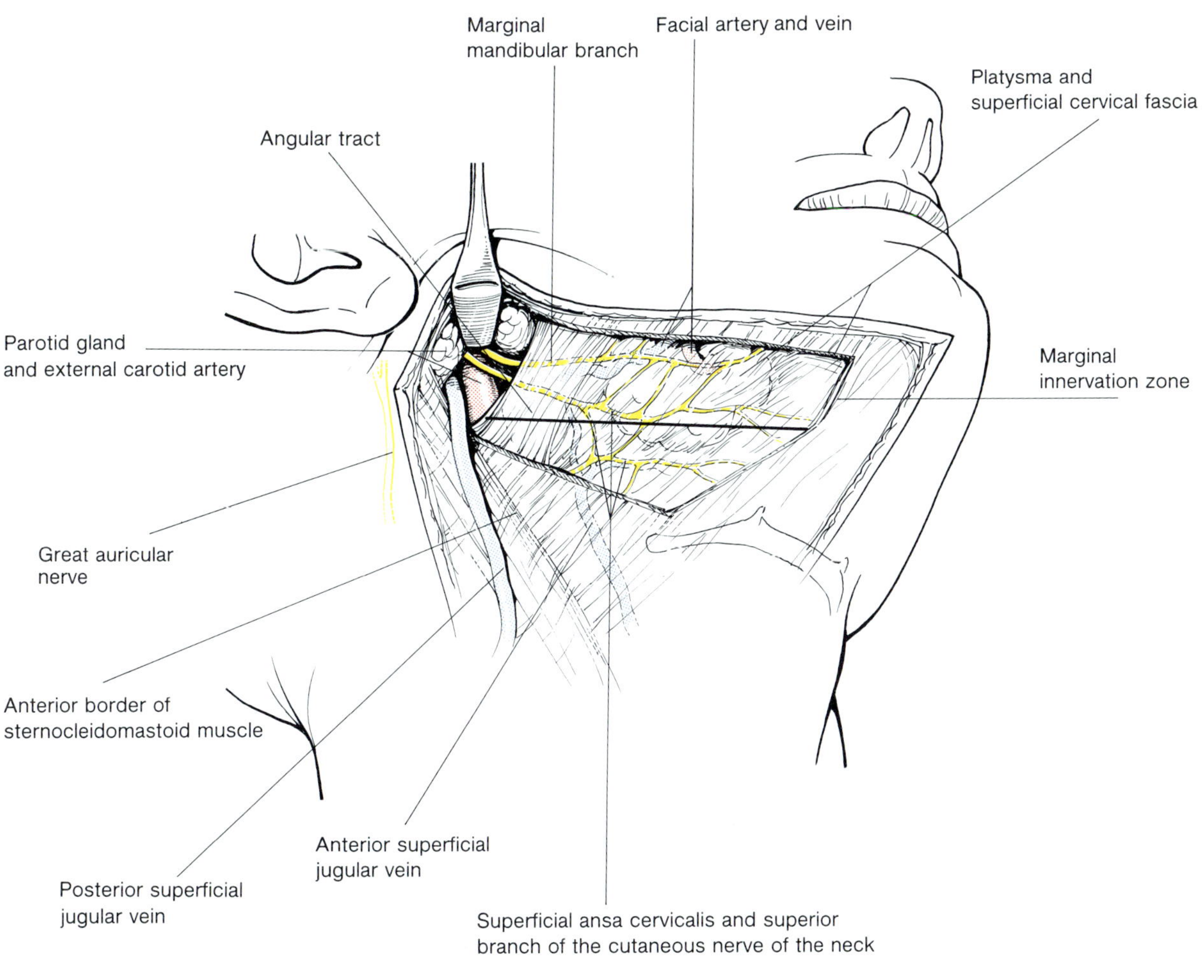

Fig. 183. Marginal and inframarginal innervation zones. The line of demarcation (heavy line) runs between the lower border of the mandible and the hyoid bone. Top: marginal mandibular branch of the facial nerve; bottom: cervical branch of the facial nerve, superficial ansa cervicalis, and cutaneous nerve of the neck

cervical fascia itself (see Fig. 182). The two connective tissue layers between the skin and platysma and between the platysma and cervical fascia form gliding layers for the platysma and accompany the underlying nerve branches. These branches are easily identified if hemostasis is carefully secured at each layer.

The fascia is clearly recognized by its light color and may be safely divided to the bare surface of the salivary gland over the length of the incision, for at this level (hyoid) the surgeon will encounter only the superficial branch of the cutaneous nerve of the neck with fibers from C3 and C4 (see Fig. 183). It is important to demonstrate the entire cut edge of the fascia, which is sharply dissected from the submandibular gland and elevated with a pair of hooks or traction sutures (Fig. 184). The scalpel blade is held against the glossy surface of the gland, which is not enclosed by a capsule but invested by a thin, transparent sheet of connective tissue. The subfascial space thus entered provides the corridor of access to the bone, which is approached along the surface of the gland.

Two special points should be noted in regard to the subfascial dissection:

1) The gland does not fill the anteriormost *angle of the digastric trigone* below the chin. Only fat and lymph nodes occur in that area, which is also devoid of facial nerve fibers. The marginal branch of the facial nerve turns upward at the extremity of the gland, crossing the mandible and passing toward the angle of the mouth (see Fig. 184a). This crossing occurs at the level of the mental foramen. If the internal fixation plate is to extend beyond that point, it will usually be necessary to lengthen the skin incision 1–2 cm toward the tip of the chin, exposing the digastric muscle surface (see the angle of the digastric trigone in Fig. 184a).
2) The superficial cervical fascia is firmly adherent to the inferior border of the mandible. But at the site where the facial artery and vein enter the face, the fascia is more loosely applied to the mandible and becomes lost in the connective tissue of the cheek. Lymph nodes are consistently found there. Very close contact should be maintained with the glandular surface during the dissection of this region.
   The connective tissue flap containing the lymph nodes and nerve branches is elevated from the gland surface with two Langenbeck retractors until the underlying bony margin can be palpated. Now a dissecting forceps is used to bluntly expose the facial vein, which is enclosed superficially by the cervical fascia (see Fig. 184b). After division of the vein it is a simple matter to ligate and divide the facial artery. At this point the mandibular border is fully accessible and can be exposed on the sub- or supraperiostal plane as needed between the mandibular angle and canine region without trauma to the soft tissues.

4.9.1.2 Paramandibular Incision

The principle of the "gridirion" incision is utilized in this approach and is made possible by the excellent mobility of the skin over the platysma. The skin in the paramandibular ara is relatively thin. During the incision the subcutaneous fat, depending on its thickness, may have to be divided in stages while bleeding is carefully controlled with a splinter forceps until the thin connective tissue over the platysma is visualized. At this point the skin is widely mobilized to the level of the hyoid bone on the connective tissue plane between the subcutaneous tissue and platysma (Fig. 185). The skin should be well elevated with Langenbeck retractors to assist the anatomic dissection and the coagulation of small arterial and venous branches. When the inferior border of the submandibular gland is reached, the same dissection technique is used to mobilize the skin anteriorly upward from that point toward the undersurface of the chin. The skin having been completely mobilized in a semicircle within the submandibular triangle, the platysma and fascia are divided close to the hyoid bone as in the sulcus incision

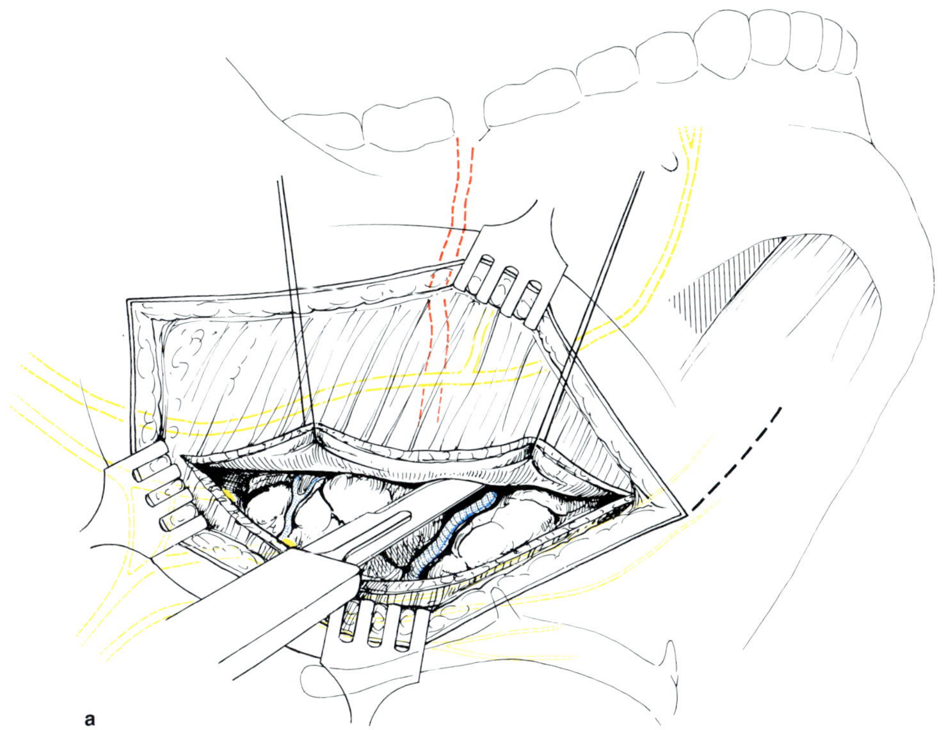

a

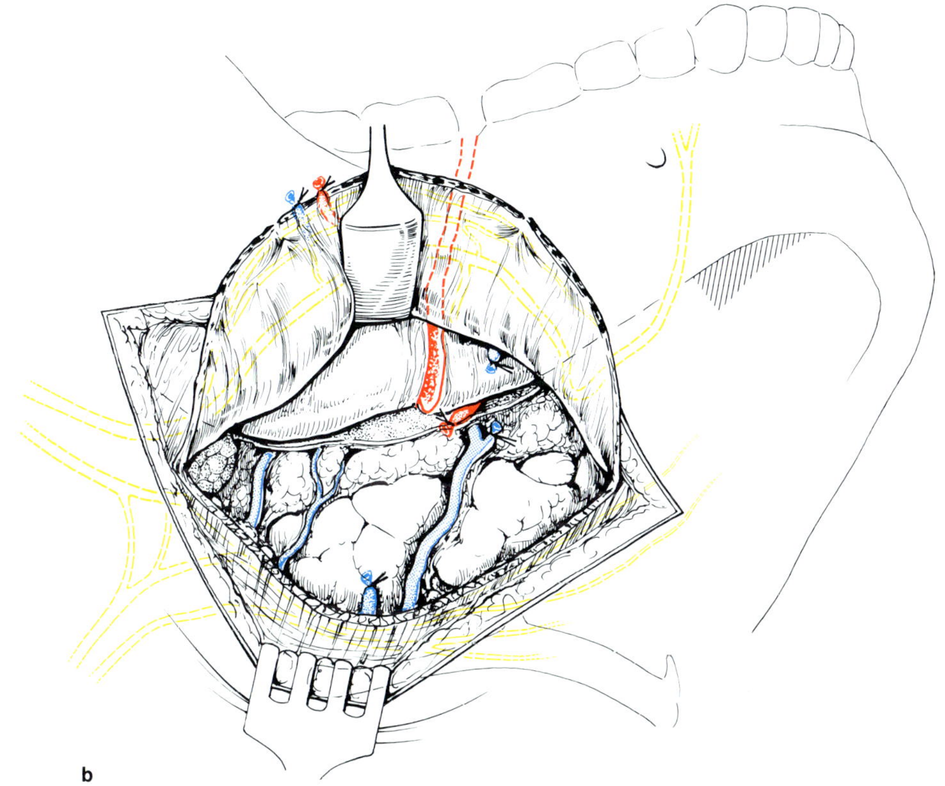

b

Fig. 184. **a** The scalpel is swept beneath the fascia on the bare surface of the submandibular gland in the direction of the mandibular border. The zone where the marginal branch of the facial nerves crosses the lower mandibular border at the anterior angle of the digastric trigone *(shaded)* is devoid of nerve fibers. **b** Note the fatty tissue between the submandibular gland and lower mandibular border. Retracting the gland medial by finger pressure makes this tissue tense and increases the separation of the marginal nerve branches. The vessels at this level are ligated, then the periosteum on the lower mandibular border is incised

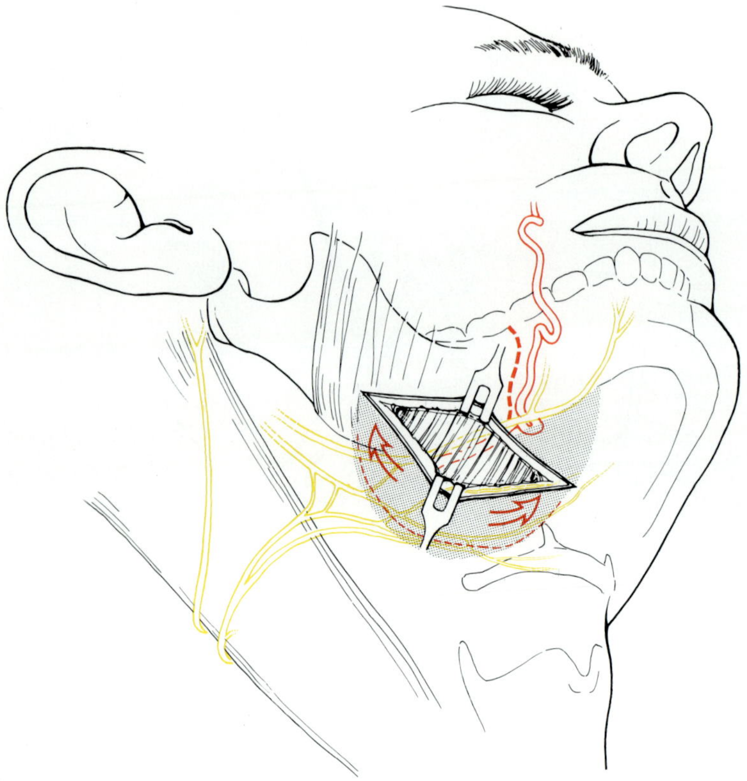

Fig. 185. Paramandibular incision and the associated semicircular mobilization of the skin between the subcutaneous tissue and platysma

(see above). At this point the subfascial or epiglandular dissection can be carried to the fractured mandible, with the advantage that the skin incision directly overlies the fracture, and the thin platysma-fascia layer can be retracted without tension.

4.9.2 Subangular Approach

Effective preservation of the facial nerve branches and adequate exposure of the mandibular angle and ramus call for an approach through the carotid triangle. With the head in the standard position (see Fig. 177), the carotid triangle presents as a skin depression between the visible borders of the sternocleidomastoid mucle, the parotid gland, and the submandibular gland. This feature, termed the *carotid fossa* (Fig. 186), represents the superior half of the carotid triangle. Both salivary glands provide key topographic landmarks for the exposure. The parotid gland partially overlies the mandibular angle and the sternocleidomastoid. The submandibular gland extends far posteriorly into the carotid trigone and covers the posterior digastric muscle belly. Thus the muscle does not provide a useful surgical landmark for approaching the mandibular angle, although it does form the anterior boundary of the carotid triangle.

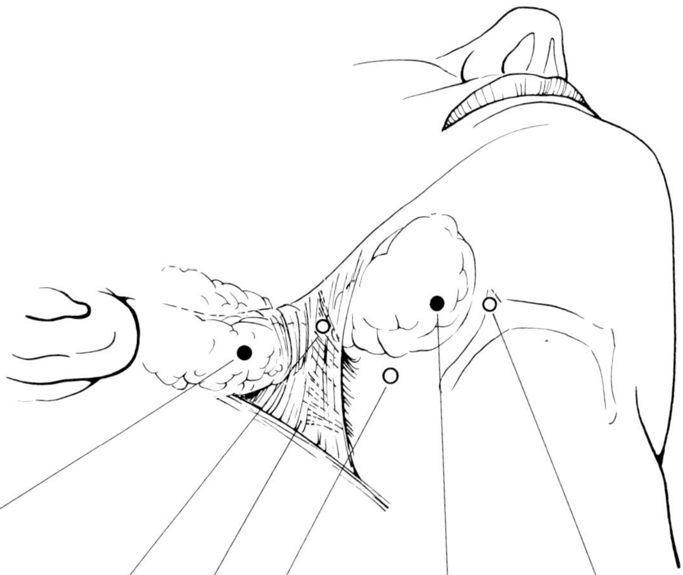

Fig. 186. Surgical landmarks useful in the subangular approach

The superficial cervical fascia encloses the sternocleidomastoid muscle by dividing into two layers that invest the superior and inferior surfaces of the muscle. At its anterior margin the fascia merges with a single sheet of connective tissue. This junction plays an important role in the subfascial dissection. In addition this site is strongly reinforced by the angular tract, which stretches between the mandibular angle and sternocleidomastoid and overlies the poles of both salivary glands (see Fig. 186).

Because of this arrangement, the division and mobilization of the fascia in the subangular approach is started at the anterior border of the sternocleidomastoid muscle. It is important to preserve the attachment between the two-layer muscular fascia (superficial and deep laminae) and the superficial cervical fascia. This is done by incising the fascia over the muscle and dissecting down around the muscle border on the subfascial plane so that the deep layer of the fascia can be elevated in continuity with the angular tract (Fig. 187).

At the pole of the parotid gland, the loose attachment of the gland to the digastric fascia is bluntly separated by spreading open the blades of a dissecting forceps. This maneuver is assisted by elevating the pole of the

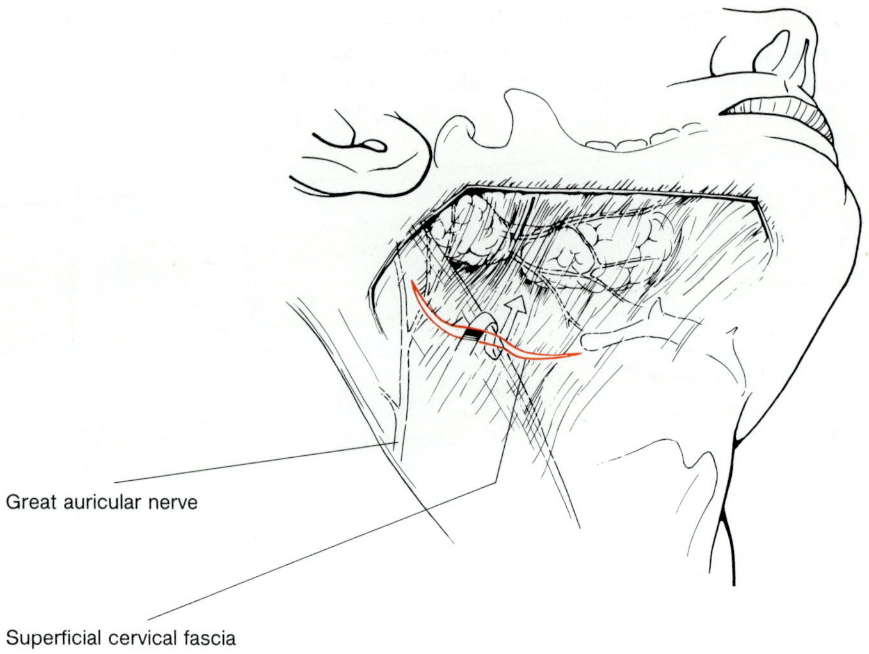

Fig. 187. Subfascial approach to the mandibular angle. The cervical fascia is opened with a curved incision *(red)* extending from the anterior border of the sternocleidomastoid muscle to the hyoid bone. The dissection is carried below the fascia and around the edge of the muscle *(arrow)*. The lower border of the mandible is approached below the angular tract. The nerve branches and pole of the parotid gland are encountered over the mandibular border

gland, taking with it the facial nerve branches emerging at its anterior margin so that the intrafascial course of the nerve fibers is not disturbed. Elevating the pole of the parotid gland gives access to the interval between the two salivary glands, whose deep borders are separated from each other by a transverse septum (this interglandular septum is part of the angular tract; it has no topographic importance in the exposure of the mandibular angle). The surface of the submandibular gland is encountered in this interval and again provides a guide plane for the subfascial or epiglandular route to the border of the mandible.

It is advantageous to perform the subangular approach in two phases: 1) mobilization of the skin and 2) dissection of the fascia.

Mobilizing the skin up to the level of the mandibular angle gives a clear view of the operative field and facilitates retraction of the soft tissues (see Fig. 187). Only the skin with the subcutaneous fat layer is mobilized in order to avoid injury to the great auricular nerve and the posterior superficial jugular vein. The skin and muscular fascia are connected in this area by strong fiber bundles, and it is difficult to separate the fat and fascia cleanly, especially if meticulous hemostasis is not achieved. Once the platysma is reached, the dissection proceeds as easily as in the submandibular trigone. The skin and subcutaneous fat are sufficiently mobilized to expose a fascial area extending from the anterior border of the sternocleidomastoid muscle down to the level of the fourth cervical vertebra and anteriorly to the hyoid bone. The first and second branches of the great auricular nerve are visualized along with the posterior superficial jugular vein; the angular tract may be appreciated as a thickened area of fascia (see Fig. 187).

Phase 2 begins with division of the fascia below the ear, the line of incision following the course of the great auricular nerve. The platysma usually begins one fingerwidth below the pole of the parotid gland. The cornu of the hyoid bone is easily palpated from the posterior aspect and provides a useful landmark. The platysma fibers and fascia are divided in stepwise fashion. When the surface of the submandibular gland is reached, it provides the topographic guide plane for the subfascial dissection, as noted above.

4.9.3 Submental Approach

The incision is made 2–3 fingerwidths below the mandibular border in the submental crease, which is usually visible. Exposure of the mandibular border presents no difficulties.

5 Closed Fractures

5.1 Definition of Terms

A "closed" fracture is one in which the mucosa and skin covering the fracture site have not been breached. It has been suggested that this term is not applicable to mandibular fractures, since fractures of the mucosa-covered mandibular bone, a derivative of the branchial arches, are generally associated with a tear in the mucosa even if a laceration is not grossly visible. Such a concept appears to be more a rationale for conservative treatment strategies than an explanation for infections in closed fractures (see p. 242). Operative treatment is concerned only with the visible mucosal wound, especially since its size correlates with the degree of contamination. This justifies a critical attitude toward use of the oral approach as an alternative to aseptic fracture treatment through an external incision. It should be stressed in this regard that not every periodontal pocket adjacent to a fracture is a direct source of infection. An additional enabling factor, such as an unstable implant, must be present in such cases for infection to occur. Thus one should be selective about removing a third molar or other tooth in the fracture line (see p. 199) and giving prophylactic antibiotics for closed fractures (see p. 132). A mandibular fracture should be regarded as closed if visual examination does not disclose an open mucosal wound in the area of the fracture (symbol: S_0).

5.2 Classification

Category	Grouping by grade of severity
F_1 S_0	I
F_2 S_0	II A
F_3 S_0	II B

5.3 Single Fracture (F_1 S_0, Grade I)

Definition: "Single" means that the mandible is fractured at only one site in the body or ramus.

The morphologic differentiation into oblique and transverse fractures on the one hand and oblique-surface fractures on the other is especially useful in single fractures, since the direction of the fracture line will dictate the most appropriate fixation method. Similar considerations apply in the fixation of multiple fractures.

Internal fixation is performed at all sites on the mandible except for the coronoid and condylar processes. That is because fractures at these sites, and especially condylar fractures, are still treated most simply and effectively by conservative means.

5.3.1 Internal Fixation of Transverse and Oblique Fractures in the Precanine Region (Median, Paramedian, and Canine Fractures)

Usually the fracture site is paramedian or at the level of the canine tooth. Most are vertical, a few oblique. On the median plane itself the bone is particularly strong because of the intersection of force trajectories in that area. Displacement on the sagittal plane tends to be minimal because of the equilibrium of muscular pulls. At most, a slight step-off deformity may be present.

5.3.1.1 Intraoral Approach: Indication for DCP

Exposure of the outer bony surface of the anterior mandible is so straightforward that the intraoral approach is widely utilized for the internal fixation of *median* and *paramedian fractures*. Because this approach violates the principle of asepsis, we continue to prefer the submental approach. However, if the intraoral approach is used, it is sufficient to expose the bone as far as the protuberance for application of a four-hole DCP between the basal arch and alveolar process. A small tension-band splint and a slightly overbent plate will provide ideal approximation and axial compression of the bone ends (Fig. 188; compare with case p. 274) as well as immediate pain relief and functional capability. Length of hospitalization is 2–3 days.

The *canine level* of the mandible is one of the most common sites for fractures. When treated by the intraoral route, these "canine fractures" require exposure of the inferior mandibular border and considerable overbending of the plate to secure approximation of the fragments on the lingual side. The curvature of the body at the cuspid level creates a site of predilection for the concentration of tensile stresses. Hence the use of a six-hole DCP is indicated (Fig. 189). It is recommended that the fixation be augmented with a small tension-band splint, as this is the best means of providing immediate pain relief and functional stability. In all cases the end of the plate must be positioned below and posterior to the mental fora-

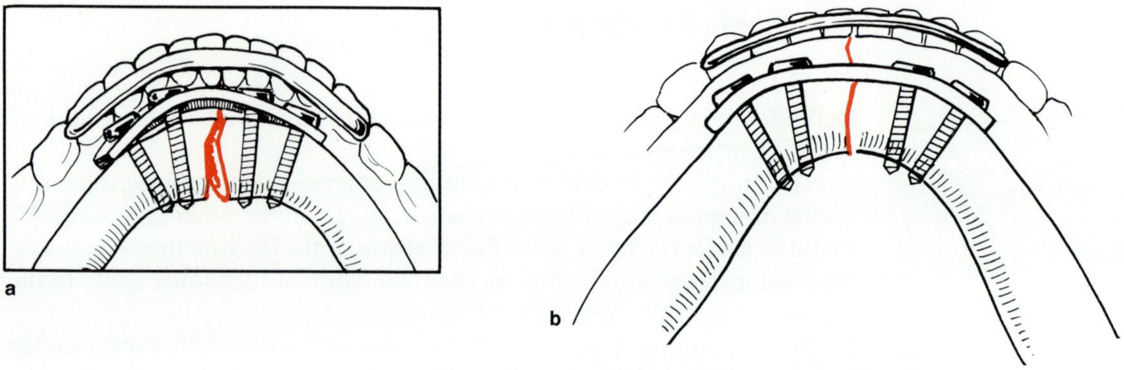

Fig. 188 a, b. Splaying on the lingual side of the fracture is eliminated by overbending the plate

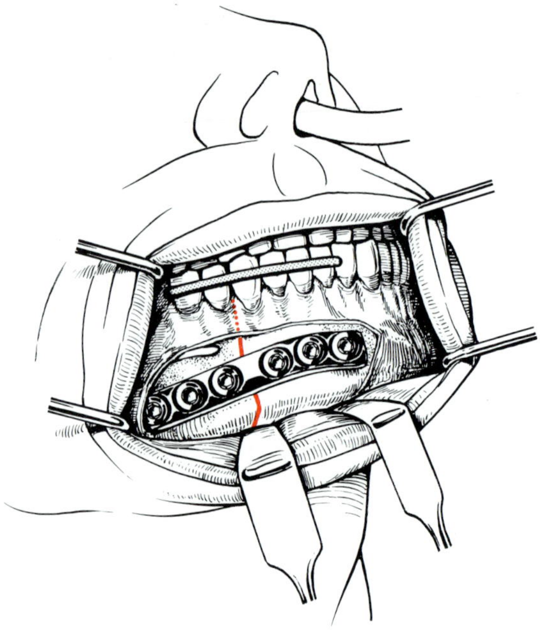

Fig. 189. Rule of thumb for fractures at the canine level: six-hole DCP and tension-band splint

men. The area about the mental foramen should be exposed sufficiently to demonstrate the site of entry of the neurovascular sheath.

The eccentric dynamic compression plate (EDCP) is contraindicated in this region. This is because the tunnel-like operating field does not give sufficient access for eccentric screw insertion, and the curve of the mandibular arch creates a biomechanical situation that is unfavorable for use of the EDCP.

5.3.1.2 Extraoral Approach: Indication for EDCP

The disadvantages of opening the fracture to the oral cavity are easily avoided by using the submental approach. The external incision is placed in the submental crease (see p. 183). The marginal plating zone can be exposed rapidly with minimal stripping of periosteum – a particular advantage in the canine area in terms of respecting the mandibular canal and mental foramen and providing free access for use of the reduction-compression forceps. The position of the plate on the outermost edge of the mandible makes it advisable to use the six-hole EDCP, which should be overbent to improve the pressure distribution on the lingual side; usually this will obviate the need for a tension-band splint. Ernst ligatures (see Fig. 53) are placed beforehand to secure the fragments in a eugnathic position.

As an alternative to the EDCP, a DCP may be used in conjunction with a small tension-band splint (see Fig. 242 b). If splinting is not possible (e.g., due to traumatic loss of the anterior teeth), a six-hole plate is used instead of a four-hole plate.The measurements of Junier (1980) indicate that tensile stresses are predominant at the border of the chin area, so that a plate applied there functions chiefly as a tension band.

5.3.2 Internal Fixation of Transverse and Oblique Fractures in the Postcanine Region (Fractures of the Lateral Mandible)

Fractures involving the premolar or molar portion of the mandible can show varying patterns of displacement. They are frequently unstable. Typically the proximal fragment is displaced upward by the elevator muscles, while the distal fragment is displaced downward by the hyoid and oral floor muscles and perhaps laterally by the force of the blow.

5.3.2.1 Extraoral Approach

The submandibular approach is better than the peroral approach (see p. 176) for fractures involving the premolar and molar regions. We draw the fracture line and inferior border of the mandible on the skin as an aid to planning the incision (Fig. 190). Space should be allowed for use of the pressure roller attachments, which are most helpful in the region between the canine and mandibular angle (see Fig. 53, p. 61).

The great value of the reduction-compression forceps in aiding the conduct of the internal fixation is itself a compelling argument in favor of the extraoral approach. This instrument makes it easy to distract the fragments for removal of any incarcerated soft tissues. The fracture is then reduced and precompressed with the handles and pressure rollers.

The technique of occlusal reduction and retention determines the selection of the internal fixation method:

1) With a *dental splint*, which serves concurrently as a tension band, one should use either the six-hole DCP (easier technique) or the EDCP as a stabilization plate (Fig. 191).
2) With *Ernst ligatures*, the pressure rollers are used to apply eccentric compression and the six-hole EDCP is applied to compensate for the absence of a tension band.
3) With *extramaxillary fixation* (see Fig. 60 c), used in the edentulous mandible when full dentures are worn, the six-hole EDCP is preferred over a DCP for transverse fractures (Fig. 192 a), although either type may be used.

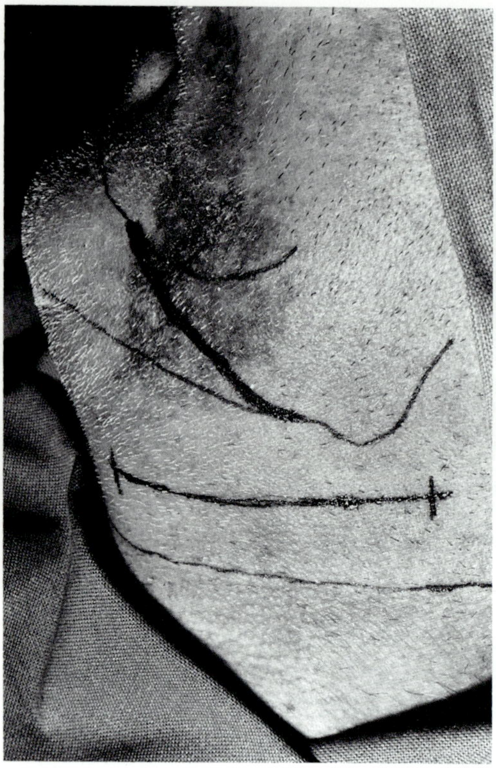

Fig. 190. The fracture line and line of incision are marked on the skin

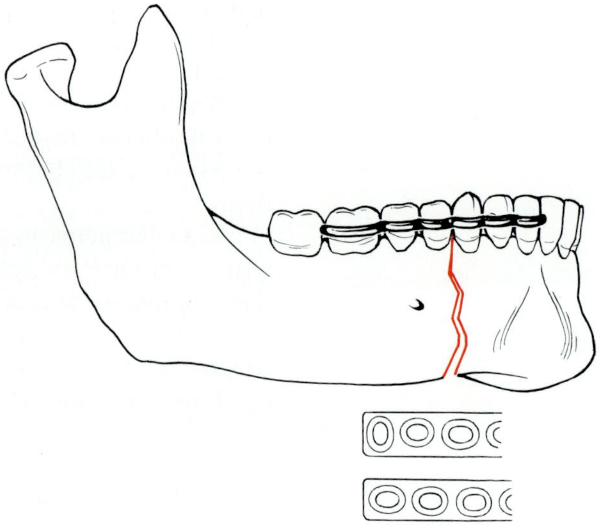

Fig. 191. A dental splint functioning as a tension band permits use of the DCP or the EDCP

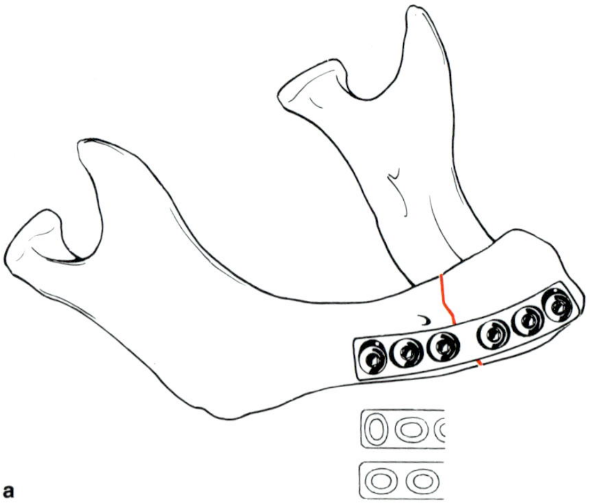

a

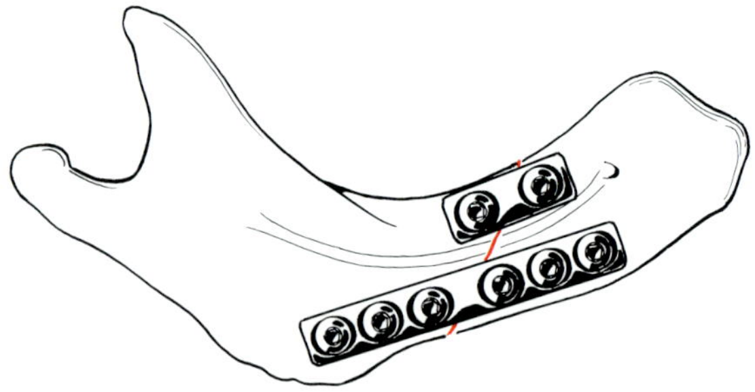

b

Fig. 192. **a** First choice for transverse fractures: EDCP, second choice: DCP. **b** The tension-band plate and compression plate combination is recommended for an oblique fracture that offers sufficient room for a tension band plate

For an oblique fracture, we recommend a two-hole tension-band plate combined with a four- or six-hole DCP in cases where the alveolar process is intact (Fig. 192b). A similar fracture in the atrophic mandible is stabilized with a reconstruction plate (see Fig. 60).

5.3.3 Internal Fixation of Angle Fractures

5.3.3.1 Statistics

The following statistics illustrate the complicating factors that may be associated with the treatment of fractures of the mandibular angle.

In a series of our own patients with anglc fractures (136 patients with a total of 327 mandibular fractures), 40% (53) had fractures of the angle *exclusively* (F_1) while 60% (83) had multiple fractures that *included* a fracture of the angle (F_2) (Litwan and Spiessl, in press).

Of the patients with multiple fractures, the majority, 71, had 3 fragments (Graph 7, a and b). Ten patients had 4-part fractures (c, d) and 2 had 5- and 6-part fractures (e). As the number of fragments increases from 3 to 6, we notice a predominance of contralateral fracture sites as a result of the contrecoup mechanism. The tendency toward contralateral involvement is especially markes in three-part fractures. The sites affected are, in order of frequency, the canine, subcondylar, molar, incisor, and angle regions (Graph 8). When more than three fragments are present, the contralateral side is invariably affected.

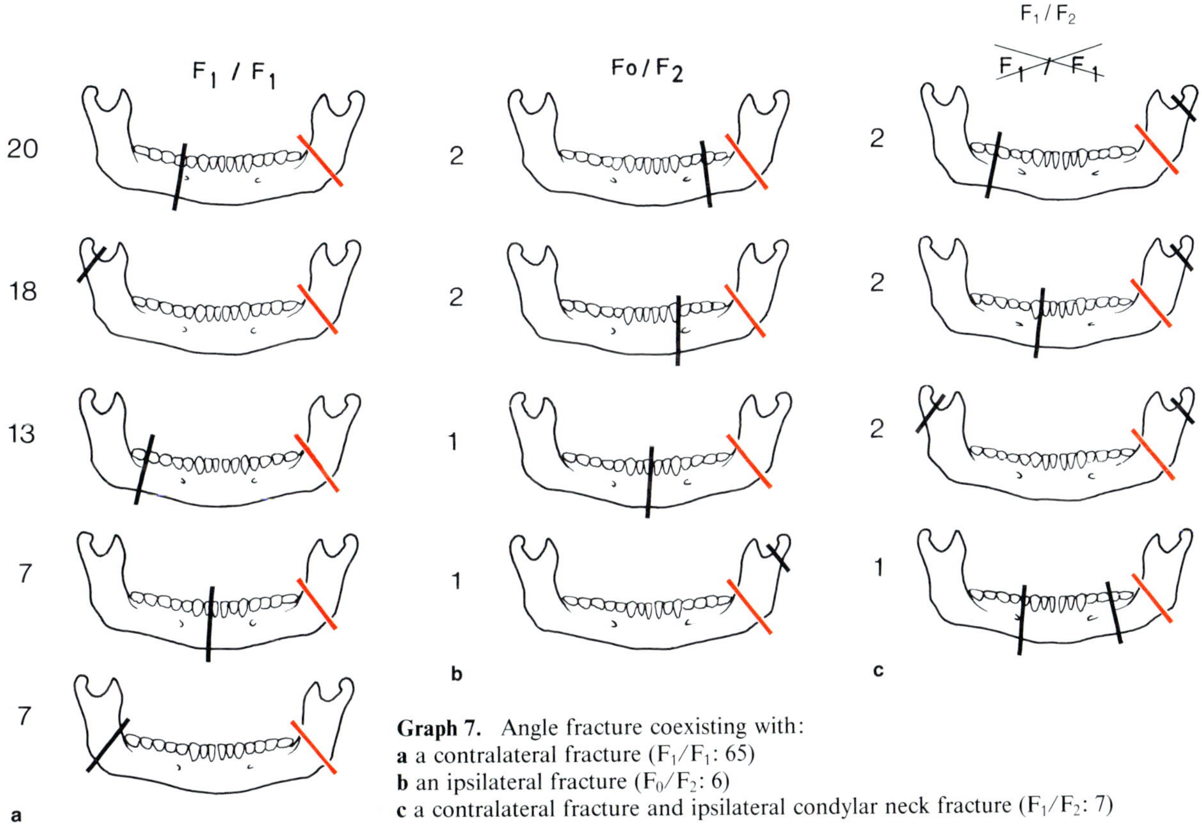

Graph 7. Angle fracture coexisting with:
a a contralateral fracture (F_1/F_1: 65)
b an ipsilateral fracture (F_0/F_2: 6)
c a contralateral fracture and ipsilateral condylar neck fracture (F_1/F_2: 7)

The surgical implications of this is that the majority of angle fractures will require treatment of a coexisting fracture on the opposite side. In addition to this, treatment of the angle fracture itself poses specific problems that relate to the anatomy of this region.

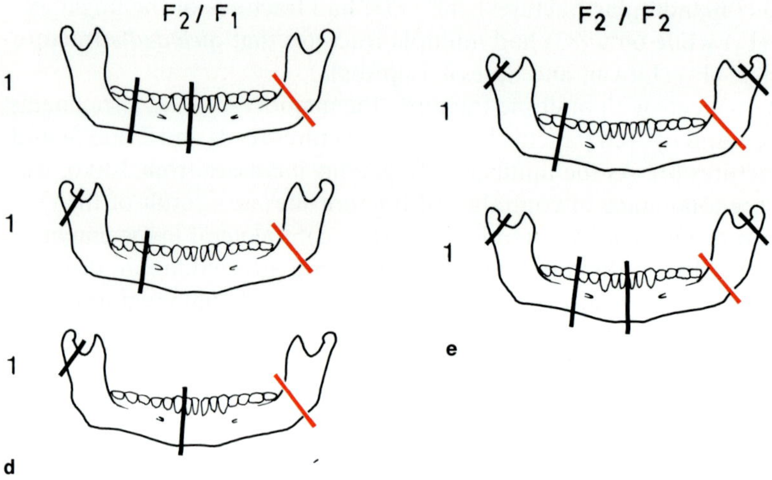

Graph 7
d a contralateral multiple fracture (F_2/F_1: 3)
e a contralateral multiple fracture and ipsilateral condylar neck fracture (F_2/F_2: 2)

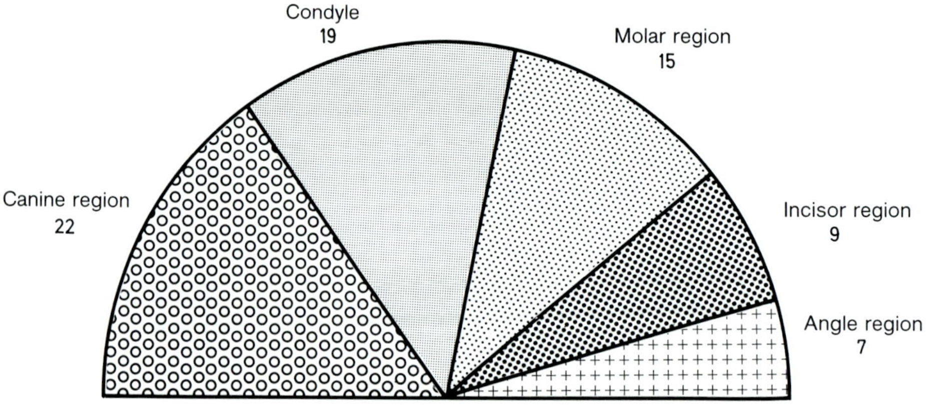

Graph 8. Frequency of contrecoup fracture sites associated with 72 angle fractures in which there is *one* accompanying contralateral fracture in the region indicated

5.3.3.2 Central Angle Fractures

Defining the surgical-anatomic boundaries of the mandibular angle: The *center* of the angle region consists of an outer and an inner angle. The region between these two angles is of practical diagnostic and surgical importance. While the apex and bisector of the angle can be determined, there is no clinically or anatomically valid method for defining the anterior and posterior limits of the angle region for surgical purposes. However, the *"three screw rule"*[6] requires us to define these limits so that the correct plate selection can be made. The apex of the mandibular angle marks the junction of the body and vertical ramus. The average apical distance between the outer and inner angle is constant even in the edentulous jaw. The three-hole length measured along the ramus and body from the outer apex establishes boundary lines that are useful in terms of fracture classification and plate selection (Fig. 193, see also Fig. 201 a, b). Fractures located within these boundaries are by definition *central* angle fractures. This region includes the alveolus of the third molar, which forms a site of predilection for the mandibular fracture[7].

[6] The average screw length is 10–12 mm for the ramus area and 14–18 mm for the body. The resulting stability difference has engendered the rule that at least 3 screws be used for plate fixation in the ramus fragment. For if one of the screw strips its thread, that hole may be left empty without destroying the stability of the fixation. This compromise is not appropriate if the loose screw is directly adjacent to the fracture, and in this case a reconstruction plate should be used.

[7] The curve between the body and ramus is a mechanical weak point and the second most frequent site, again due largely to the presence of the wisdom tooth. The third molar shows a direct relation to the fracture line in 70% of our patients with angle fractures.

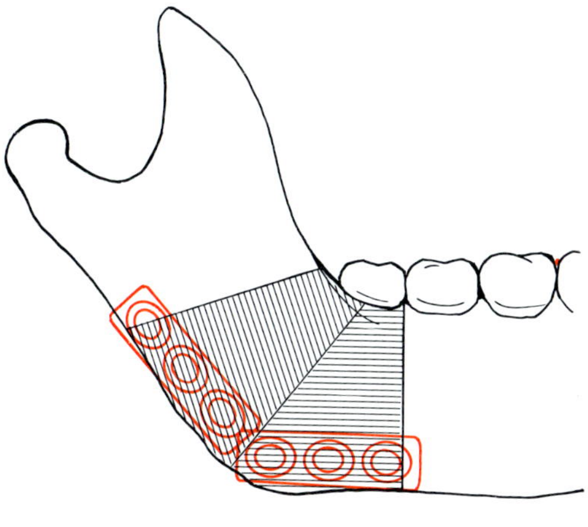

Fig. 193. Defining the surgical-anatomic boundaries of the mandibular angle.
- The inner angle encompasses the third molar and retromolar fossa.
- The angle bisector extends from the apex of the outer angle to the midpoint of the inner angle (both points can be identified on the orthopantomogram and at operation).
- The anterior and posterior boundaries of the mandibular angle are measured from the apex.
- The unit of measurement is the three-hole width of the DCP, measured from the apex of the outer angle. The resulting boundaries (anterior and posterior) define the *central* angle region

If the three-hole distance (from the apex of the mandibular angle) marks the end of the angle region, fractures within that region cannot be adequately stabilized with a straight plate (DCP, EDCP). The third hole will be too close to the mandibular border to provide a secure hold for a screw (Fig. 194), and the plate will be stabilized mainly by the screw adjacent to the fracture (see p. 108).

The alternative of using a more limited exposure and applying a shorter plate (two holes on each side) would require a perfectly placed tension band at the inner angle of the mandible (oblique line). The lack of space plus other constraints (see p. 200) make it difficult to place an effective tension band in that area.

Experience has shown that the reconstruction plate is the only device that will permit the stable insertion of three fixation screws on each side of a central angle fracture (Fig. 195).

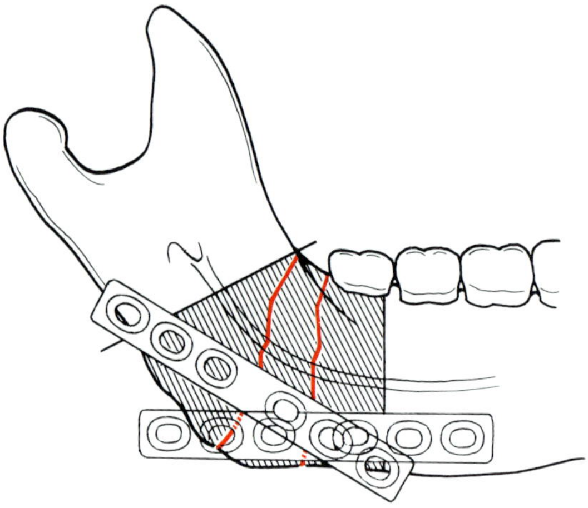

Fig. 194. Here there is not enough room for three screws in each fragment when a straight plate is used, regardless of how the plate is oriented on the bone

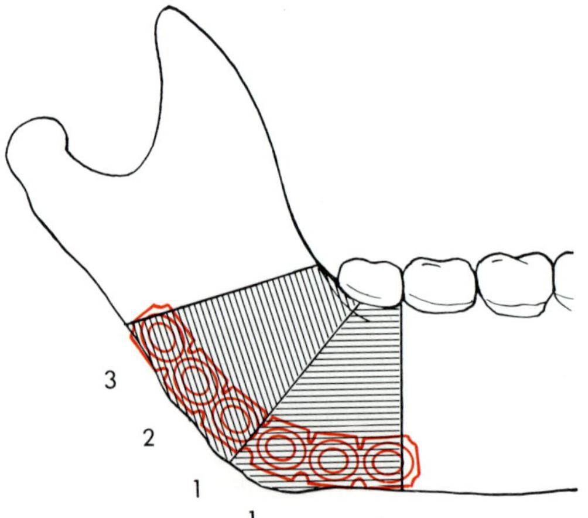

a

Fig. 195. **a** The problem in Fig. 194 can be solved by using the reconstruction plate, inserting the screws in the sequence 1, 2, and 3. **b** Apical fracture distal to the third molar (apex is "closed" to the fracture line). **c** Stabilization of the fracture with a six-hole reconstruction plate is consistent with the three screw rule. **d** Status after implant removal

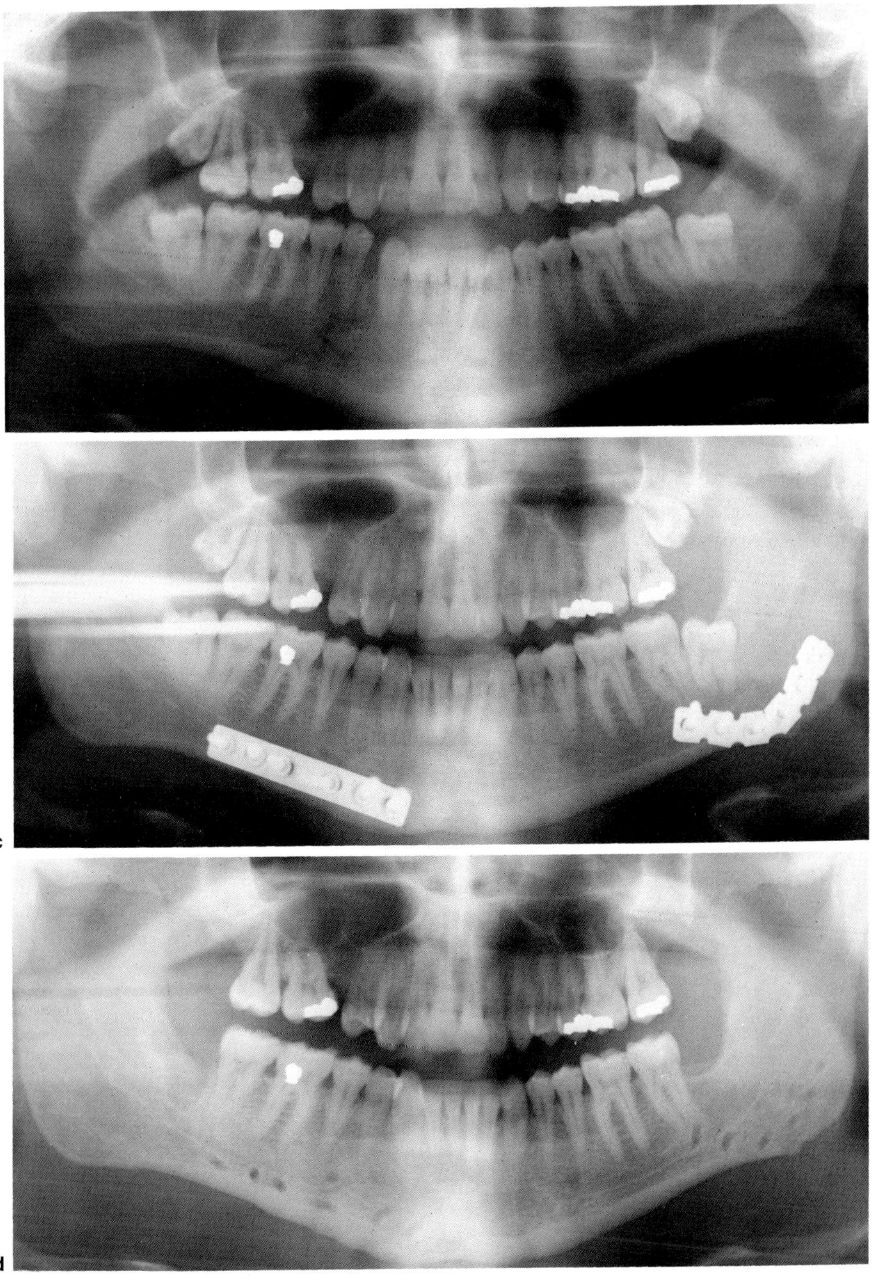

b

c

d

Fig. 195 b–d

Besides the fact that the ramus is considerably thinner than the body, the presence of a closed muscular sling around the mandibular angle also influences treatment planning. If the fracture is at the center of the muscular sling and shows little or no displacement owing to the equilibrium of muscle pulls, fixation with a single lag screw may be satisfactory (see Fig. 38).

5.3.3.3 Peripheral Angle Fractures (Angle-Body and Angle-Ramus Fractures)

The mandibular angle marks the junction of the body with the ramus, which ascends obliquely on the sagittal plane. Thus, the angle region includes portions of the body and the ramus, and so a postcanine fracture that extends back into the angle region or a supra-angular fracture that extends down into that region is still considered to be an angle fracture (Fig. 196). We call this type of fracture a *peripheral* angle fracture. The body or ramus component of the fracture presents its own treatment problems, as the following case illustrates (see also Fig. 173).

Peripheral angle fracture on the left side with an incomplete basal wedge fragment in an edentulous mandible (Fig. 197).

Fracture formula:	F_1 L_4 (see Fig. 173)
Clinical category:	F_1 S_0
Grade of severity:	I B

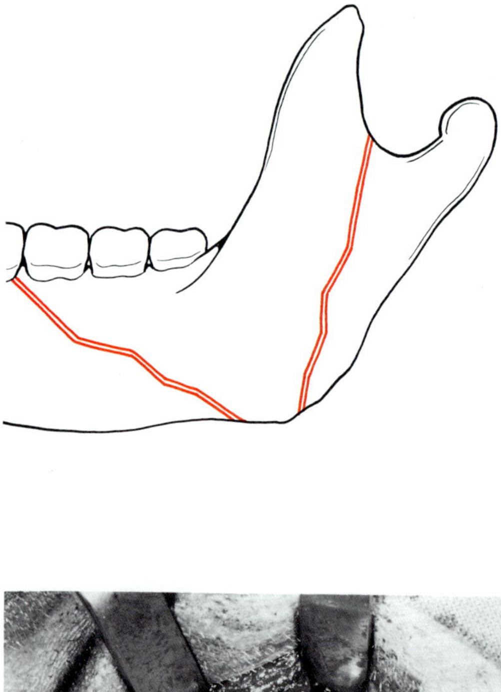

Fig. 196. The *peripheral* angle fracture involves a portion of the body or ramus

a 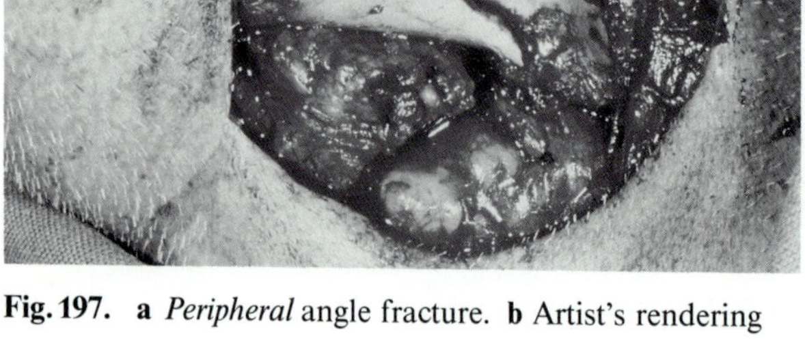

b 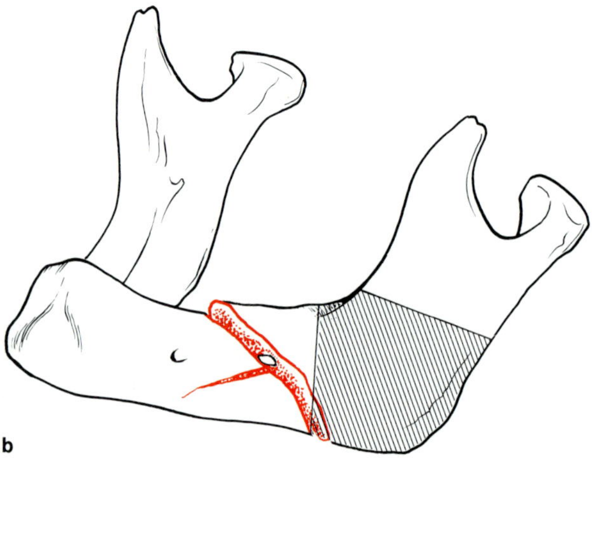

Fig. 197. **a** *Peripheral* angle fracture. **b** Artist's rendering

Problem of Treatment

Because no teeth are available for the placement of a dental splint, a tension-band plate is indicated. Eliminating this plate (by using an EDCP) poses a risk of instability due to the obliquity of the fracture line. The solution is illustrated in Figs. 198 and 199.

a
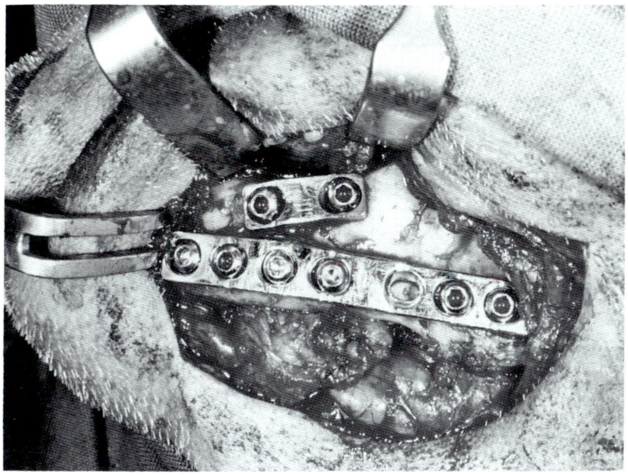

b
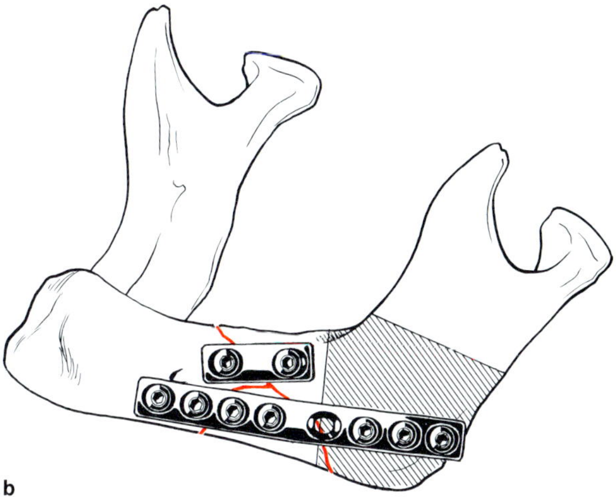

Fig. 198 a, b. Small tension-band plate used in conjunction with a long eight-hole buttress plate. The peripheral component of the angle fracture makes it possible to obey the three screw rule

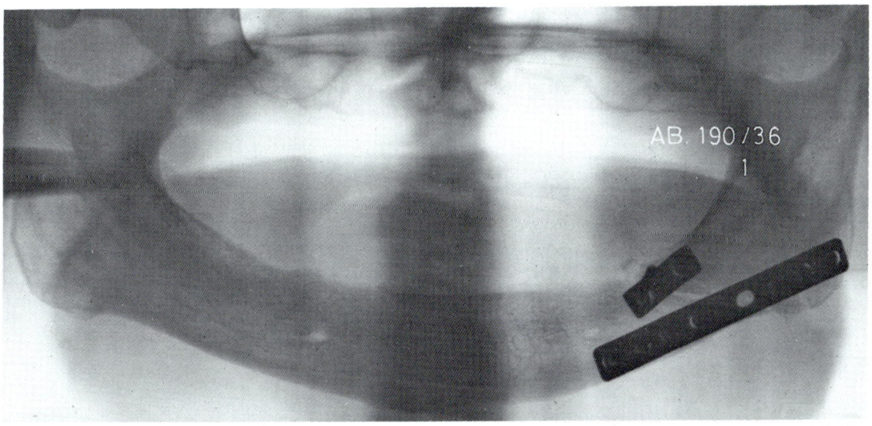

a

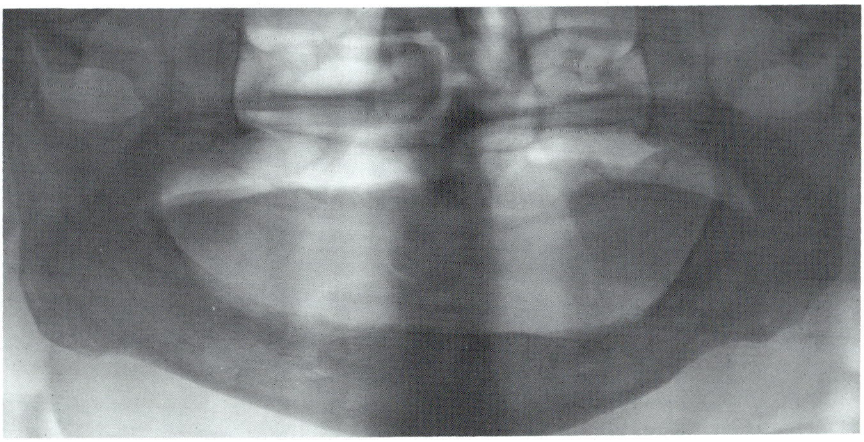
b

Fig. 199 a, b. Status postoperatively and after plate removal

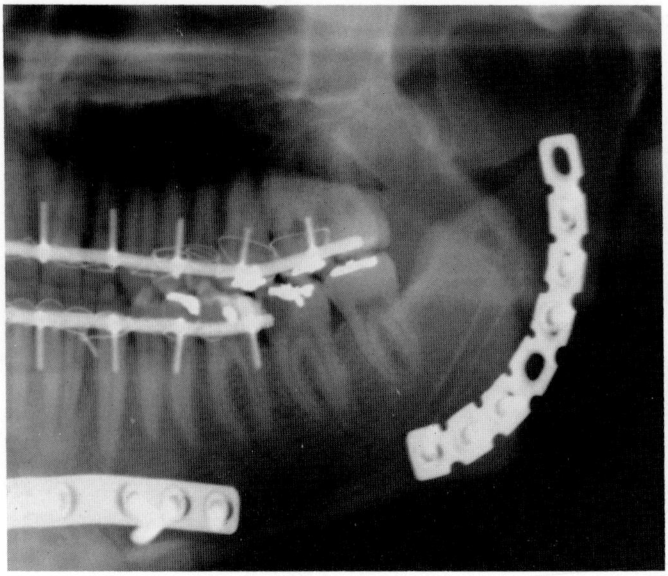

a

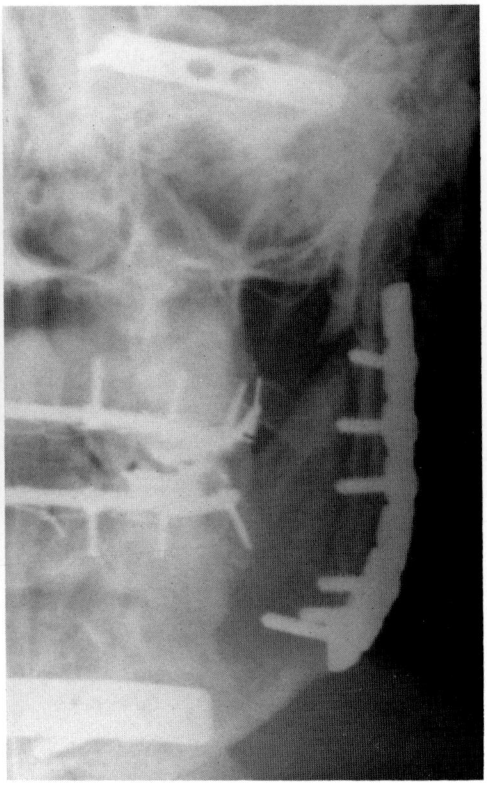

b

Fig. 200 a, b. Peripheral angle fracture with extension to the semilunar incisure. A reconstruction plate is indicated for this type of injury. Fracture of the coronoid process requires IMF for two weeks

The peripheral angle fracture with extension to the semilunar incisure is managed differently (Fig. 200). A straight plate would be unsuitable in this case, so the fracture is stabilized with an individually adapted reconstruction plate that extends to the semilunar incisure.

5.3.3.4 Marginal Angle Fractures (Pre- and Supra-angular Margin Fractures)

For lack of a clear definition, a fracture at the level of the second molar is included in the category of angle fractures. The immediate proximity of the angle justifies this. But from the standpoint of plate selection, it is helpful to use a specific term like *preangular* and *supra-angular* margin fracture (Fig. 201 a, b). The preangular margin fracture offers at least enough space to accommodate a three-hole DCP or EDCP length on each side of the fracture line.

Many supra-angular margin fractures are amenable to fixation with a tension band. Usually there is sufficient space for a two-hole or four-hole plate (Fig. 201 c). Occasionally a six-hole plate may be applied to the basal side (Fig. 201 b). Plate selection is aided by the orthopantomograph, on which the outer and inner angles of the mandible and the bisector can be drawn close to actual size. The preangular and supra-angular zones are easily identified using this technique (Fig. 202) and the

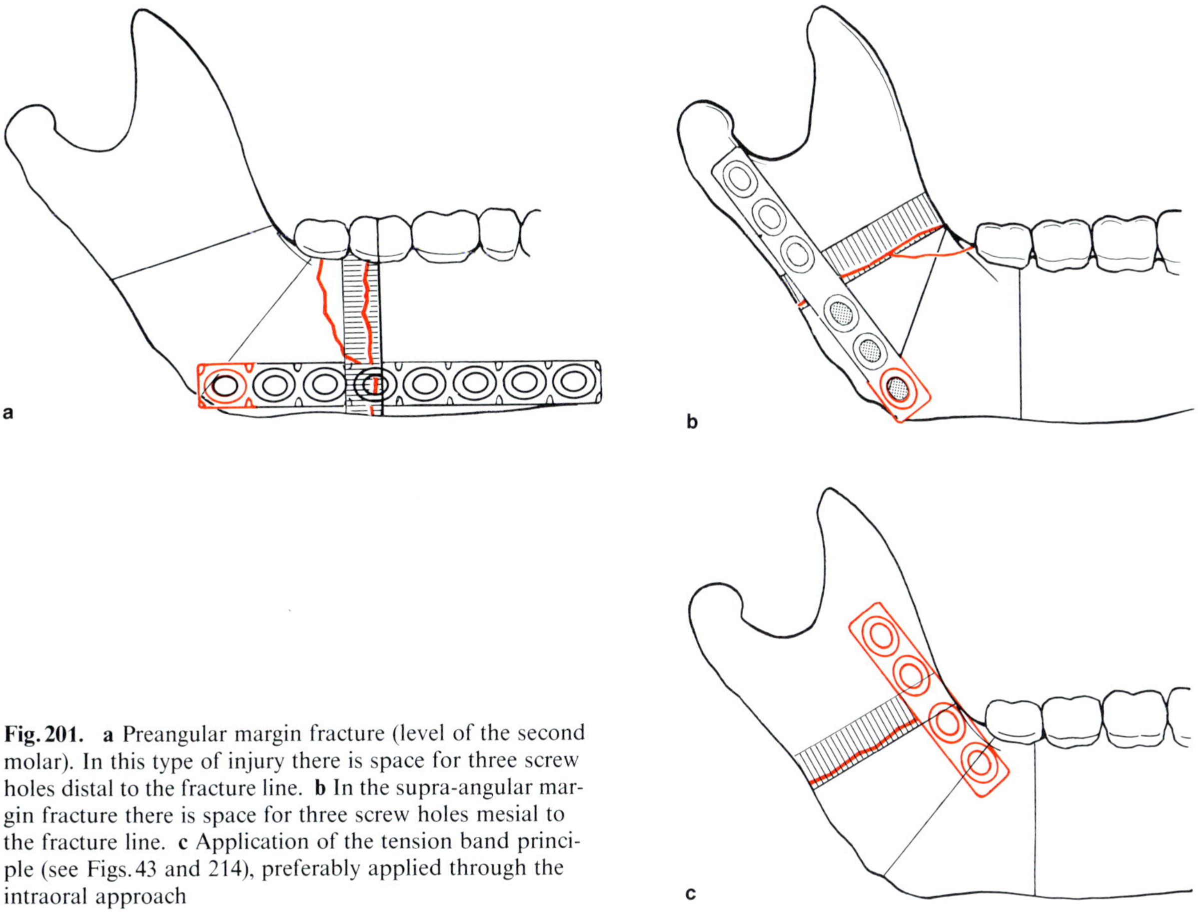

Fig. 201. **a** Preangular margin fracture (level of the second molar). In this type of injury there is space for three screw holes distal to the fracture line. **b** In the supra-angular margin fracture there is space for three screw holes mesial to the fracture line. **c** Application of the tension band principle (see Figs. 43 and 214), preferably applied through the intraoral approach

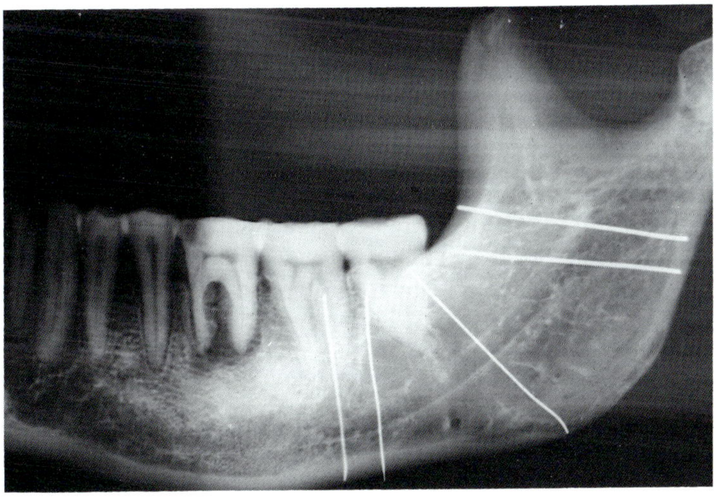

Fig. 202. The orthopantomograph as an aid to the preoperative classification of pre- and supra-angular margin fractures and optimum plate selection

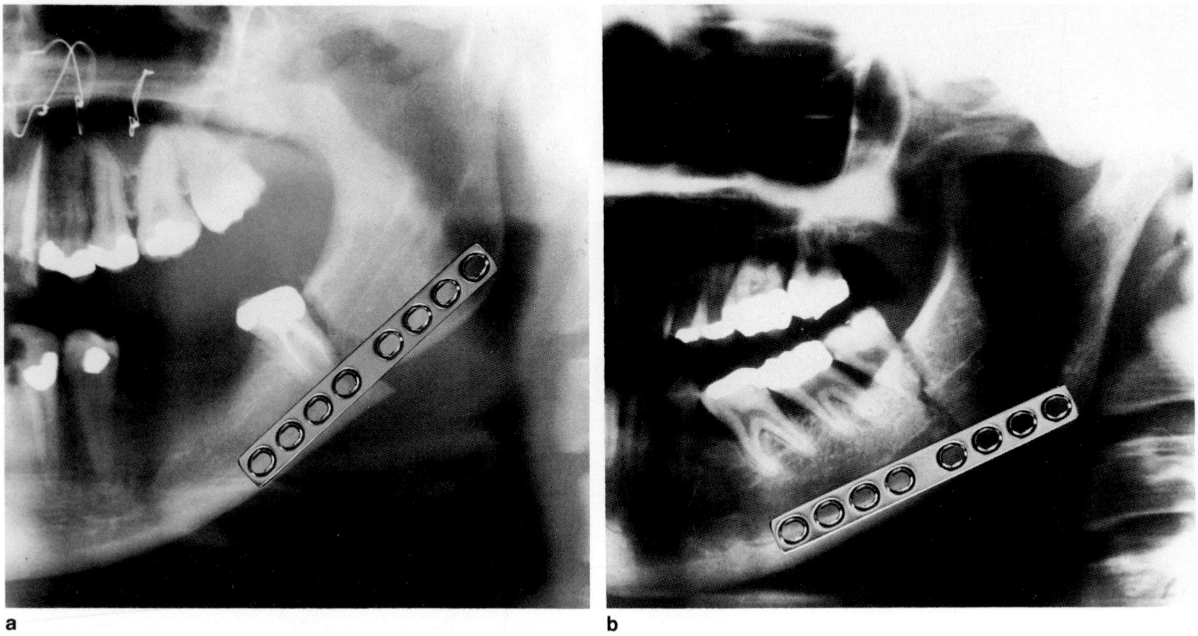

Fig. 203. **a** A trial eight-hole plate is overlaid on the orthopantomogram to determine whether the three screw rule can be statisfied. If there is *space for four holes distal to the fracture line on the radiograph, a six-hole CDP or EDCP should be used.* **b** If there is *space for just three holes distal to the fracture line, a reconstruction plate should be used*

Trial eight-hole plate to determine the three screw rule (Fig. 203):

We utilize an eight-hole plate in conjunction with the orthopantomogram as an aid to preoperative planning. The magnification factor of the film is 1.2. Therefore, if there is room for four plate holes on each side of the fractureline on the radiograph (Fig. 203 a), there will be space for *three* screws on the actual bone. A six-hole DCP or EDCP would be used.

The rule may be stated as follows: *Four plate holes on the OPG correspond to three plate holes in the mandible. If there is not room for four holes* (Fig. 203 b), *the reconstruction plate* (prebent) *is indicated* (see Figs. 194, 195, and 225).

5.3.3.5 Rules for Electing the Internal Fixation of Angle Fractures

A systematic approach to the classification of angle fractures makes it easier to select an appropriate internal fixation technique. Thus:

1) The *central* angle fracture (within the defined region of the mandibular angle) (see Fig. 193) is stabilized with:
   - a preshaped reconstruction plate with 6 or more holes, or
   - a single lag screw (see Fig. 38).
2) The *peripheral* angle fracture (starting outside the angle and terminating at the base of the angle region, see Fig. 196) is stabilized with:
   - a preshaped reconstruction plate with 6 or more holes, or with a basal plate and alveolar tension band (e.g., Fig. 198) or with an EDCP (e.g., Fig. 240 b).

3) The *marginal* angle fracture (see Fig. 201) is stabilized with:
- a DCP or EDCP with 6 or more holes in a *preangular* margin fracture (Fig. 201 a)
- a tension band plate with 2 or more holes (preferably applied through the intraoral route) in a *supra-angular* margin fracture (Fig. 201 c).

5.3.3.6 Problems Specific to the Mandibular Angle

5.3.3.6.1 Relation of the Third Molar to the Fracture Line

Removal of the third molar is associated with a number of undesired effects, including

- the conversion of a closed fracture to an open one,
- loss of the bony buttress on the tension side,
- loss of the possibility for inserting a tension band plate.

Uncritial routine extraction is to be condemned, therefore.

Extraction of the erupted third molar is indicated when:
- the apex is "open" to the fracture line (Fig. 204 a),
- the root is fractured (Fig. 204 b),
- the third molar is partially erupted (cryoptogenic infection or dentitio difficilis).

Extraction is not indicated for:

- an apex that is "closed" to the fracture line (Fig. 205),
- an unerupted or impacted third molar (to avoid creating an open fracture and to preserve the alveolar buttress).

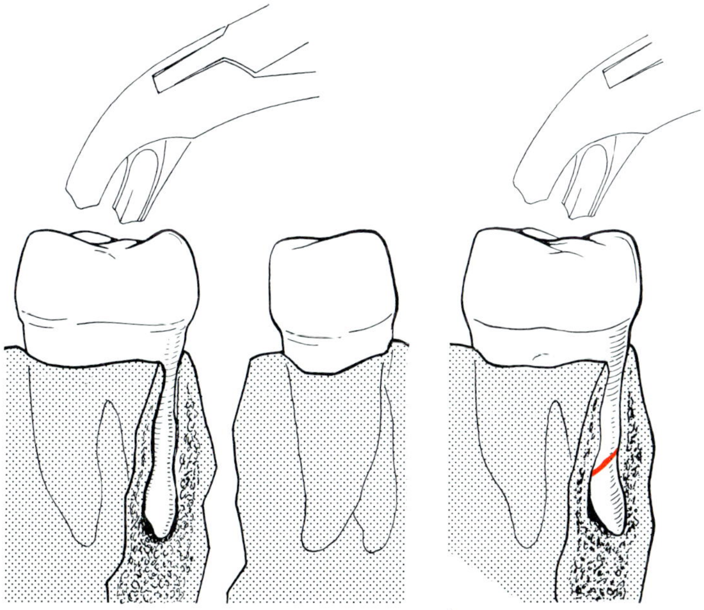

Fig. 204 a, b. Extraction of the third molar is indicated **a** for an exposed apex and **b** for a fractured root

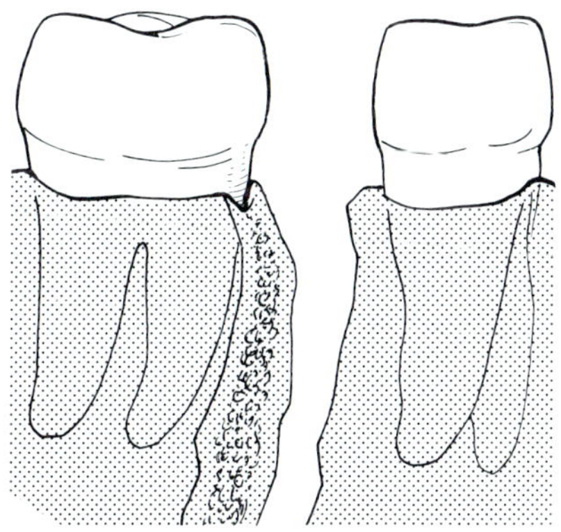

Fig. 205. The tooth may be retained if the apex is closed

5.3.3.6.2 Lack of Space on the Tension Side

It is important to consider the use of a tension band because of the very high tension stresses that are imposed upon the inner angle of the mandible. This assessment is best made preoperatively with the aid of an orthopantomogram in order to avoid unnecessary removal of periosteum.

Lack of space is usually most critical in the preangular area. This is due to the presence of the second and third molars (or their empty alveolae) and the mandibular canal.

1) Often the first obstacle on the tension of the angle is the third molar, which may be erupted, impacted, or unerupted. It is possible to drill through the root or neck of the tooth under aseptic conditions (e.g., extraoral approach) if this is deemed necessary for the placement of a critical screw. Generally this will not result in clinical problems. The stability imperative is a greater concern here than the iatrogenic insult to the wisdom tooth. Later, at the time of implant removal, the tooth may be left alone in the asymptomatic patient. Generally the question of drilling the third molar comes up only in connection with single lag-screw fixation (see p. 202); most angle fractures per se would call for use of the reconstruction plate (see p. 192).
2) In principle, the second molar could be handled similarly if no forensic objections were raised. This is especially in preangular margin fractures (see Fig. 201 a), where the second molar poses a true obstacle to the attachment of a tension band plate. The EDCP (see Fig. 232) or the lag screw (see Fig. 228) offers an alternative in these cases.
3) An effective obstacle may be posed by the empty alveolus of the third molar (see above), by an area of retromolar comminution, or by a pathologic process such as a cyst or apical focus in the adjacent tooth. Here one should follow the principle that it is better to dispense with a tension-band plate than insert an initially or potentially loose screw. The reconstruction plate offers an effective solution (see Rules for Electing Internal Fixation, p. 198; Figs. 2, 276 b, and 353).
4) Finally, the mandibular canal may pose an obstacle to a tension band when the alveolar process is atrophic. The EDCP or reconstruction plate are the methods of choice for these cases (see Figs. 210 and 211).

5.3.3.7 Technique of Internal Fixation of the Angle

The primary considerations are:

- classification of the injury as a prelude to correct patient selection (see above);
- the approach, as a factor that influences patient selection.

When operative fixation has been decided upon, it remains to establish the technical principles of the fixation. Two basic options exist:

1) *Interfragmental* compression by means of a
   - tension band,
   - tension band and stabilization plate,
   - EDCP,
   - single lag screw,
   - lag screw combined with a neutralization plate.

2) Osseous *splinting* by means of
- a reconstruction plate,
- external skeletal fixation.

5.3.3.7.1 Internal Fixation of Central Angle Fractures

The most common error made in treating the central, apical angle fracture is to use a four- or six-hole DCP instead of a reconstruction plate. The four-hole DCP violates the "three screw rule" (see p.6 and p.191), while a six-hole DCP placed across the mandibular angle leaves precarious "edge holes" that do not afford a secure hold for bone screws.

The preoperative orthopantomogram is an excellent guide to patient selection and treatment planning. A straight eight-hole plate is overlaid on the film just as if it were being applied to the fracture itself. If four plate holes can fit between the fracture and the posterior border of the mandibular angle (see Fig. 203a), a six-hole (E)DCP will be adequate on the actual bone. If four plate holes cannot be accommodated on the film, a reconstruction plate should be used (see Fig. 195a).

For central angle fractures (see Fig. 194), the curvature of the bone dictates the fixation method. The only acceptable options are the reconstruction plate, owing to its universal malleability, and the single lag screw.

5.3.3.7.1.1 Reconstruction Plate Utilized as a "Stabilization Plate" or "Osseous Splint"

The *stabilization plate,* when used as one component of a plate and tension-band system, requires the concomitant use of a small tension band. This depends on the degree of displacement and the space available at the inner angle of the mandible. If the reduction requires that the fracture be exposed as far as the inner angle, a tension band can be applied, and the space available will determine whether a short or longer plate is used. The advantage of the tension-band plate is its efficacy as an antidistraction device. It permits an accurate reduction and enables effective precompression to be applied with the reduction-compression forceps. A contoured reconstruction plate will then afford excellent stabilization (e.g., Fig. 2c).

Osseous splinting is indicated for the minimally displaced or undisplaced angle fracture. These fractures are easy to reduce and do not require exposure of the inner angle. They are stabilized with a six- or eight-hole reconstruction plate applied with the screws in the neutral position to avoid distraction on the tension side and possible overriding of the bone ends. Ernst ligatures are satisfactory for occlusal retention. The length and thickness of the plate are sufficient to create a stable splint that will permit immediate, painless function of the jaw (e.g., Fig. 225b). One week of hospitalization is required.

5.3.3.7.1.2 Single Lag Screw Fixation of the Inner Angle (Percutaneous Screw Fixation of the Intraorally Exposed Fracture)

The transverse fracture across the oblique line, retromolar fossa, and the vestibular and lingual expansions of the mandible creates a broad fracture surface that is amenable to fixation with a single lag screw. The advantage of this method, introduced by Niederdellmann (1980), is the ability to effect a functionally stable internal fixation with a minimal amount of material and with no external scar (Fig. 206, see also Fig. 38). The screw functions by creating interfragmental compression on the tension side of the bone. The single screw (2.7 mm) is strong, long, and elastic enough to transform residual bending forces into compressive stress during mandibular function. The fragments must be intact and able to transmit compression to ensure that an effective buttress is present. This may require drilling through the third molar rather than extracting it (see p. 200). The single lag screw can be used in a multiple fracture if a good basal buttress is established (Fig. 207); for the technique of single lag screw, see p. 49 ff.

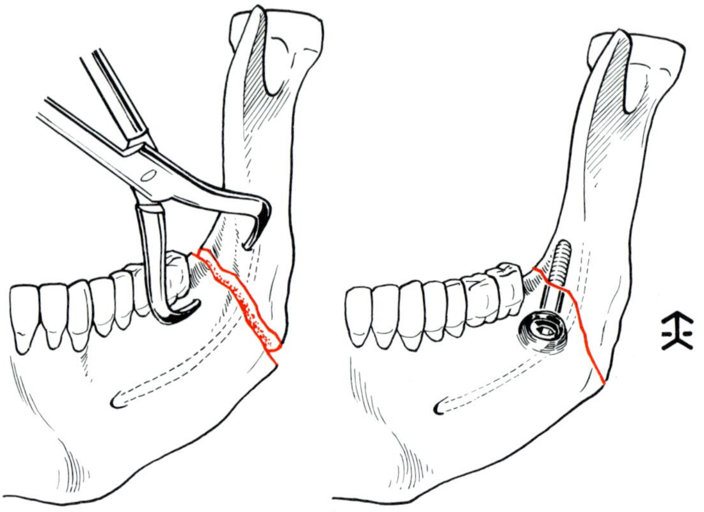

a b

Fig. 206. a Anatomic reduction and retention of the intraorally exposed fracture (for safety, prior intermaxillary retention of the occlusion with Ernst ligatures is advised). **b** Single lag screw introduced percutaneously by the technique of Niederdellmann (1980). (The screw head should be well countersunk in the cortex so that the screw can be angled correctly relative to the fracture plane)

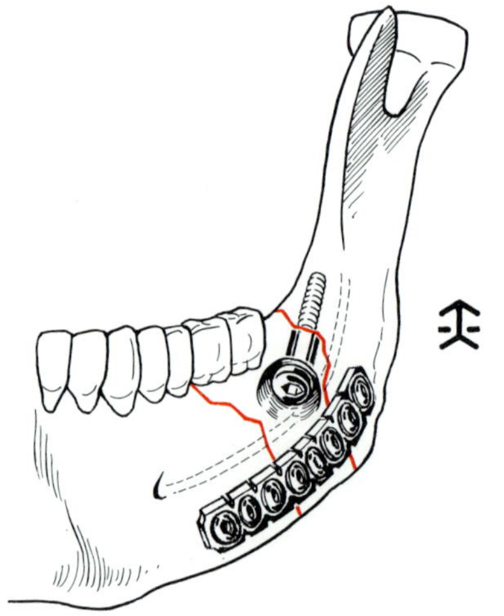

Fig. 207. Single lag screw "protected" by a reconstruction plate placed primarily to buttress the segmental fracture

5.3.3.7.2 Internal Fixation of Peripheral Fractures (Angle-Body and Angle-Ramus Fractures)

In peripheral angle fractures (see definition p.194), the course of the fracture line in the angle region largely determines the choice of the fixation method. These are radial fractures that are centered at the mandibular angle. The oblique fracture line can become a problem when axial compression is applied due to the tendency of the fragments to slip and override (Fig.208). This is a general problem that has led to implementation of the "antiglide principle" in the form of the "one-hole antiglide plate" (Brunner and Weber 1981). The spiked end of the lower fragment is engaged with a lag screw, and as the screw is driven home, a contoured washer beneath the screw head is pressed against the fragment to prevent its displacement (Fig.209). The fragments can then be united under pressure with an eight-hole DCP. Fragment gliding can also be prevented by occlusal retention with rigid splints, so in many cases it is unnecessary to use a separate antiglide washer.

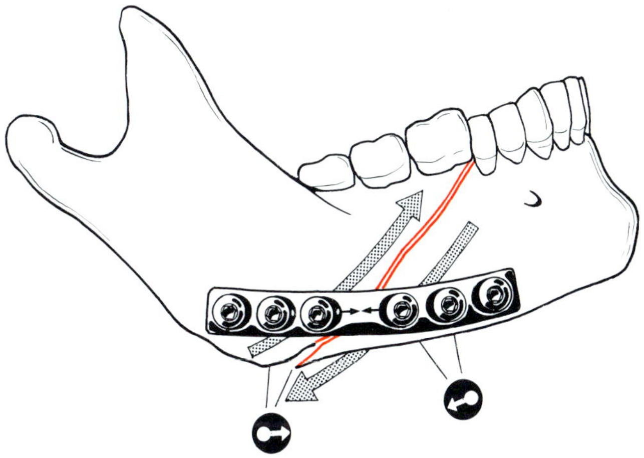

Fig.208. The self-compressing action of the DCP can cause fragment overriding in the peripheral angle fracture: *iatrogenic displacement*

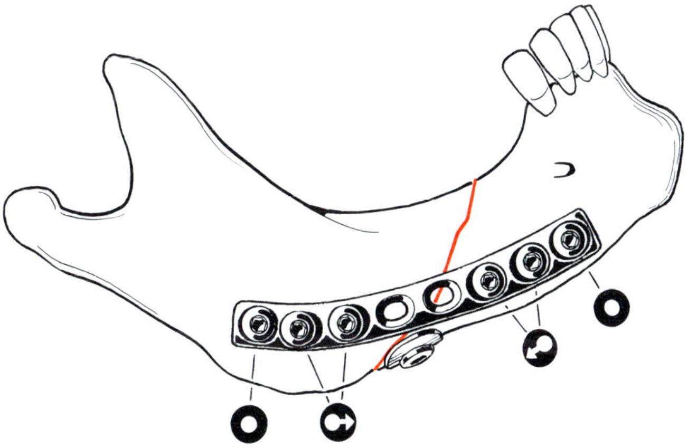

Fig.209. An "antiglide" washer keeps the fragments in place while interfragmental compression is applied

An alternative to interfragmental compression is to create a rigid buttress (osseous splint) by means of a reconstruction plate (Fig. 210).

The oblique fracture line poses a special problem in the edentulous and atrophic mandible that cannot be solved adequately by conservative methods. Even in the severely atrophic "pipestem" mandible, plate fixation is still the best option for problem cases of this kind. Besides observing the three screw rule, care should be taken that one or two plate holes over the oblique fracture line are left vacant. This means that at least an eight-hole reconstruction plate will be needed (Fig. 211). With this method a slightly imperfect reduction can be tolerated without jeopardizing stability.

Implant removal is an important concern and should be done no later than *one* year after the internal fixation to avoid the bone loss and structural changes that can result from stress protection (see p. 33). The findings of Gautier (1984) are of interest in this regard. They indicate that steel plates produce the least rarefaction of bone in comparison with elastic implants (e.g., a polyacetal plate). No doubt the best method in a physiologic sense is external skeletal fixation, but this modality is reserved for very specific indications (see p. 69 and p. 92).

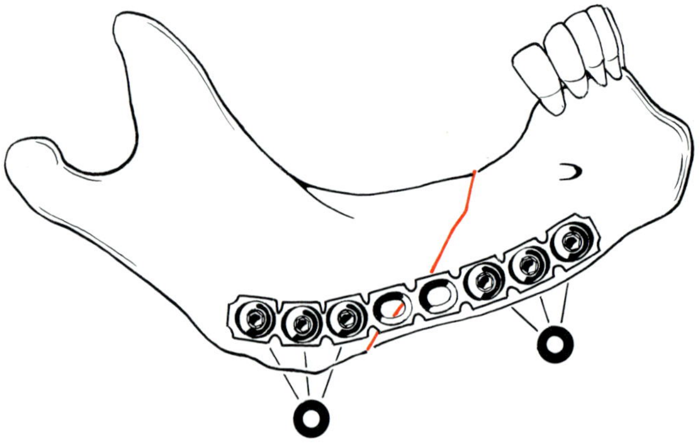

Fig. 210. The fracture may be buttressed with a reconstruction plate as an alternative to compression plating

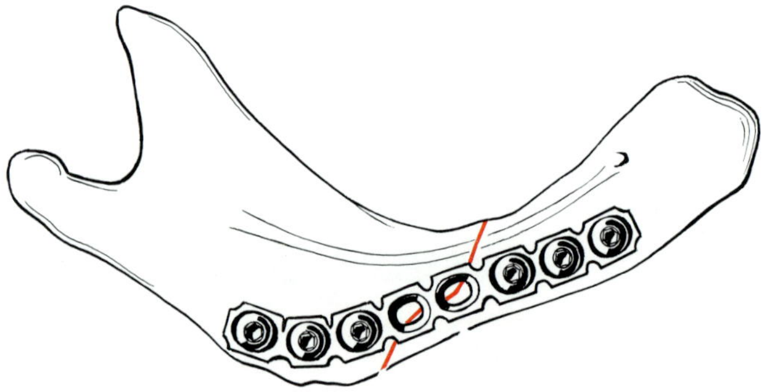

Fig. 211. Peripheral angle fracture in the atrophic mandible stabilized with the eight-hole reconstruction plate

5.3.3.7.3 Internal Fixation of Marginal Angle Fractures

5.3.3.7.3.1 Use of the EDCP and Reconstruction Plate

If there is not enough space for a tension-band plate in a preangular margin fracture (see p. 200), the six-hole EDCP offers a possible solution (Fig. 212). It should be noted that the terminal screw in the oblique outer hole of the plate can compensate for the missing tension band only if the screw has a solid bony anchorage. This can be a problem when the end of the plate aligns with the posterior border of the ramus, leaving insufficient space for the secure placement of a screw through the terminal hole. The bone is no more than 5–6 mm thick in this region. The reconstruction plate is consistently the implement of choice for the management of these cases.

If it is necessary to extract the third molar from the fracture line, this often entails sacrifice of the bony buttress on the alveolar side. The EDCP is inappropriate in the absence of an alveolar buttress, and the best solution is osseous splinting with the reconstruction plate (Fig. 213).

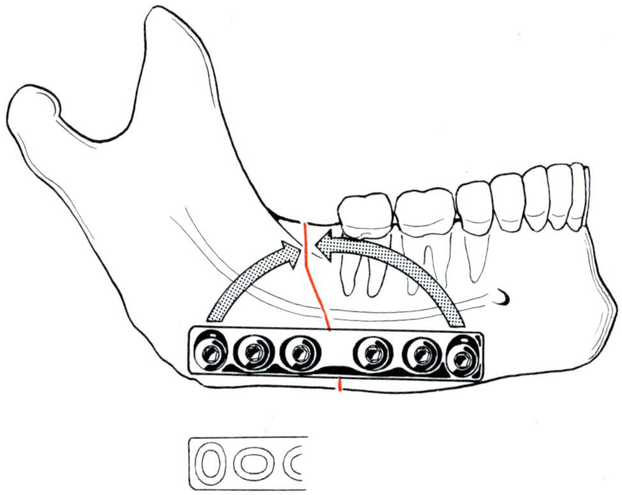

Fig. 212. Preangular margin fracture stabilized with a six-hole EDCP (there is insufficient space for a tension-band plate)

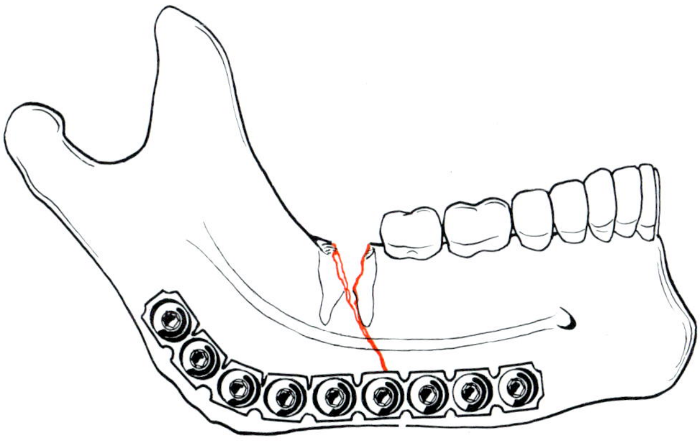

Fig. 213. Preangular margin fracture stabilized with a reconstruction plate (EDCP cannot be used due to the lack of a buttress in the alveolar process)

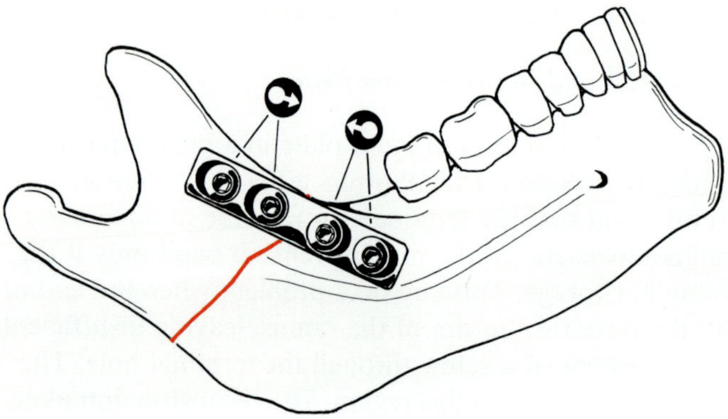

Fig. 214. The supra-angular margin fracture is the classic indication for the tension-band plate (a two-hole plate may be used in the smaller mandible)

5.3.3.7.3.2 Classic Application of the Tension Band Plate

The superior angle margin fracture is identical to a transverse fracture of the ramus (Fig. 214). It is one of the few fractures that can be stabilized in classic fashion with a simple tension band. The margin of the ramus is exposed intraorally, and a four-hole DCP is attached. The holes have to be drilled obliquely, but this is not a problem since the screw can be angled through the DC plate hole (25° axial and 7° transverse) and still exert its compressive action (see p. 107).

5.3.4 Internal Fixation of Oblique-Surface Fractures

Definition of Terms

The oblique-surface fracture is a shear fracture whose surface is orientied *longitudinally* with respect to the bone axis. It differs from the oblique fracture, which is a bending fracture oriented *at right angles* to the bone axis. The surface area of the latter fracture is small.

Owing to its obliquity and large surface area, the oblique-surface fracture is ideally suited for fixation with lag screws. The lag screw, the simplest internal fixation device with the greatest effect (greater than that of plates), is often given too little consideration during treatment planning. In any case its applications in the dentulous mandible are limited by the teeth and nerve canal (Fig. 215).

The ideal indication is the oblique-surface fracture in the edentulous mandible. A good example is shownin Fig. 216. The fracture is compressed with four lag screws inserted below the plane of the mental nerve (Fig. 217). The advantage of this method is that it achieves a maximum of stability in a very small space with a minimum of fixation material. Most fractures of this kind can be adequately stabilized with three well placed lag screws. Even when spaced very close together, the screws produce a static force sufficient for good functional stability in all directions without a tension

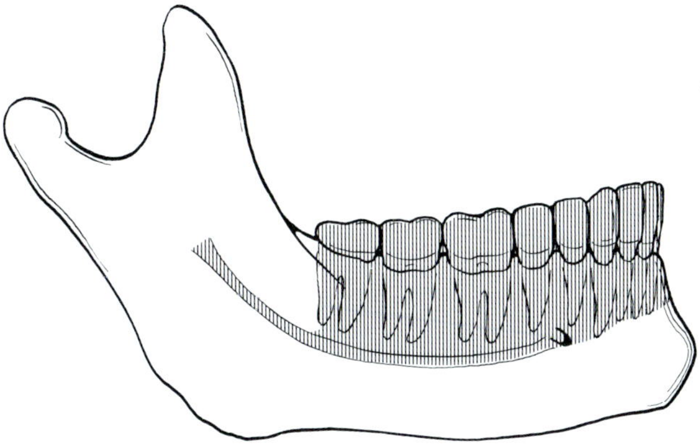

Fig. 215. Only a limited area is available for functionally stable internal fixation of the mandible. The technical principle of lag screw fixation imposes further constraints

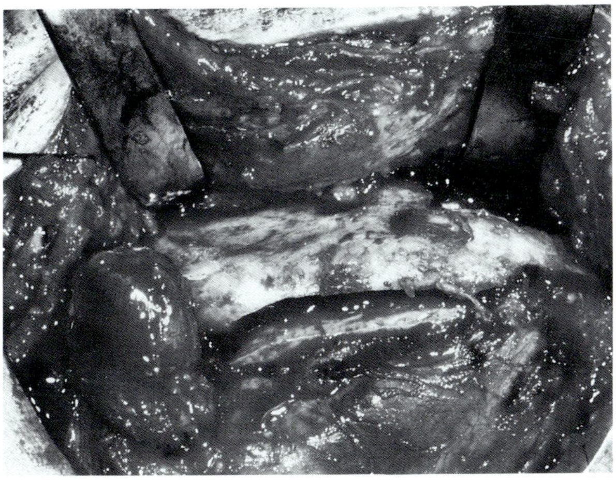

a

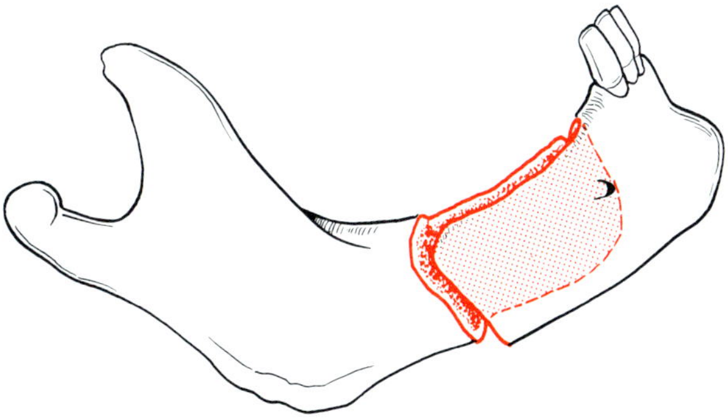

b

Fig. 216 **a** Oblique-surface fracture. **b** Artist's rendering of the injury

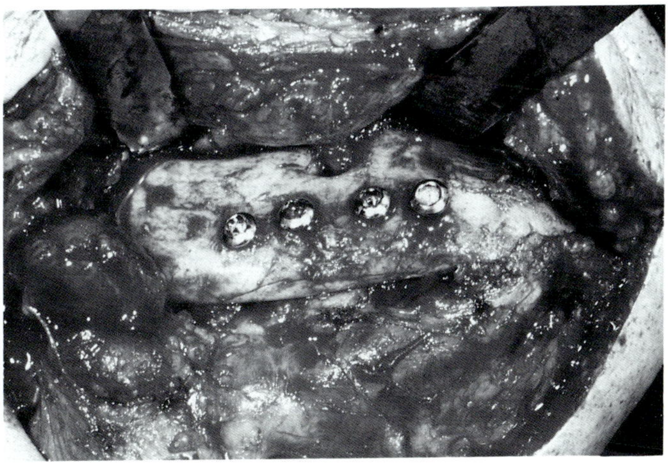

a

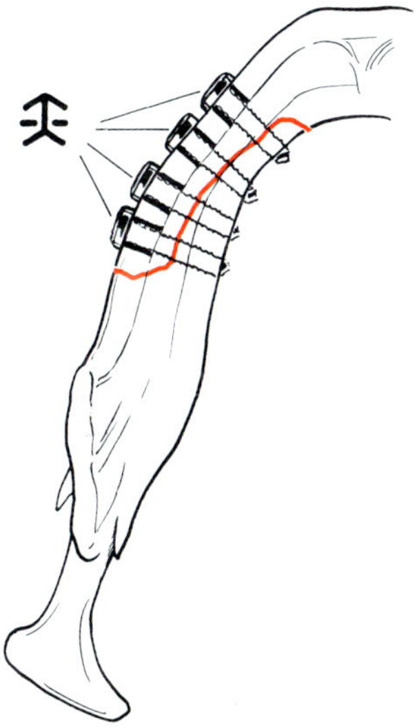

b

Fig. 217. **a** The mental foramen provides a landmark for insertion of the four lag screws. **b** Horizontal section on the plane of the lag screws

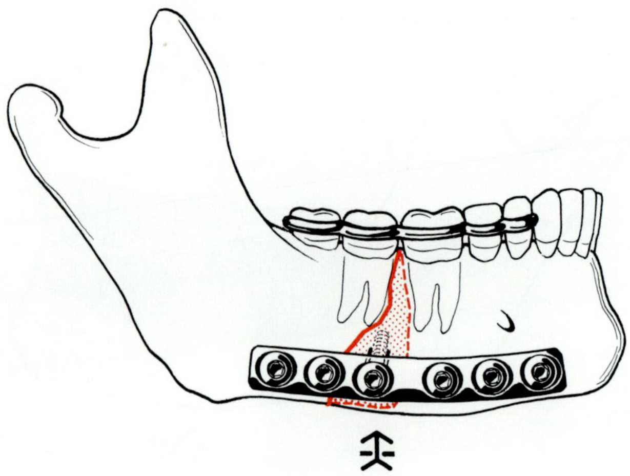

Fig. 218. Transverse fracture with an oblique surface stabilized by a lag screw inserted through the compression plate

band (see p. 219). If there is not enough space for a third screw, a rigid splint can be placed on the teeth adjacent to the fracture as compensation. If only one lag screw is used, it must be "protected" with a neutralization plate. The screw may be placed outside or inside the plate (Figs. 218 and 237).

5.4 Multiple Fractures (F_2 S_0, Grade II A)

5.4.1 Internal Fixation of a Double Fracture in the Dentulous Mandible

5.4.1.1 Indications

Most double fractures occur as a result of direct and indirect mechanisms. One hemimandible is fractured in the postcanine region while the other is fractured through the angle or below the condyle (see p. 189). The instability of the central fragment hampers both the reduction and the fixation. It is particularly difficult to reestablish the preinjury occlusion if conservative treatment is attempted, and intermaxillary fixation will prove difficult if there is a coexisting fracture of the maxilla. In such cases the advantages of open reduction and functionally stable fixation support the application of ASIF principles.

5.4.1.2 Techniques of Internal Fixation

The key to preoperative planning in the doubly fractured mandible is the recognition that the biomechanical and technical principles applied to the internal fixation of the single fracture are also applicable to the fixation of multiple fractures. Thus, each side will require its own procedure in terms of approach, method, and technique. There is no firm rule as to which fracture should be stabilized first, although most surgeons begin on the right side. One may wish to begin with the fracture that appears to be the simpler of the two.

The various indications and techniques of internal fixation will be illustrated by individual case reports using the following scheme: diagnosis, classification, treatment, and course.

Double fracture: *Postcanine and condylar neck* (Fig. 219)

Fracture formula:	$F_1\ L_3/F_1\ L_6\ 0_1$
Clinical category:	$F_2\ S_0$
Grade of severity:	II A

Intraoral Procedure

The maxilla and mandible are splinted, and intermaxillary fixation is applied to retain the occlusion.

Extraoral Procedure

A six-hole EDCP is used due to the distal weakness of the tension-band splint (attached only to the second molar; Fig. 220). The EDCP provides the stability necessary for postoperative functional therapy of the condylar

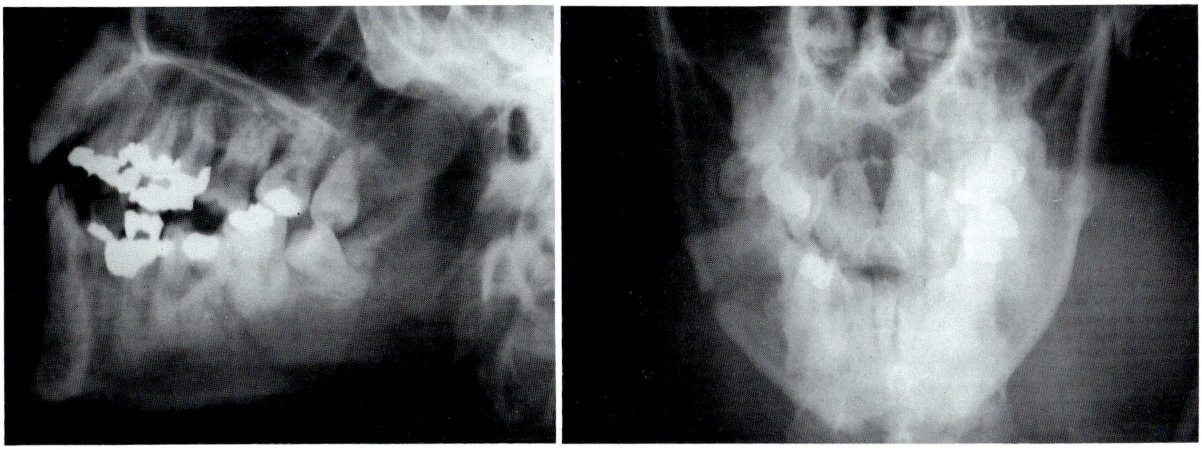

a **b**

Fig. 219. **a** Postcanine fracture. **b** Condylar neck fracture

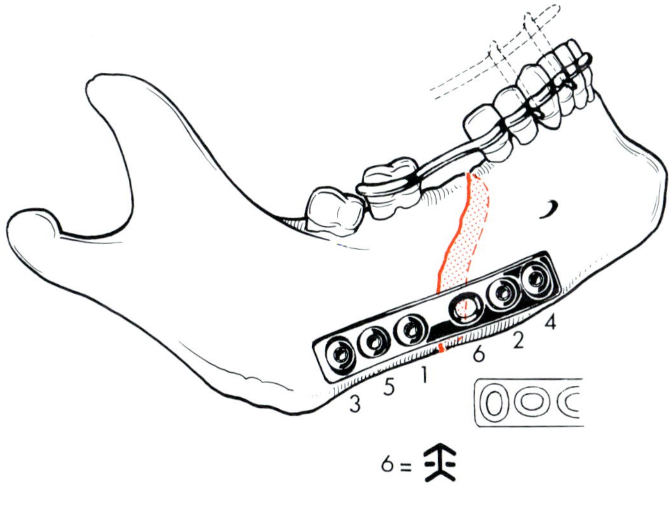

Fig. 220. EDCP used in conjunction with a weak dental splint. The sixth screw is inserted as a lag screw

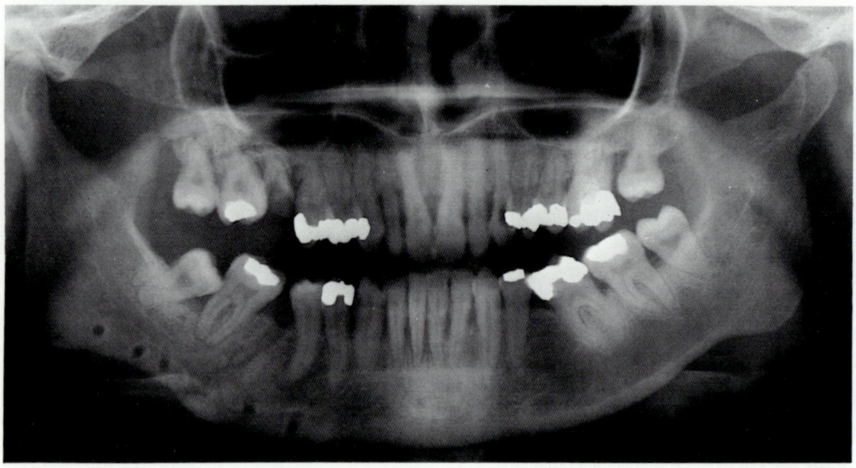

Fig. 221. Status after implant removal

neck fracture. Because the fracture is of the oblique-surface type, the sixth screw is inserted as a lag screw. Figure 221 shows the status after removal of the fixation material.

Oblique-surface fracture[8] in the edentulous, precanine[9] portion of the mandible on the right side and bilateral subcondylar fractures (Fig. 222)

Fracture formula	$F_1\ L_6\ F_1\ L_2/F_1\ L_6\ O_1$
Clinical category:	$F_2\ S_0$
Grade of severity:	II A

Intraoral Procedure

A prosthetic splint with bite rims is necessary for correct intermaxillary fixation, and two weeks' immobilization of the bilateral subcondylar fractures is required.

[8] See Fig. 166
[9] See Fig. 173

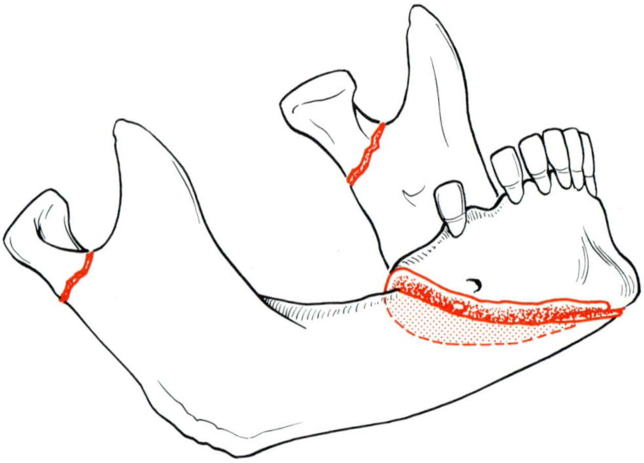

Fig. 222. Oblique-surface fracture in the edentulous precanine region with associated bilateral subcondylar fractures

Extraoral Procedure

The fracture is reduced *anteriorly* and held together with the reduction forceps while four lag screws are inserted across the fracture site. The screws are oriented in different directions (Fig. 223).

Functional treatment of the subcondylar fractures is initiated at two weeks postoperatively.

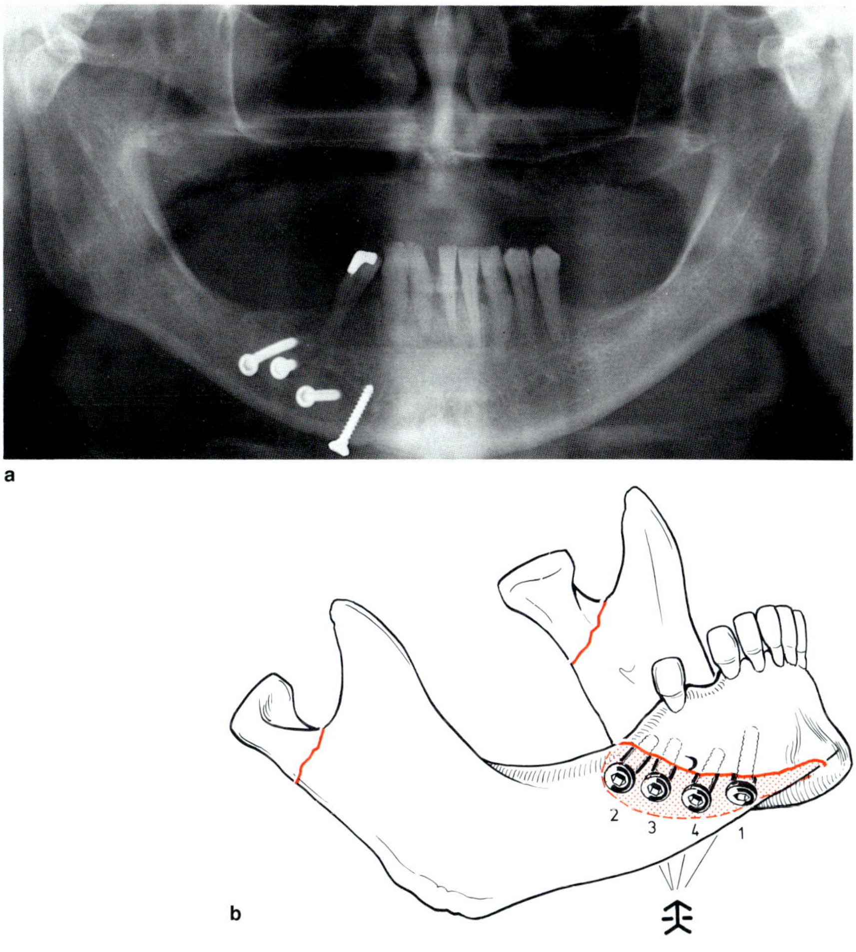

Fig. 223 a, b. Fixation of the oblique-surface fracture with lag screws

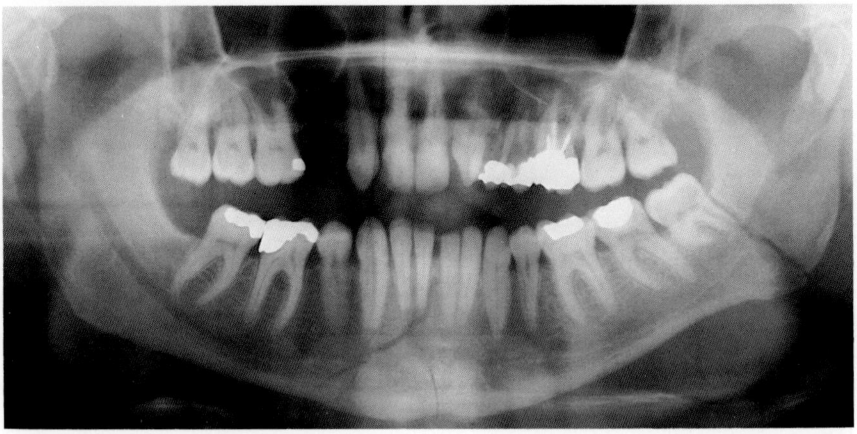

Fig. 224. Closed double fracture

Closed double fracture: *Right postcanine oblique fracture extending to the midline, typical central fracture of the left angle (apical fracture) with lack of space at the inner angle, and left condylar neck fracture* (Fig. 224)

Fracture formula:	F_1 L_2/F_1 L_4 F_1 L_6 O_1
Clinical category:	F_2 S_0
Grade of severity:	II A

Intraoral Procedure
The maxilla and mandible are splinted, and occlusion is retained for two weeks with intermaxillary wires (standard procedure for condylar fractures).

Extraoral Procedure (Fig. 225)
Right side:
Four-hole DCP (stabilization plate combined with the tension-band splint).
Left side:
Six-hole reconstruction plate, since the fracture involves the apical part of the angle, and a straight plate would violate the three screw rule (see p. 191 ff.).

Postoperative Care
Functional therapy for the condylar neck fracture was instituted at two weeks postoperatively using a monoblock. Figure 226 shows the status after operation (a) and after implant removal (b).

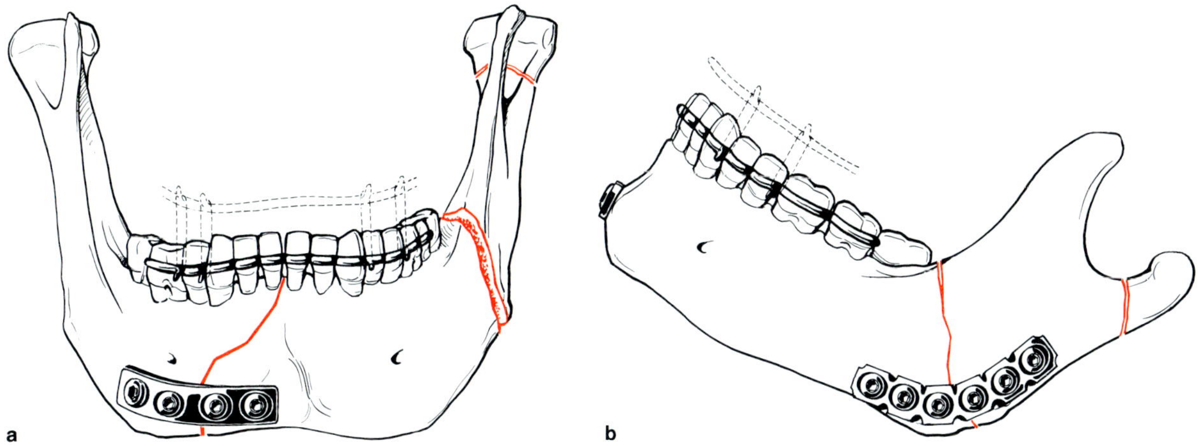

Fig. 225. **a** Four-hole DCP in conjunction with a tension-band splint. **b** Malleable reconstruction plate

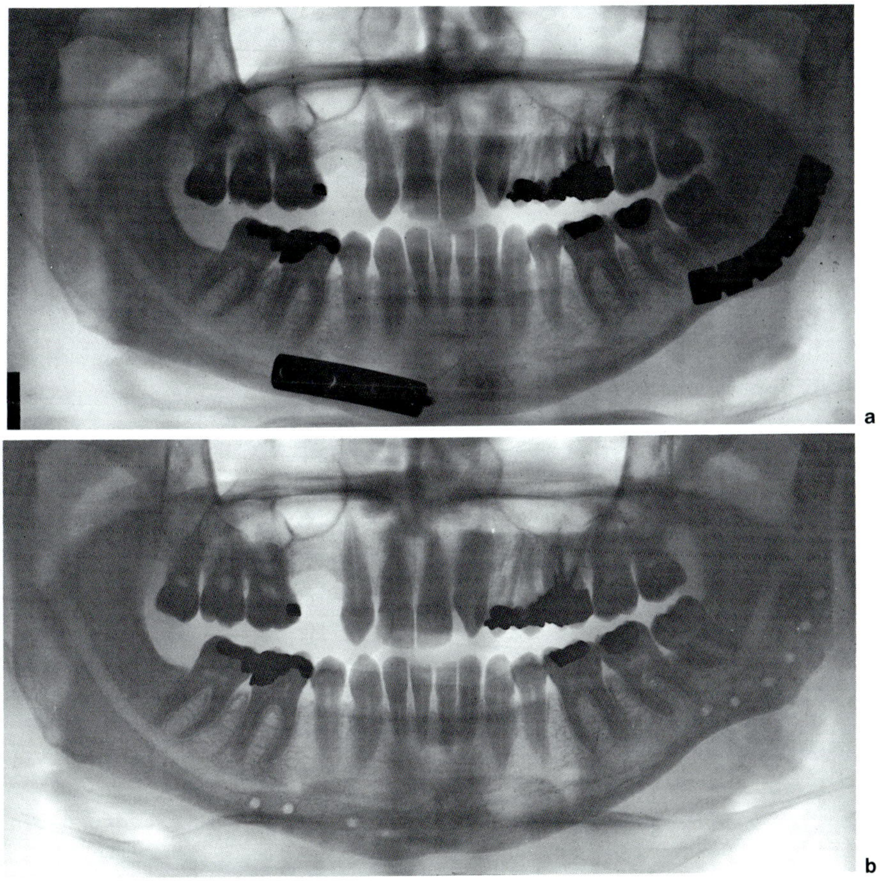

Fig. 226 a, b. Status after **a** operation and **b** implant removal

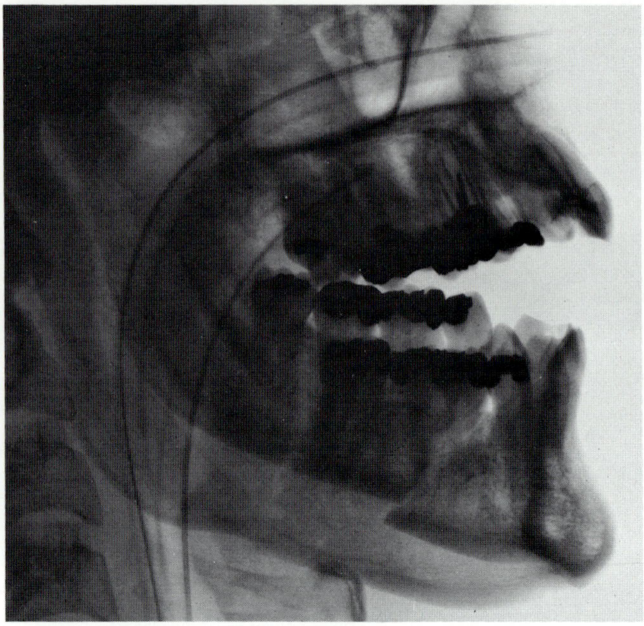

Fig. 227. Unstable double fracture

Closed, extremely unstable double fracture in a patient with multiple trauma: *Oblique-surface fracture of the right mandibular angle and a left postcanine oblique fracture* (Fig. 227)

Fracture formula:	$F_1\ L_4/F_1\ L_3\ O_1$
Clinical category:	$F_2\ S_0$
Grade of severity:	II A

Intraoral Procedure

The extreme instability of the fracture necesitates maxillomandibular splinting and intermaxillary retention of the occlusion.

Extraoral Procedure

Right side: (Fig. 228 a)

The first lag screw is placed on the tension side so that the basal reduction of the oblique-surface fracture can be adjusted. Afterward the remaining lag screws are inserted in positions 2 and 3 (see Fig. 228 a).

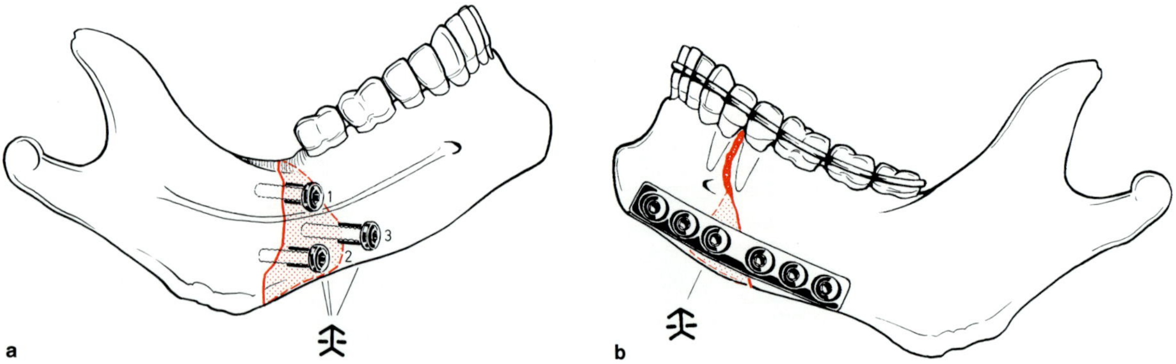

Fig. 228. **a** Lag screw 1 is placed first so that the basal reduction can be adjusted. Then lag screws 2 and 3 are inserted. **b** Six-hole DCP as part of a plate and tension-band system (see text)

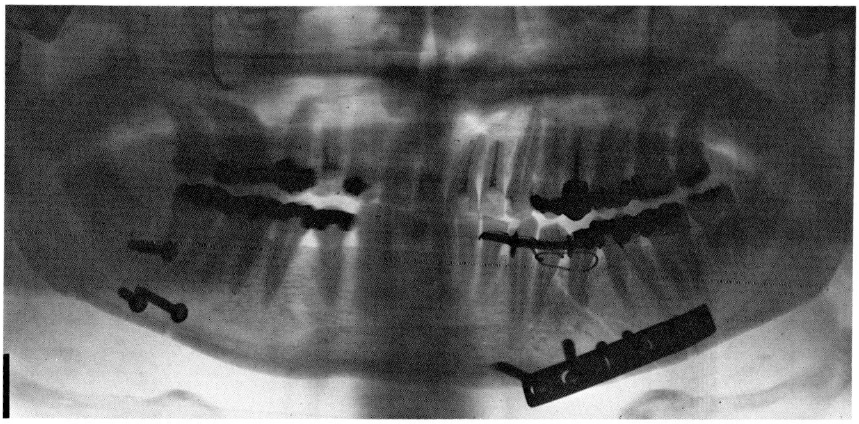

Fig. 229. Status after operation

Left side: (Fig. 228 b)
A six-hole DCP is placed in conjunction with the mandibular splint because of the anterior site of the fracture (between the first and second premolars) and the pronounced obliquity of the fracture line. The pointed end of the distal fragment is not favorable for the placement of a screw; hence a six-hole plate is selected a priori, and the screw adjacent to the fracture is inserted as a lag screw (see p. 208).

Figure 229 shows the status after operation.

Closed double fracture: *Right preangular margin fracture next to the alveolus of the unerupted third molar, whose apex is closed to the fracture; also an oblique postcanine fracture on the left side* (Fig. 230)

Status of occlusion:	O_1/O_1 (open bite)
Fracture formula:	$F_1\ L_4/F_1\ L_3$
Clinical category:	$F_2\ S_0$
Grade of severity:	II A

Intraoral Procedure (Fig. 231)

1) Tension-band splint on the left molar side and occlusal reduction
2) Retention of the third molar to avoid iatrogenic opening of the fracture (see p. 199)
3) Retention of the occlusion with Ernst ligatures (see Fig. 53)

Extraoral procedure (Fig. 232)
Right side:
Six-hole EDCP (preangular margin fracture, three screw rule is applicable).
Left side:
Four-hole DCP applied in conjunction with the tension-band splint.

Figure 223 a shows the postoperative status and 233 b the status following implant removal.

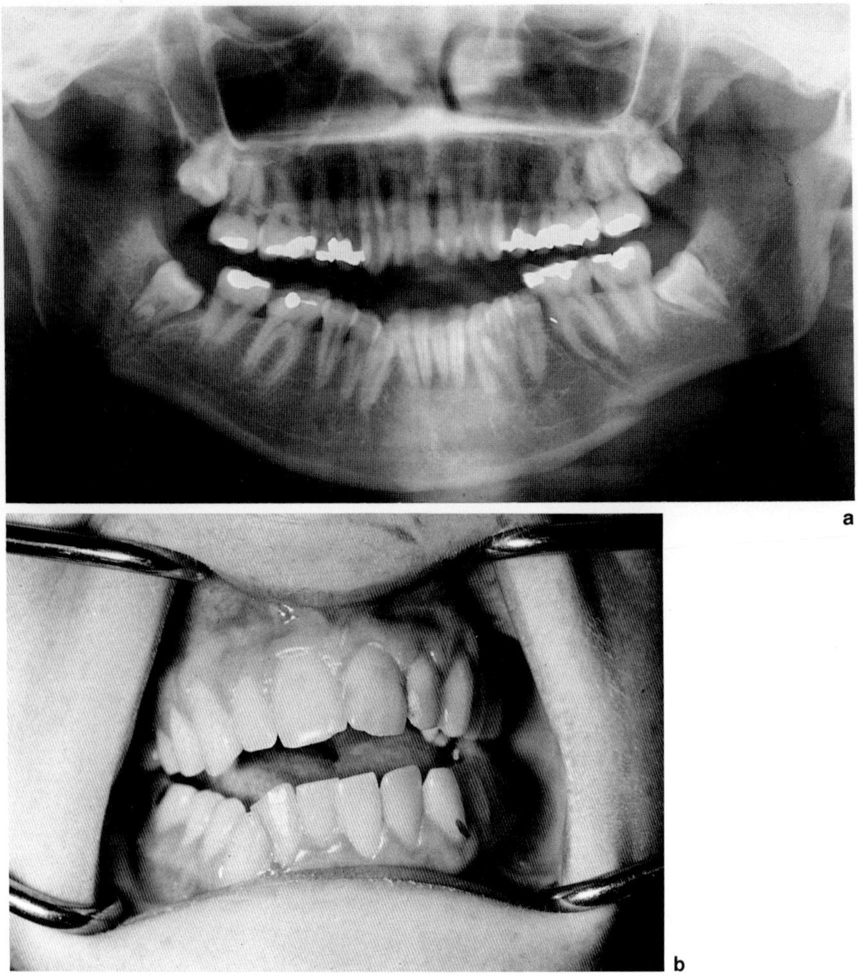

a

b

Fig. 230. **a** Preangular margin fracture and postcanine oblique fracture. **b** Occlusal status

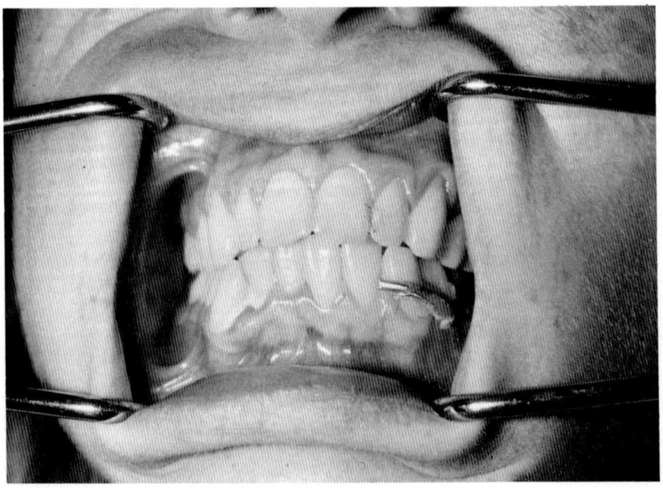

Fig. 231. Tension-band splint (barely visible)

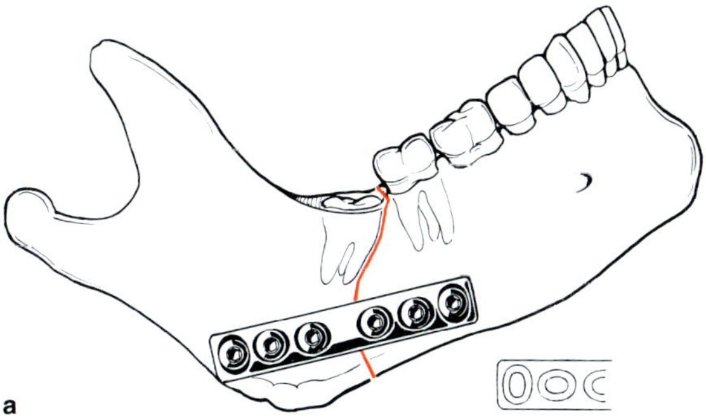
a

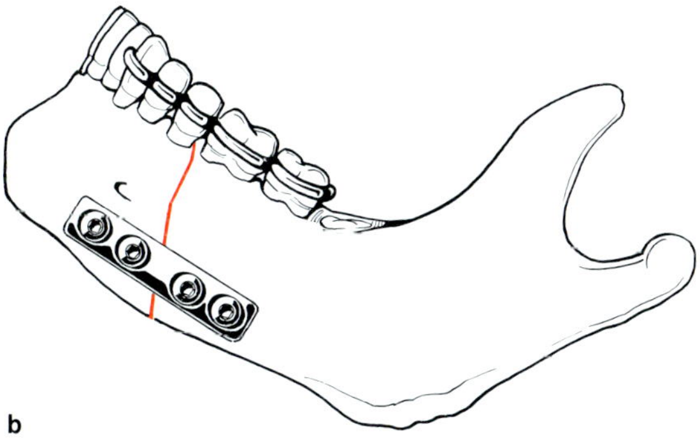
b

232. **a** Application of this EDCP is consistent with the three screw rule (see footnote 6 p. 191).

b Plate and tension-band system comprising a four-hole DCP and a dental splint (see p. 58)

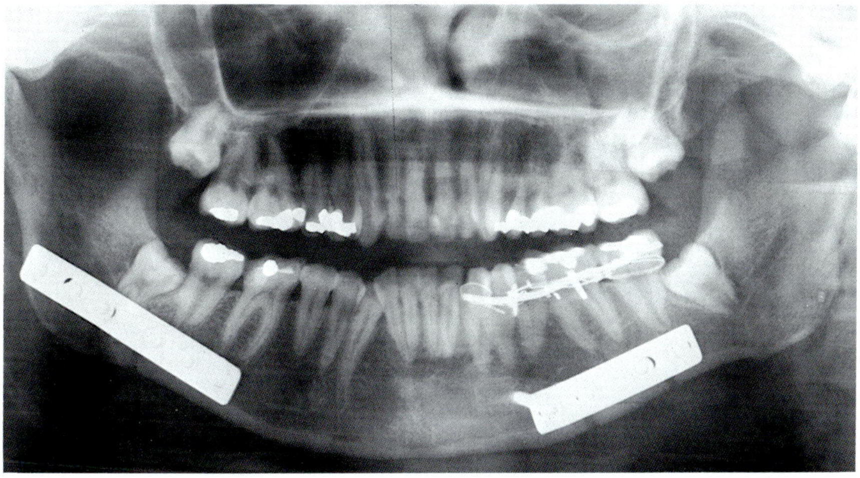
a

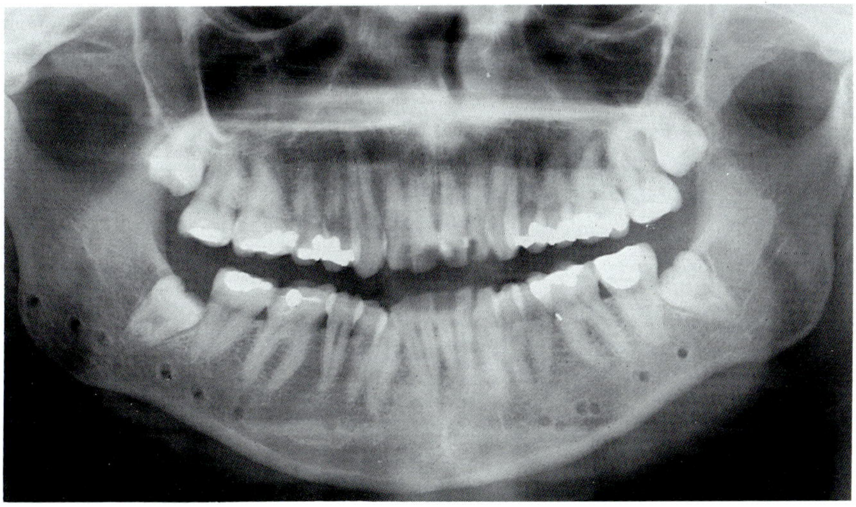
b

Fig. 233 a, b. Status after **a** operation and **b** plate removal

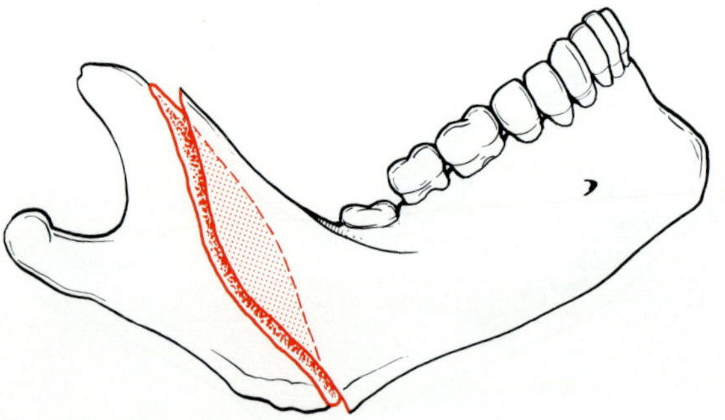

Fig. 234. Peripheral angle-ramus fracture with an oblique surface

Closed double fracture: *Peripheral angle-ramus fracture with an oblique surface in the right ramus (Fig. 234); transverse postcanine fracture on the left side* (see Fig. 235 c)

Fracture formula:	$F_1\ L_4/F_1\ L_3\ O_1$
Clinical category:	$F_2\ S_0$
Grade of severity:	II A

Intraoral Procedure

A full mandibular splint is applied and the occlusion retained with Ernst ligatures.

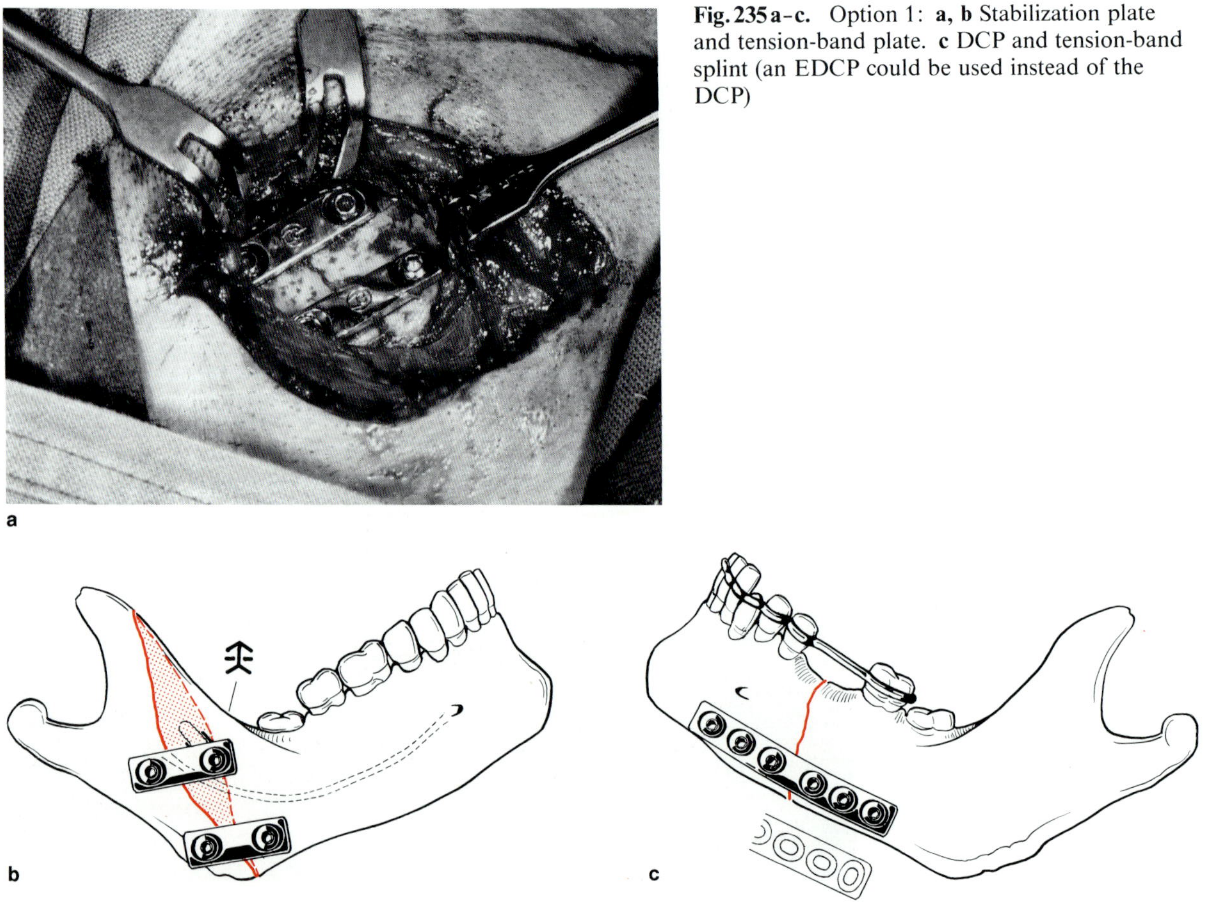

Fig. 235 a–c. Option 1: **a, b** Stabilization plate and tension-band plate. **c** DCP and tension-band splint (an EDCP could be used instead of the DCP)

Extraoral Procedure

Right side:

Option 1 (Fig. 235 a, b):

A plate and tension-band plate system is constructed within the angle region using two long two-hole DCPs placed in the supra-angular and apical zones. Screw 1 crosses the racture site and functions as a lag screw.

Left side: (Fig. 235 c)

Six-hole DCP applied in conjunction with a mandibular tension-band splint (alternative: six-hole EDCP if the splint cannot be anchored securely to the last molar).

Figure 236 shows the status after implant removal at three years postoperatively.

The following options may also be considered:

Option 2 (Fig. 237):

A lag screw placed on the tension side and a two-hole buttress plate is placed in the apical zone to protect the lag screw (see p. 208).

Option 3 (Fig. 238):

Fixation with three lag screws (see p. 206). This requires exposing the fracture higher on the coronoid process.

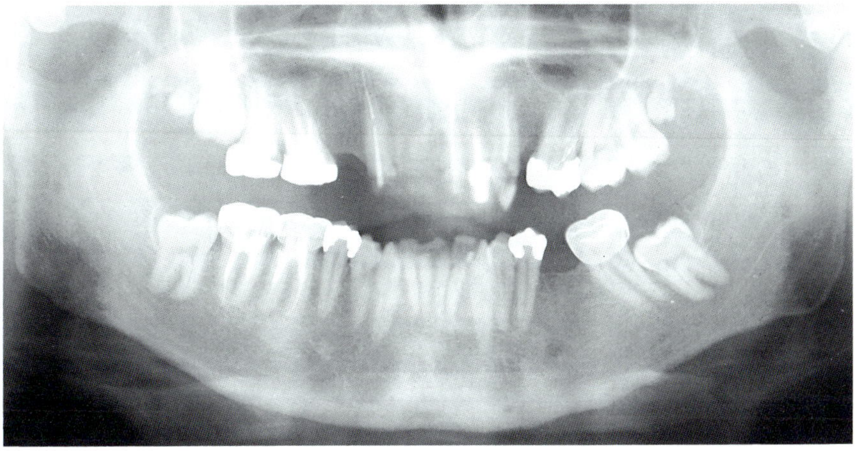

Fig. 236. Status at three years postoperatively

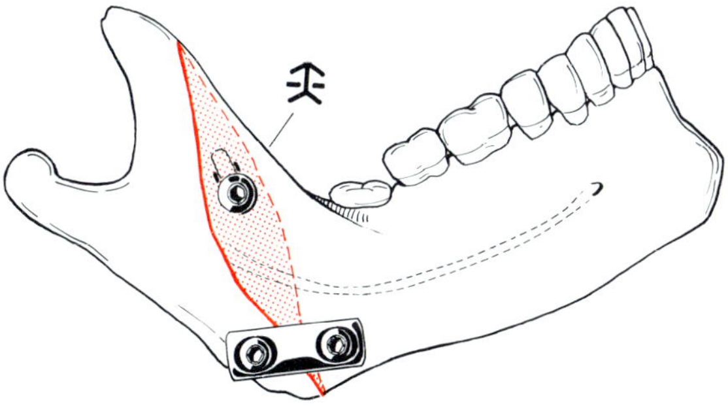

Fig. 237. Option 2: A lag screw protected with a stabilization plate

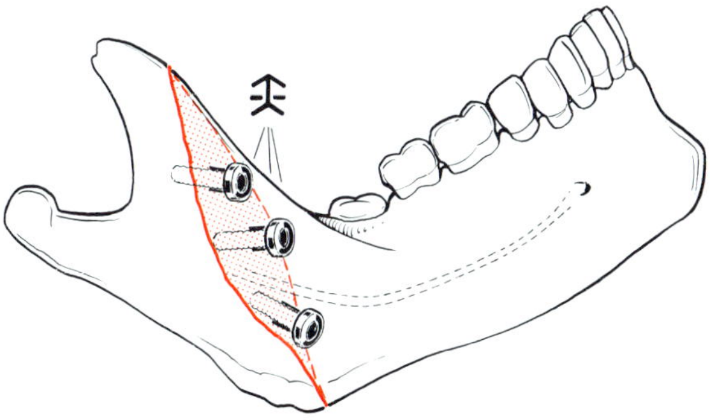

Fig. 238. Option 3: Fixation with multiple lag screws

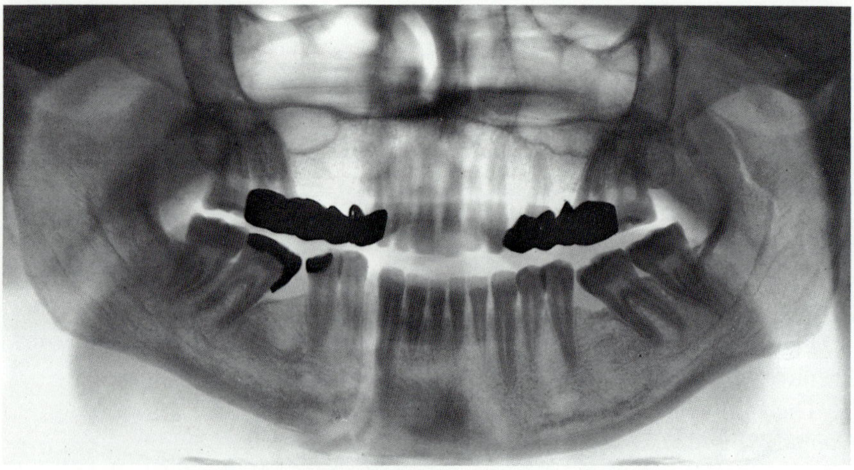

a

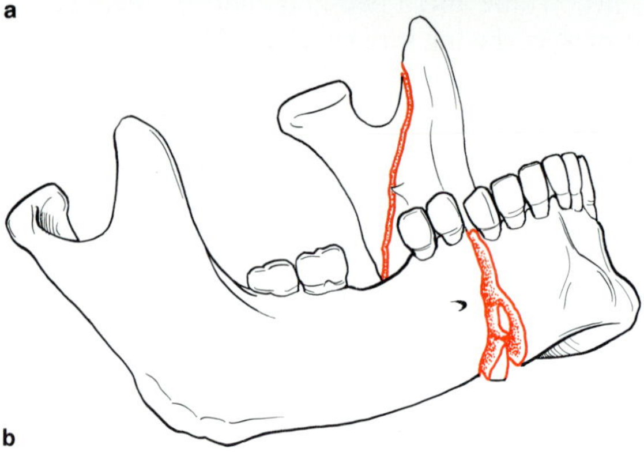

b

Fig. 239 a, b. Postcanine transverse fracture and peripheral angle fracture

Closed double fracture: *Right postcanine fracture and left peripheral angle-ramus fracture* (Fig. 239)

Fracture formula:	$F_1\ L_3/F_1\ L_4\ O_1$
Clinical category:	$F_2\ S_0$
Grade of severity:	II A

Intraoral Procedure
Tension-band splint on the right mandibular teeth and occlusal retention.

Extraoral Procedure (Fig. 240)
Right side:
Six-hole DCP applied in conjunction with the tension-band splint. The wedge-shaped intermediate fragment is interposed when the reduction-compression forceps is activated (Fig. 240 a).
Left side:
The four-hole EDCP substitutes for a tension band in spite of it, it violates the "three screw rule". This requires releasing only the lower insertion of the masseter, so the beneficial splinting action of the muscle sling is essentially preserved (Fig. 240 b).

Both sides of the internal fixation are shown in Fig. 240 c.

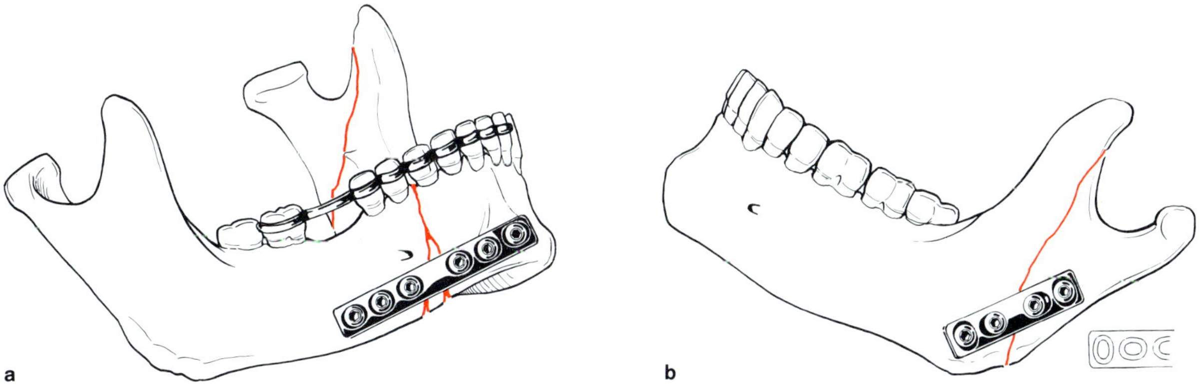

a b

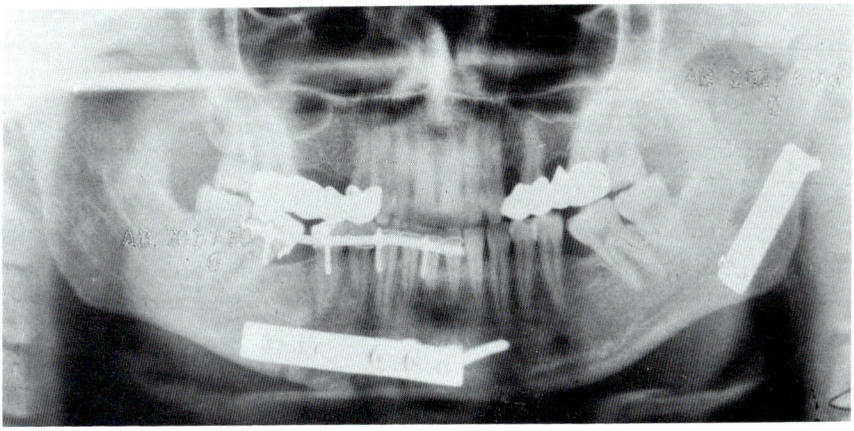

Fig. 240. **a** Six-hole DCP combined with a tension-band splint. **b** Replacement of the tension band by an EDCP (see text) **c** General view of the fixation

c

Double fracture: *Central angle fracture with a wedge fragment and an ipsilateral paramedian fracture with tooth loss in a multiple trauma patient* (Fig. 241)

Fracture formula:	$/F_1\ L_4\ F_1\ L_1\ O_1$
Clinical category:	$F_2\ S_1$
Grade of severity:	II B

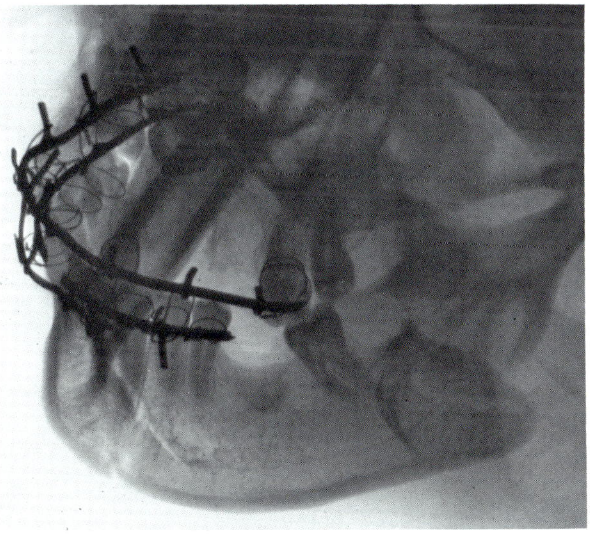

a

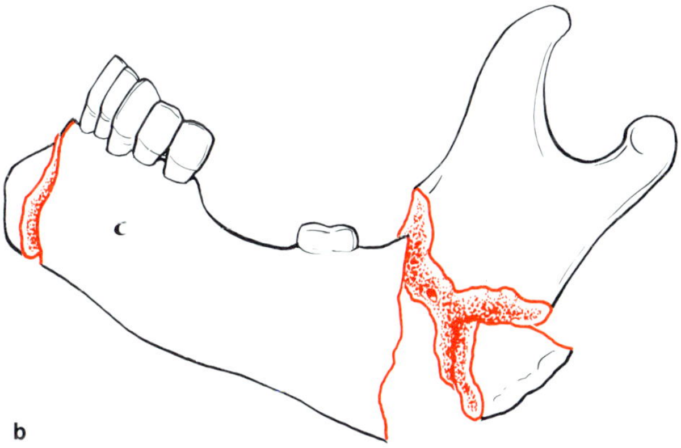

b

Fig. 241. **a** Three-part angle fracture with an associated paramedian fracture. **b** Artist's rendering

Intraoral Procedure
Nonsalvagable teeth are removed, maxillary and mandibular splints are applied, and the occlusion is retained with intermaxillary wires.

Extraoral Procedure (Fig. 242)
The paramedian fracture, being the easier to treat, is stabilized first with a four-hole DCP in conjunction with the tension-band splint. The 2 × 2 cm wedge fragment is reduced, and a ten-hole reconstruction plate is applied to stabilize the angle and bridge the fracture site.

Figure 243 shows the status after removal of the fixation material. Apparently the wedge fragment did not become revascularized and underwent partially necrosis and resorption. Usually this results in infection and sequestration. The absence of this complication in the present case presumably relates to the stabilizing effect of the internal fixation.

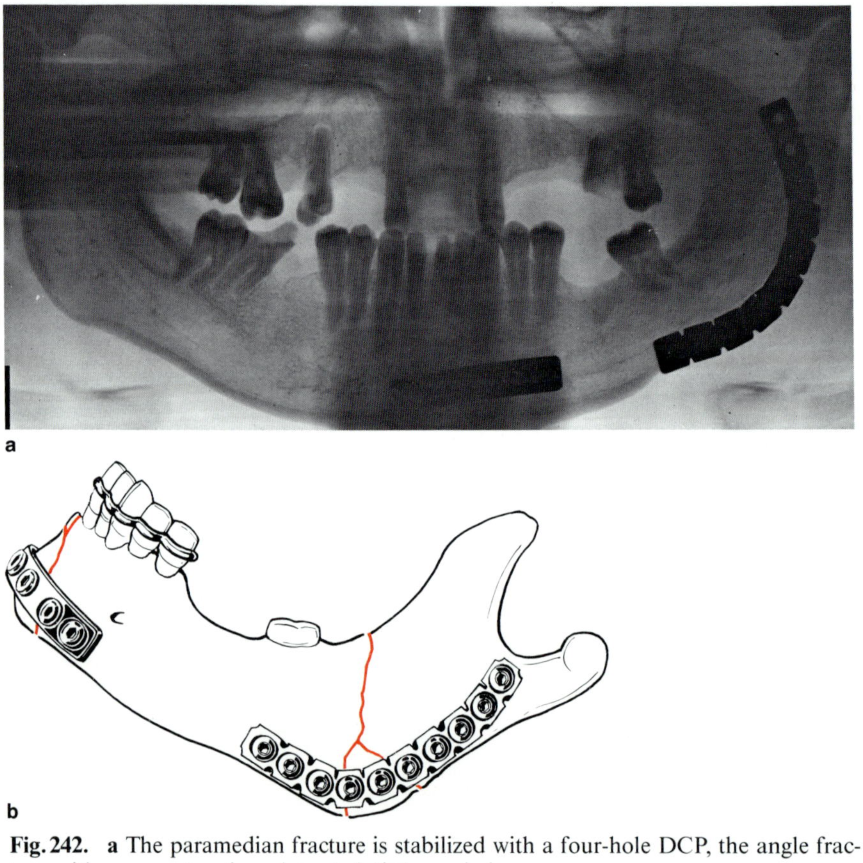

Fig. 242. a The paramedian fracture is stabilized with a four-hole DCP, the angle fracture with a reconstruction plate. **b** Artist's rendering

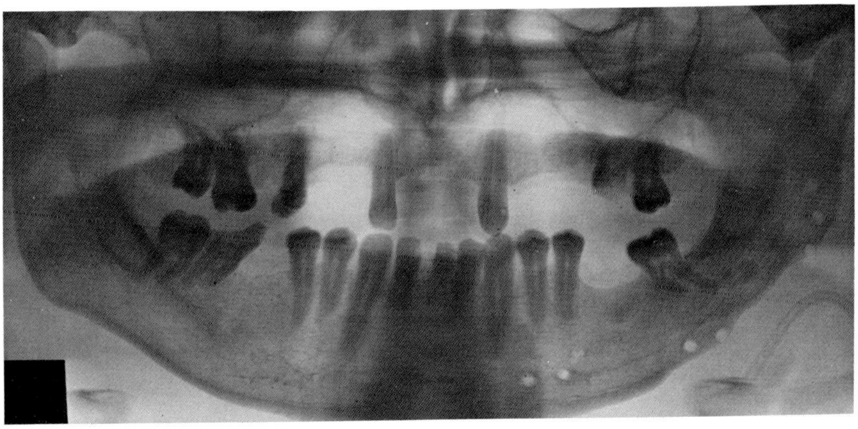

Fig. 243. Status after implant removal

5.4.2 Internal Fixation of a Double Fracture in the Edentulous Mandible

5.4.2.1 Indications

Double fractures of the edentulous mandible are often symmetrical. The unstable central fragment is difficult to reduce and stabilize by non-operative means, which also are very uncomfortable for the patient (e.g., Gunning-type splint, circumferential wiring, wire sutures). Thus, the replacement of unsatisfactory intermaxillary fixation by a functionally stable internal fixation represents a significant advance.

5.4.2.2 Techniques of Internal Fixation

Atrophy and osteoporosis are often the major problem in the edentulous jaw. They result in a deficiency of compressive strength at the ends of the fragments and around the screw holes. Axial compression with a plate is not the primary method of choice in this type of mandibule. It is preferable to span and support the symmetrical fractures with a single reconstruction plate. A plate of this type extending from one angle of the mandible to the other will provide sufficient extra holes in the event that one or more threads become stripped when the screws are inserted (see p. 64 ff.).

The disadvantage of extensive removal of periosteum is obvious in this situation and is avoided by *leaving the periosteum in place*. Despite the pressure from the plate, large areas of the preserved periosteal sheath will retain their vascular supply (see p. 31). Later it may be advantageous to perform bone grafting at the time of plate removal.

The following case presentations will serve to illustrate the technical principles:

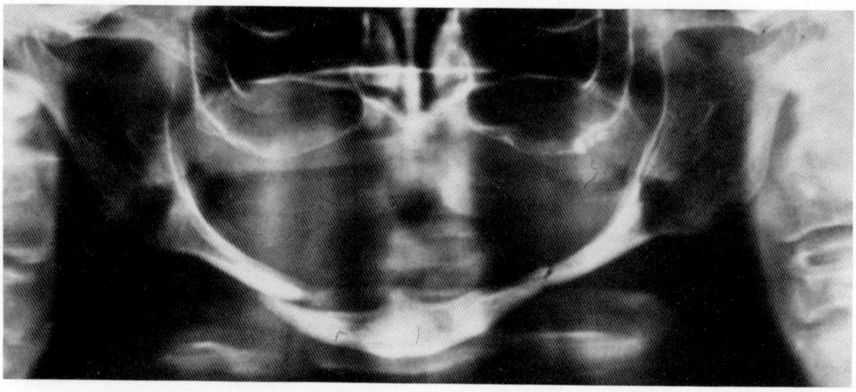

Fig. 244. Double fracture in the severely atrophic mandible

Double Oblique Fracture in the Pipestem Mandible (Fig. 224)

Fracture formula:	$F_1\ L_3/F_1\ L_3$
Clinical category:	$F_2\ S_0$
Grade of severity:	II A

Intraoral Procedure (Fig. 245)
The fractures are stabilized intraorally with occluding dentures that are held in approximation with anterior and lateral extramaxillary clamps. The anterior clamp engages the bony nasal floor and the basal edge of the mandible.

Extraoral Procedure (Fig. 246, see also Fig. 60c)

1) The soft tissue are carefully dissected from the periosteum, which is left attached to the bone, especially in the areas away from the fracture lines.
2) The eighteen-hole reconstruction plate is contoured to the mandible with the aid of a malleable templats. Both fractures are stabilized with this one plate (in this instance interfragmentary pressure is not possible because of the oblique fracture lines).

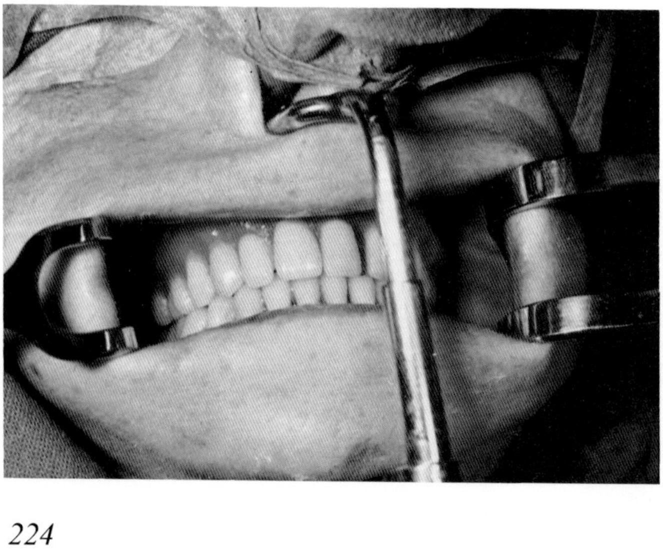

Fig. 245. The occluding dentures are retained with intermaxillary clamps

Fig. 246. **a** Appearance at operation (see text). **b** Postoperative radiograph

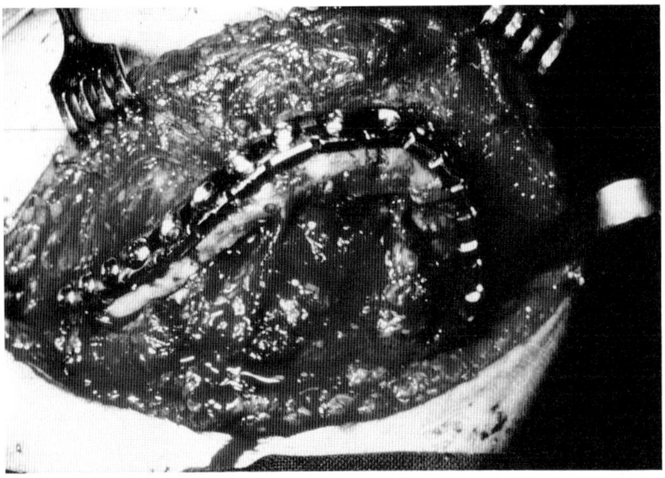
a

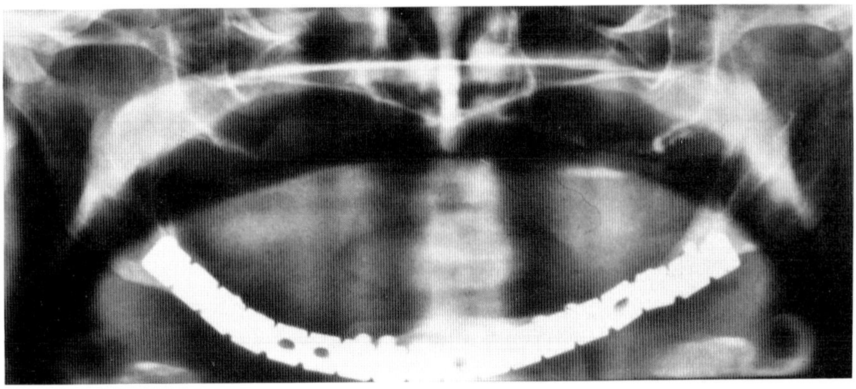
b

Bone grafting at the time of plate removal one year later (Fig. 247)
At implant removal one year after the primary operation, the atrophic mandible is augmented with bilateral split rib grafts. Utilizing the existing screw holes, the bone grafts are fixed to the pipestem mandible under pressure with lag screws.

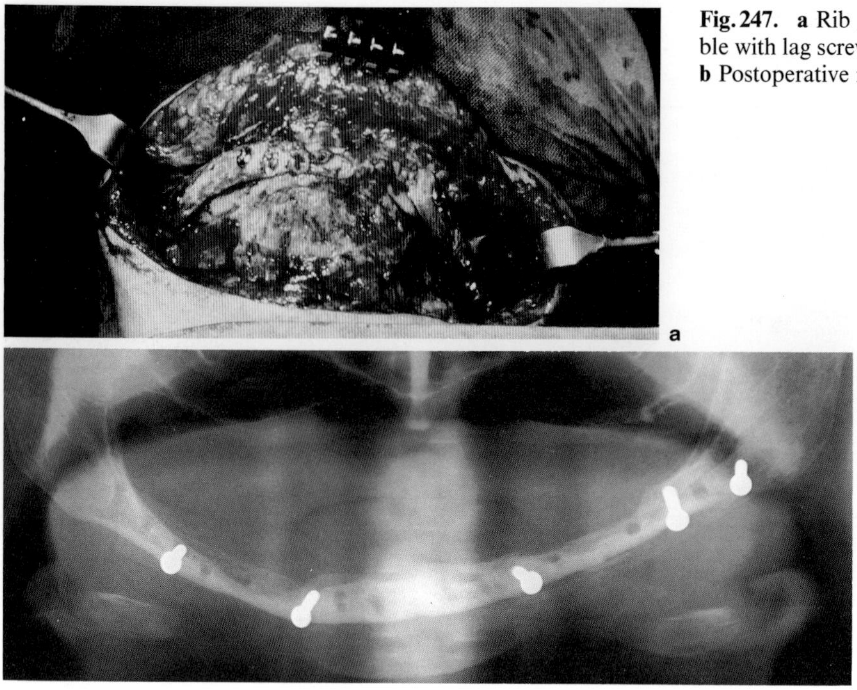

a

b

Fig. 247. **a** Rib grafts are attached to the mandible with lag screws (at the time of plate removal). **b** Postoperative radiograph

Transverse postcanine fracture on the right side with a severely atrophic alveolar ridge (Fig. 248 a) **and a postcanine nonunion on the left side (result of an untreated fracture sustained 3 months before the current fracture)** Fig. 248 b)

Fracture formula:	$F_1\ L_3/F_1\ L_3$
Clinical category:	$F_2\ S_0$
Grade of severity:	II A

Intraoral Procedure
Intermaxillary fixation with extramaxillary clamps holding the dentures in occlusion (see Fig. 245).

Extraoral Procedure (Fig. 249)
This is an exception to the rule of using a single appliance to stabilize symmetrical fractures (see p. 225), because the lesion of the left side is a nonunion. Interfragmental compression is necessary in order for the nonunion to consolidate. (Induction of intermediate osteogenic tissue (see p. 35). This pressure would be more difficult to generate with a long reconstruction plate than with a separate six-hole DCP, which may be overbent slightly (see p. 45) to maximize its effect.
Left side:
The initial step is to stabilize the nonunion with a six-hole DCP. It is unnecessary to freshen the fragments, since the fracture was sustained only 3 months earlier (see p. 285).
Right side:
The transverse fracture is stabilized with a six-hole DCP. A four-hole DCP might be inadequate because of the atrophy and osteoporosis.

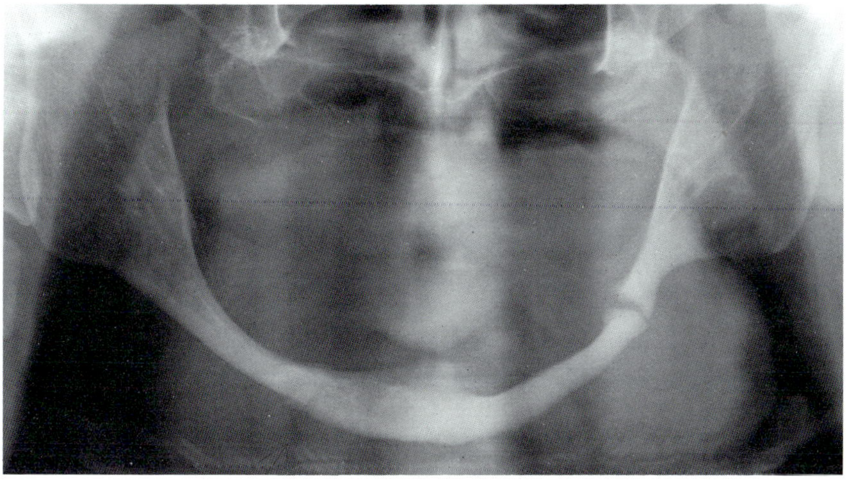

a

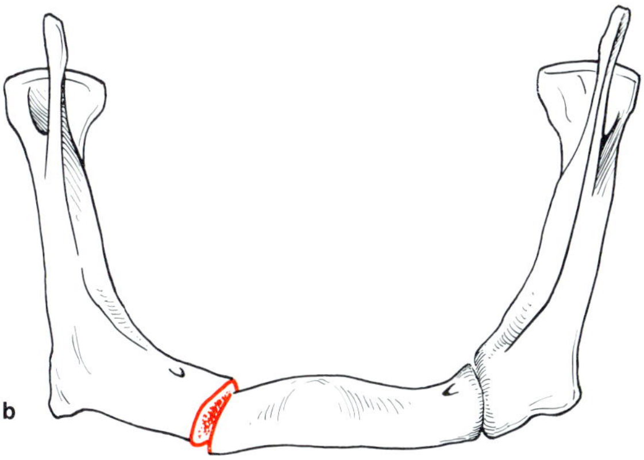

b

Fig. 248. **a** Fresh transverse fracture on the right side, "elephant foot" type of nonunion on the left side. **b** Artist's rendering

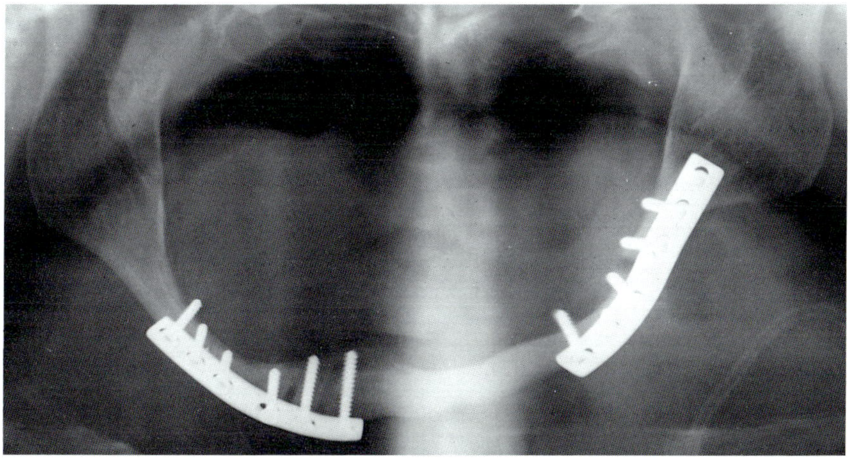

Fig. 249. The nonunion is stabilized by interfragmental compression alone (see text)

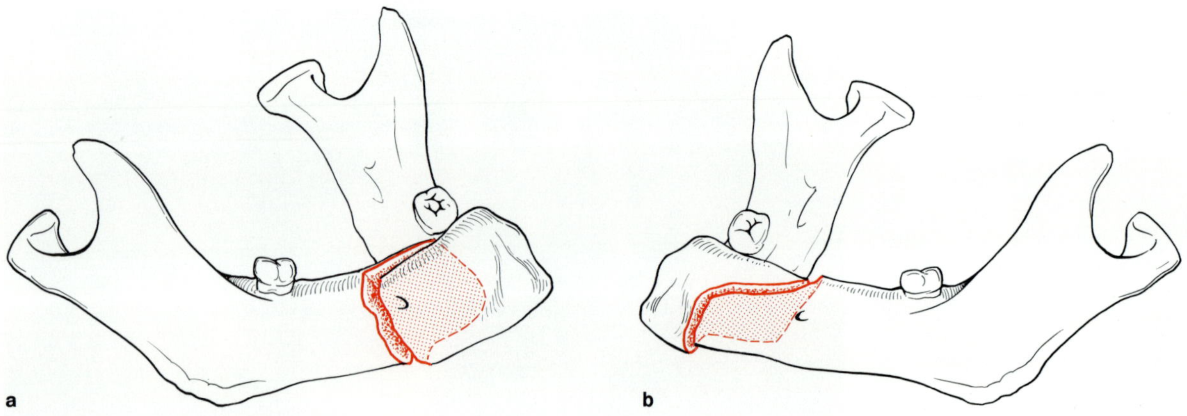

Fig. 250 a, b. Double oblique-surface fracture

Double Oblique-Surface Fracture (Fig. 250)

Fracture formula:	$F_1 L_3/F_1 L_1$
Clinical category:	$F_2 S_0$
Grade of severity:	II A

The lines of cleavage run in opposite directions, i.ke., the sheared cortical plate is directed posteriorly on the right side and anteriorly on the left. Because of this and the large fracture area, the jaw is relatively stable. The fractures are easy to reduce, and intraoral retention is not required.

Extraoral Procedure (Lag Screw Fixation) (Fig. 251)
Right side:
The interdigitating fragments are easily reduced with a sharp forceps and three lag screws are inserted basally.
Left side:
The upper part of the cortical plate is too thin for a lag screw, and only two lag screws are inserted to avoid the risk of cracking the fragment. As the static compression of lag screws is greater than that of a DCP, adequate stability is achieved in this precanine position of the fracture.

The postoperative status is shown in Fig. 252 a, b.

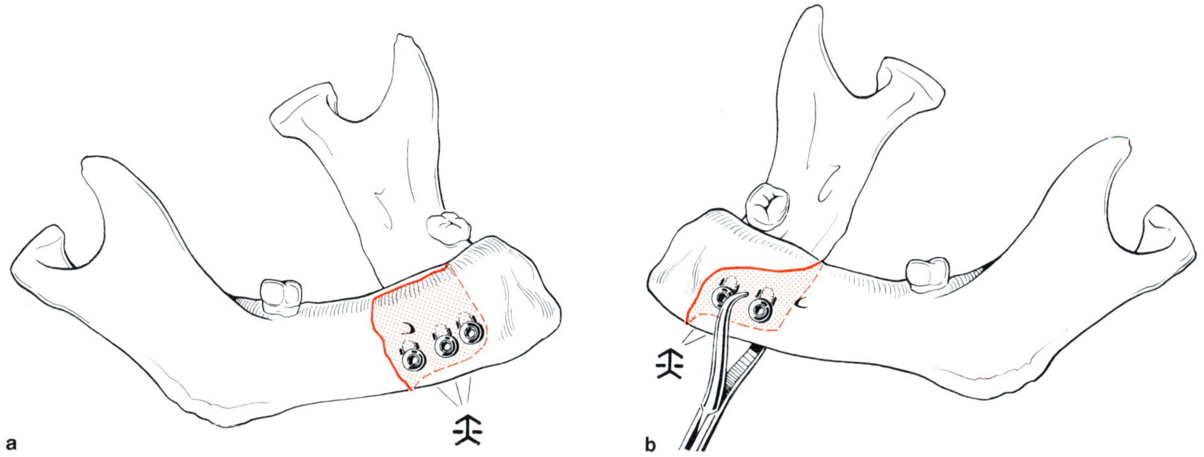

Fig. 251 a, b. Lag screw fixation

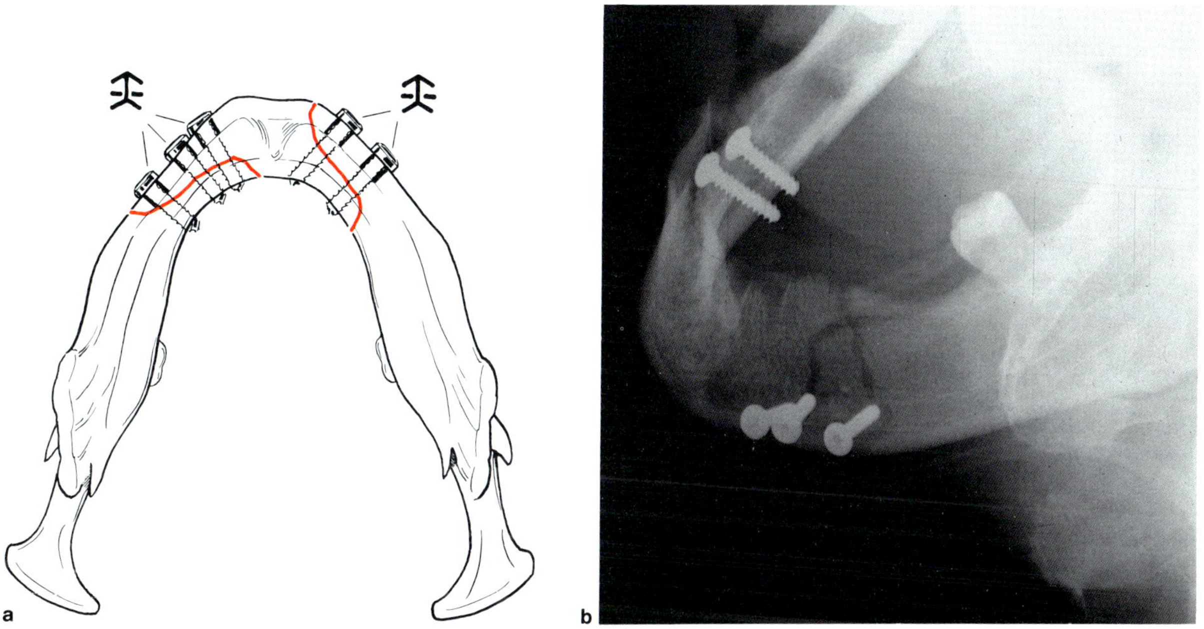

Fig. 252 a, b. Status after the internal fixation (**a** drawing, **b** radiograph)

5.4.3 Unilateral Segmental Fracture

A segmental fracture of the mandible refers to two or more successive fracture lines involving one half of the mandible (see definition p. 153 ff.). The sequential arrangement of the fracture lines results in the presence of mobile intermediate segments.

This fracture is comparable to the "bilevel" fracture in a long bone, and its management is just as complex. The unstable intermediate segment makes it difficult to establish the "axis" of the mandible during the fixation. Immobilization of both fracture sites on the same side stands or falls with the quality of the intraoral splinting. Even a single tooth remaining in the fragment will aid the internal fixation by making it easier to manipulate and reposition the segment. This is illustrated by the multiple trauma case below:

Closed, unilateral precanine and postcanine segmental fracture on the left side (the intermediate segment is completely unstable, and the remaining dentition is heavily involved by caries) (Fig. 253)

Fracture formula:	$/F_1\ L_1\ F_1\ L_3$
Clinical category:	$F_2\ S_0$
Grade of severity:	II A

Emergency internal fixation is undertaken in the multiply injured patient to facilitate intensive care.

Intraoral Procedure (Fig. 254)

1) Divided mandibular splints are applied at the fracture sites to aid the reduction and retention of the segmental fragment.
2) The occlusion is retained with Ernst ligatures (see p. 61) and with a bridging ligature [see Fig. 254 (2)] stiffened with acrylic resin.

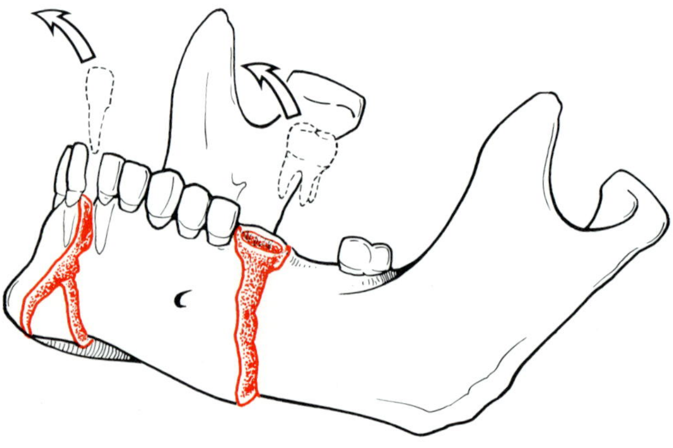

Fig. 253. Unilateral segmental fracture

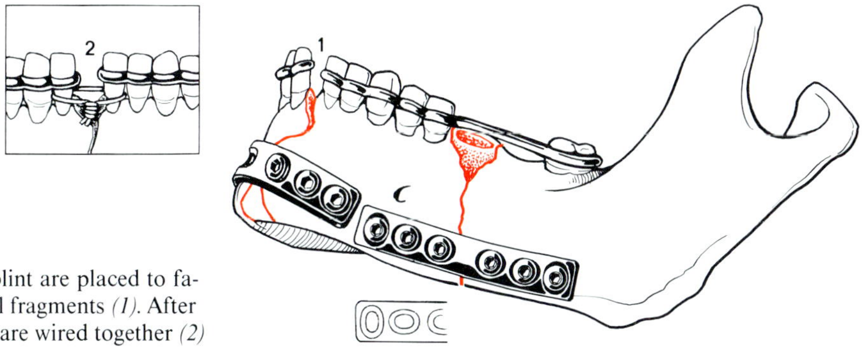

Fig. 254. Divided mandibular splint are placed to facilitate reduction of the segmental fragments *(1)*. After the reduction, the divided splints are wired together *(2)*

Extraoral Procedure (Fig. 255)
Precanine fracture:
This fracture is stabilized with an eight-hole DCP in conjunction with the mandibular splint (the loose marginal fragment is fit into position but not separately fixed). One screw hole over the fracture site is left empty.
Postcanine fracture:
The oral splint holds the fracture together rather loosely and so permits the EDCP to exert its eccentric comression (tension-band splint without a locking action, see p. 57).

Figure 256 shows the roentgenogram after implant removal.

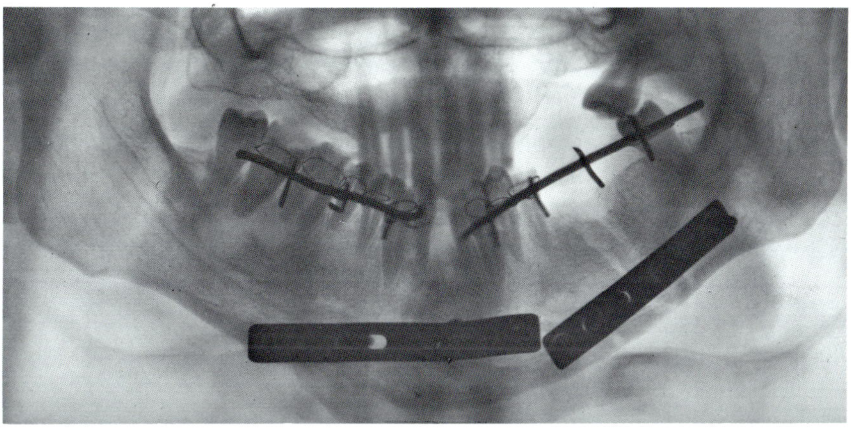

Fig. 255. See text

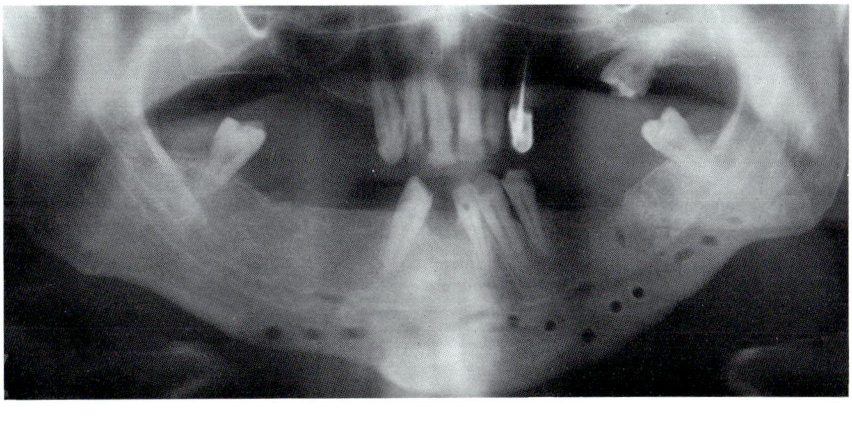

Fig. 256. Radiographic status after removal of the plates and splints

5.4.4 Unilateral Segmental Fracture and Contralateral Single Fracture

This is a complex fracture characterized by *bilateral* instability and displacement of the segments (see definition p. 153 ff.). *Treatment should always begin with the simplest fracture.* This principle is often violated, because radiographic coverage may be inadequate to give a true picture of fragment displacements. Evaluation is expecially difficult in multiple trauma cases where X-ray projections centered on the mandible usually cannot be obtained. In such cases the exploratory exposure of all fracture sites is the only definitive way to establish which site can be stabilized most easily (Fig. 257). This is particularly important in edentulous patients, in whom intraoral measures usually cannot be employed to retain the individual oral fragments. Their dentures are either lost or fractured, as the following case illustrates:

Right-sided segmental fracture (Fig. 258 a) **and contralalteral transverse fracture** (Fig. 258 b) **in the edentulous atrophic mandible. Outstanding feature: complete instability**

Fracture formula:	$F_1\ L_3/F_1\ L_3$
Clinical category:	$F_2\ S_0$
Grade of severity:	II A

Intraoral Procedure
Intraoral measures are not possible due to absence of the dentures and multifocal instability.

Extraoral Procedure (Fig. 259)
Left side:
The more favorable fracture side is on the left side. The central fragment is displaced like a butterfly but terminates on the right side in an oblique surface that is easily reduced against the adjacent fragment with a pointed forceps. Treatment begins with the left fracture, which can be ideally reduced and stabilized with a four-hole DCP (Fig. 259 a). At this point the anterior fragment is in an orthograde position.
Right side:
The completely mobile segment is fixed with a retention screw (Fig. 259 b), and the segmental fracture is buttressed with a ten-hole reconstruction plate (Fig. 259 c). A single reconstruction plate extending from angle to angle, as shown on p. 225, would be too complicated because of the displacement of the fragments. It is better to fix the fracture sites separately, using a four-hole plate on the side of the single fracture (Fig. 259 d).

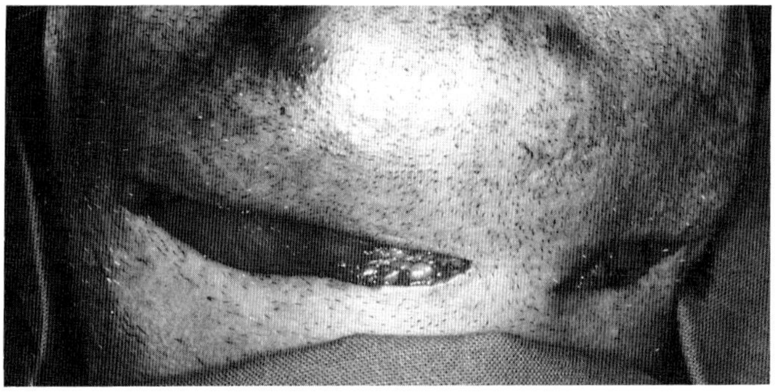

Fig. 257. Bilateral incisions for evaluating the relative grades of severity of the fractures on each side

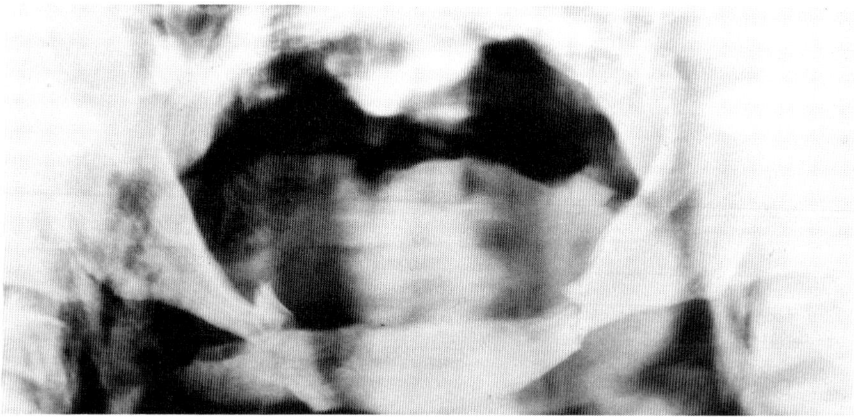

a

b

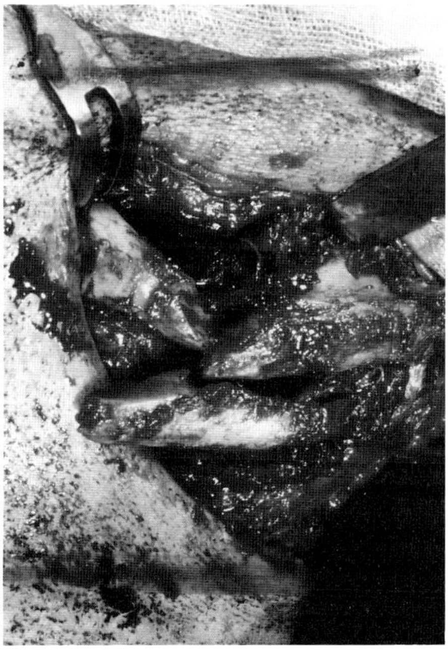

Fig. 258. **a** Segmental (double) fracture on the right side and contralateral transverse fracture. **b** Site of operation on the right side

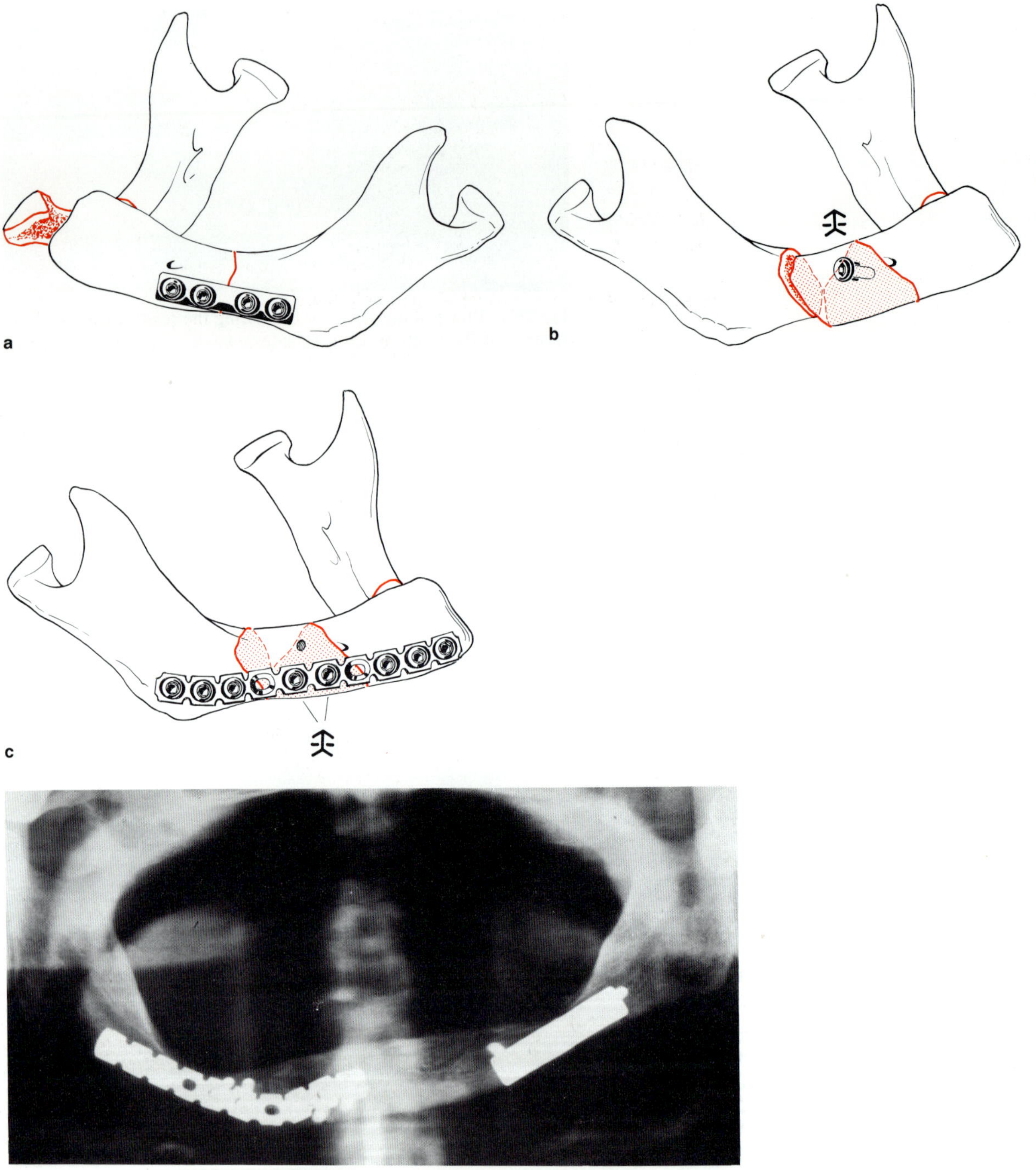

Fig. 259. **a** First the single fracture is stabilized with a four-hole DCP. **b** Preliminary fixation of the central segment with a lag (retention) screw. **c** The segmental fracture is bridged with a reconstruction plate; two lag screws are inserted through the oblique fracture surface (see p. 208). **d** General view of the fixation

5.5 Comminuted Fractures (F_3 S_0)

A comminuted fracture of the mandible may consist of a segment broken into larger individual fragments or a circumscribed area of smaller fragments that have been splintered from larger segments. This *localized* fragmentation (see definition p. 153 ff.) differs from the short comminuted fracture in the diaphysis of a long bone, for example, where an *entire* segment is broken into many small pieces. Most of these fractures are managed by bone grafting the site and bridging it with a plate. In the comminuted mandible, by contrast, we generally see larger pieces of cortex broken from the lateral or lingual aspect of the bone or perhaps a circumscribed splintering of the inferior margin. Sufficient peripheral continuity of the cortex remains, in cross-section, to make possible an anatomic reduction and interfragmental compression.

Not infrequently, one or two of the fragments are large enough to fit back into the gap between the bone ends.

The technical principles of internal fixation are illustrated by the following case reports:

Closed, comminuted fracture with a large basal wedge fragment, a third molar in the fracture line, a splintered alveolar process, and a contralateral condylar neck fracture (Fig. 260)

Fracture formula:	F_3 L_3/F_1 L_6 O_1
Clinical category:	F_3 S_0
Grade of severity:	II B

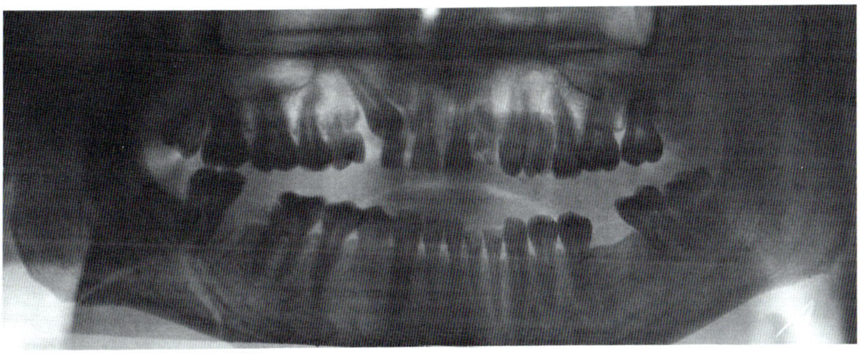

a

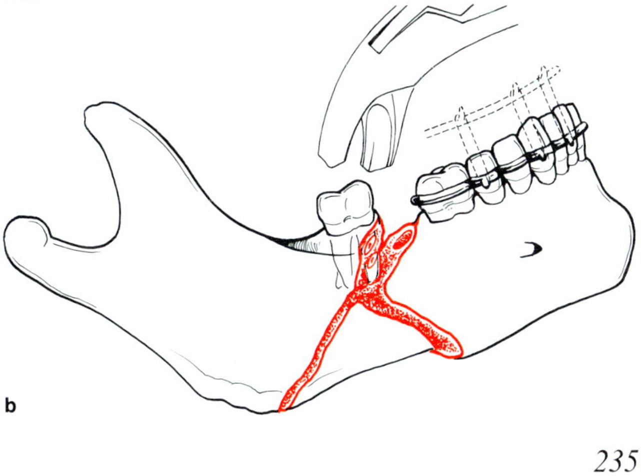

b

Fig. 260. **a** Closed comminuted fracture. **b** Tooth in the fracture line is extracted and the anterior part of the mandible is retained in occlusion using intermaxillary wires

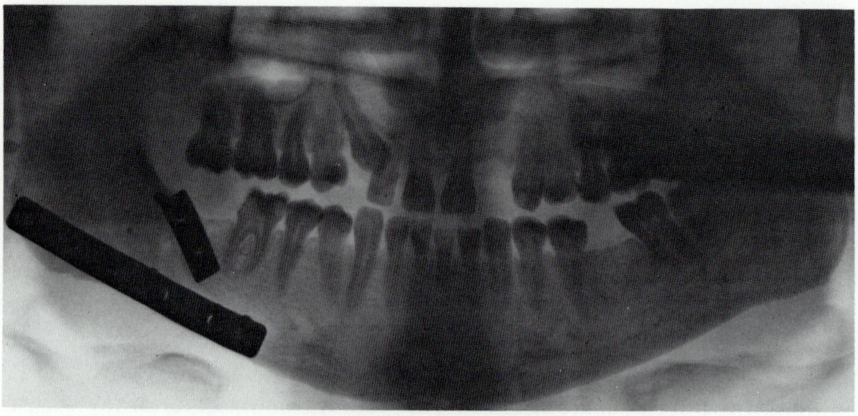

a

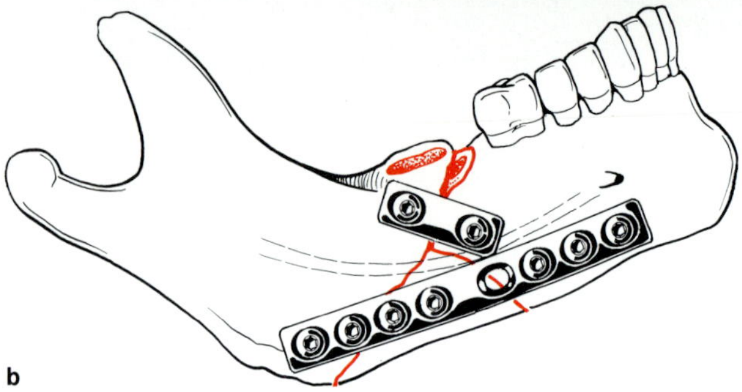

b

Fig. 261. **a** Plate and tension-band system, with the stabilization plate attached to the wedge-shaped basal fragment. **b** Artist's rendering

Intraoral Procedure
The bone splinters and third molar are removed from the line of fracture, the mucosa is closed using a flap technique, maxillary and mandibular splints are applied, and the jaws are retained in orthograde occlusion using intermaxillary wires (see Fig. 260 b).

Extraoral Procedure (Fig. 261)
The tension side of the fracture is secured with a two-hole DCP applied as a tension band (Fig. 261 a), and interfragmental compression is effected with an eight-hole DCP attached to the main fragments and also to the basal wedge-shaped fragment (Fig. 261 b).

Comminuted fracture on the left side and postcanine transverse fracture on the right side (Fig. 262)

Fracture formula:	$F_1\ L_3/F_3\ L_1\ L_3$
Clinical category:	$F_3\ S_0$
Grade of severity:	II B

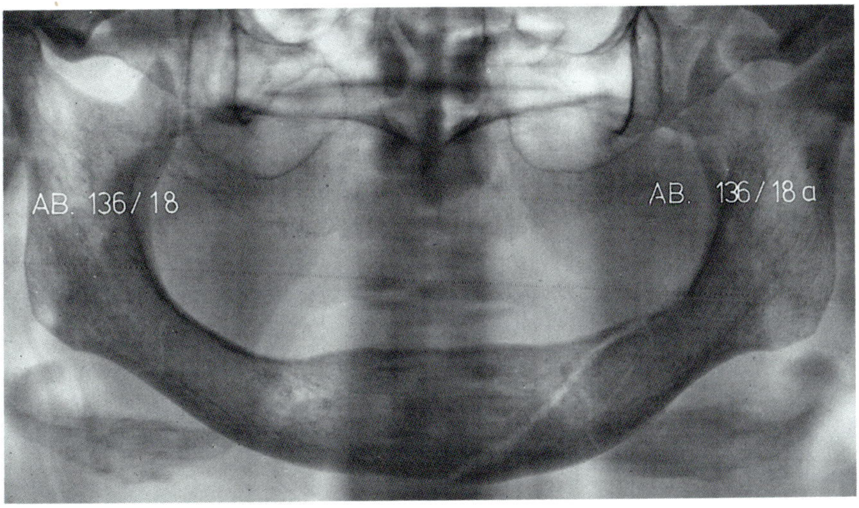

a

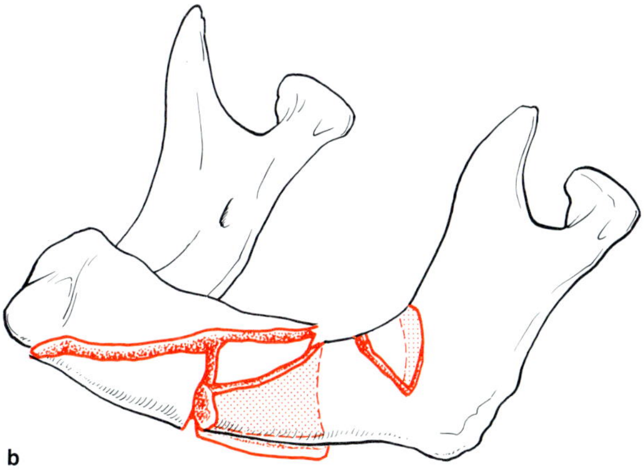

b

Fig. 262. **a** Comminuted fracture on the left side and transverse fracture on the right. **b** Artist's rendering of the comminuted fracture

Extraoral Procedure
To minimize devascularization (see p. 131), the fracture is exposed and fixed through separate subangular and submental incisions (Fig. 263 a).

In this case the operation is begun on the left side[10] where the fracture surfaces are large and are easily reduced and fixed with lag screws. The anterior oblique fracture through the mental foramen is bridged with a six-hole CDP (Fig. 263 b, c).

Right side:
The smooth, transverse fracture is stabilized with a six-hole DCP (Fig. 263 d).

Figure 264 shows the status at eight years postoperatively, following removal of the implants.

[10] It is recommended that the less experienced operator begin on the right side (see p. 232 ff).

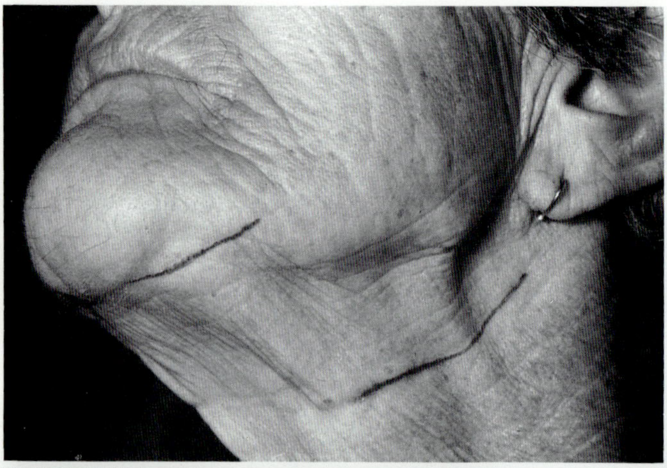

a

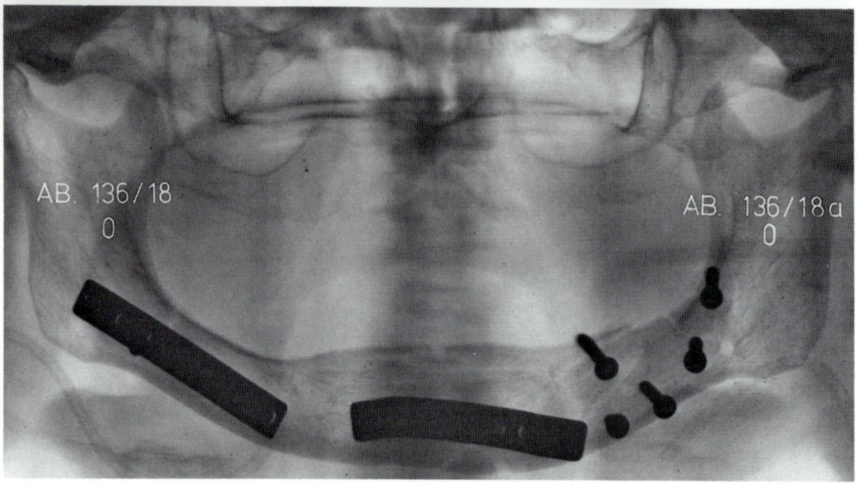

b

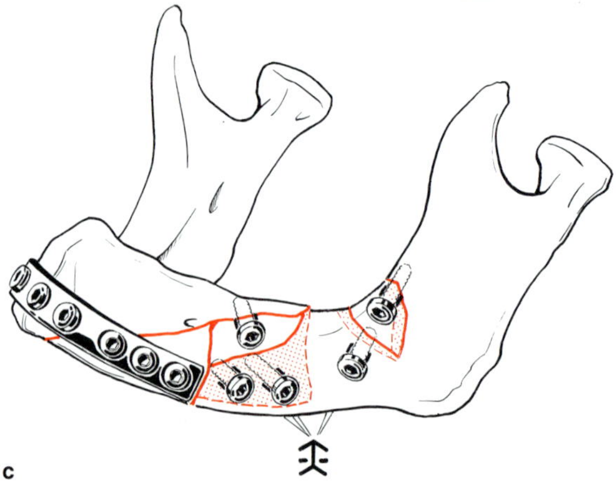

c

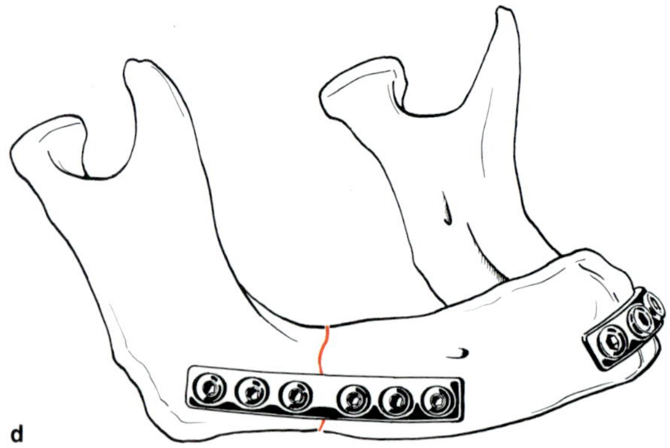

d

Fig. 263. **a** Devascularization is minimized by using two separate approaches: submental and subangular. **b** The comminuted fracture is fixed first with lag screws and a six-hole DCP. **c** Artist's rendering. **d** Six-hole DCP stabilizing a preangular margin fracture

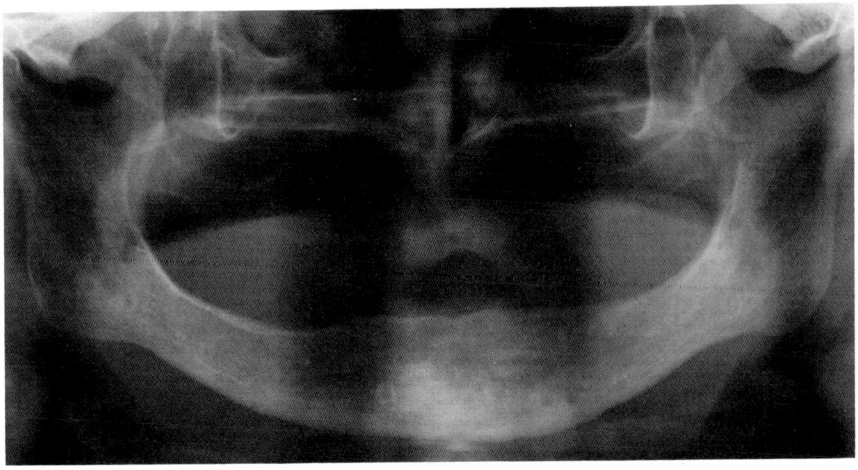

Fig. 264. Status after implant removal

Comminuted fracture of the left angle and ramus (Fig. 265)

Fracture formula:	$/F_3\ L_{4/5}$
Clinical category:	$F_3\ S_0$
Grade of severity:	II B

Intraoral Procedure
Occlusal alignment is reestablished and retained with Ernst ligatures.

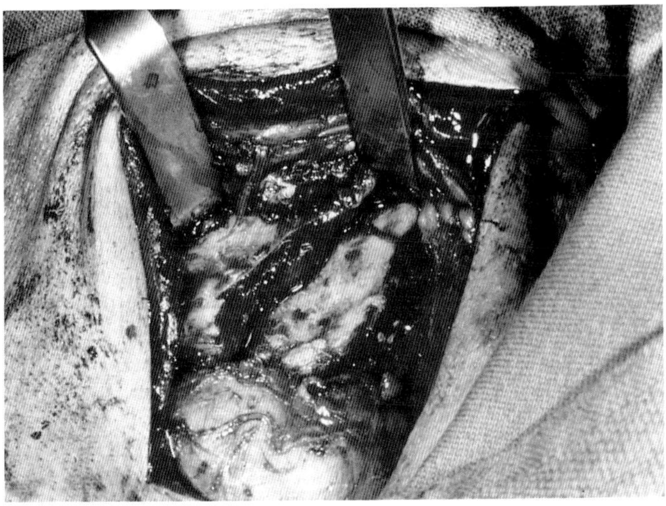

Fig. 265. Operative view of part of the comminuted fracture

Extraoral Procedure (Fig. 266)
First the largest fragment of the comminuted articular segment is fixed to the main mandibular fragment with a two-hole DCP, using the maximum compression displacement on both sides *(0.8 mm + 0.8 mm)*. This is necessary because the fragment edges cannot be perfectly aligned by instrumentation. The plated fragments provide a solid base for fixation of the condylar process (small two-hole plate) and as such require additional basal stabilization with a five-hole DCP. (A reconstruction plate would also be advantageous in this situation.) Two holes over the comminuted part of the angle are left empty. Screws 1, 2, and 3 unite the articular segment with the main fragment to create a functionally stable assembly (see Fig. 266 b).

The status after removal of the plates is shown in Fig. 267.

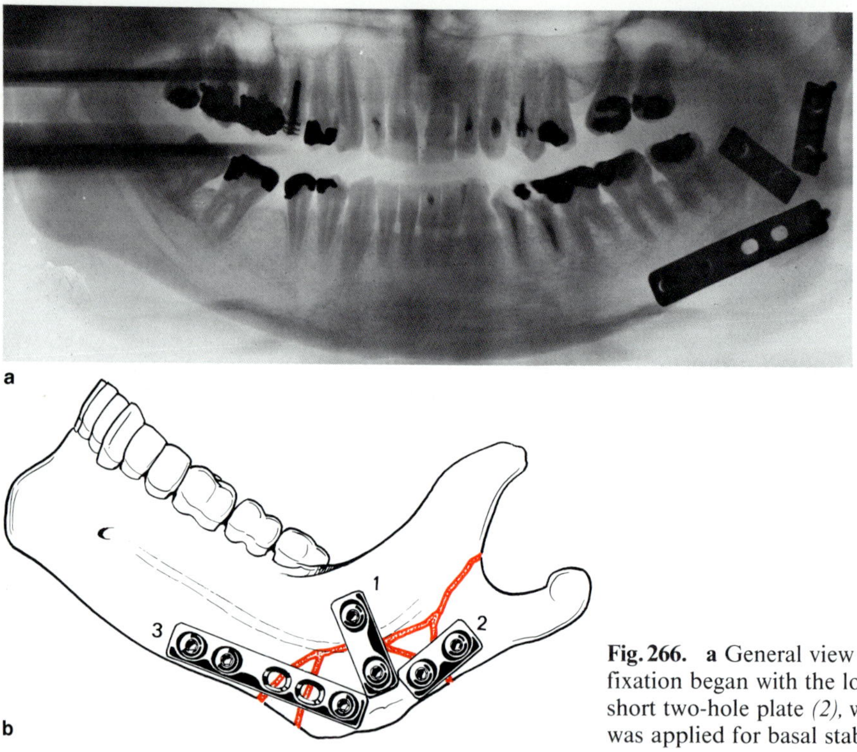

Fig. 266. **a** General view of the internal fixation. **b** The fixation began with the long two-hole DCP *(1)* and the short two-hole plate *(2)*, whereupon the five-hole plate *(3)* was applied for basal stabilization

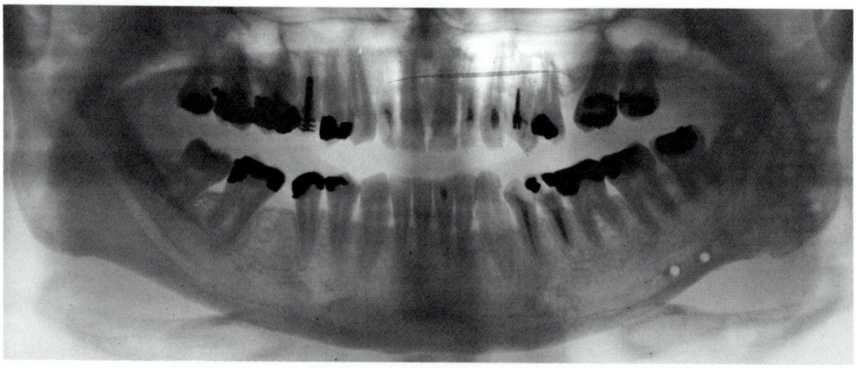

Fig. 267. Status after removal of the plates

6 Open Fractures

6.1 Definition of Terms

The hallmark of the open fracture is an open soft-tissue injury in proximity to the fracture, with a potential for infection of the bone. Frequently the term "open" implies the presence of a severe vascular disruption in addition to critical contamination of the wound.

6.2 Classification

Grades of Severity
An open fracture of the mandible may be classified by severity as Grade III or Grade IV (see also p. 159).

Grade III: Single or multiple fractures that are open intraorally (S_1 F_1/F_2)
Single or multiple fractures that are open extraorally (S_2 F_1/F_2)
Single or multiple fractures that are open intraorally and extraorally (S_3 F_1/F_2)
Grade IV: Comminuted fracture open intraorally (S_1 F_3)
Comminuted fracture open extraorally (S_2 F_3)
Comminuted fracture open intraorally and extraorally (S_3 F_3)

Summary

Category		Grade of severity
F_1/F_2	S_1/S_2	III A
F_1/F_2	S_3	III B
F_3	S_1/S_2	IV A
F_3	S_3	IV B

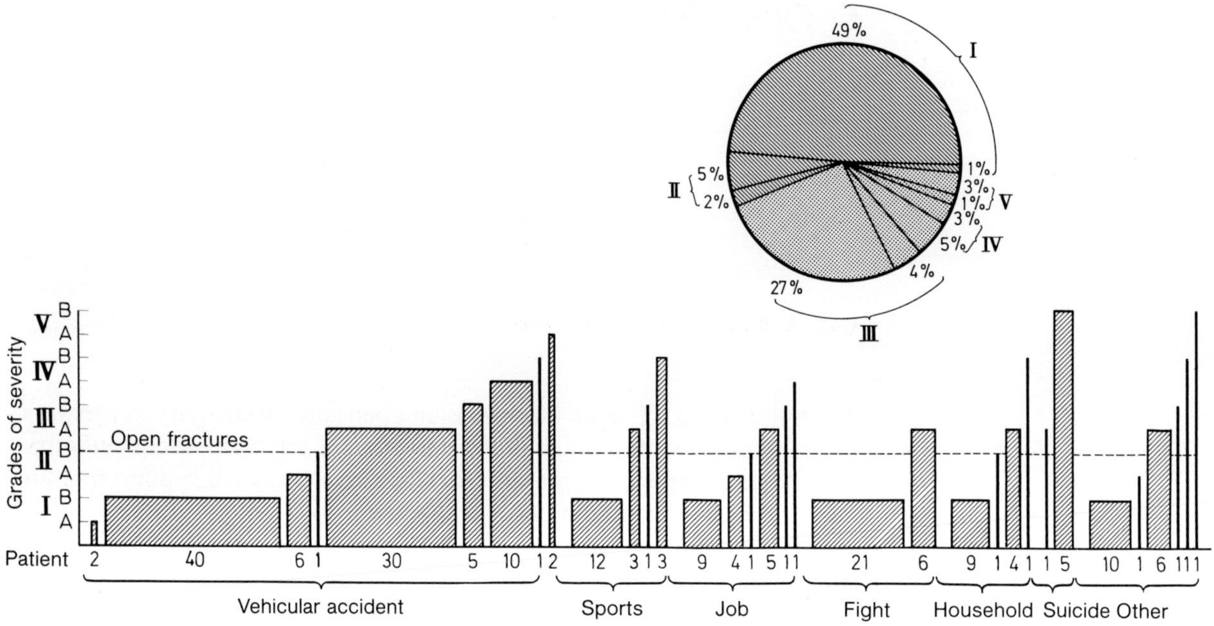

Graph 9. Series of 205 mandibular fractures (Philps 1986) divided into closed (I A–II B, 57%) and open fractures (III A–V B, 43%) and arranged by cause of injury

6.3 Statistics

Statistics indicate that open fractures are only slightly less prevalent than closed fractures. For example, of 205 cases that were seen at our hospital from 1976 to 1982, 87 were treated as open fractures and 118 as closed fractures. Thirty-five of the open fracture cases showed evidence of an oral mucosal wound, 33 had external (extraoral) soft-tissue wounds, and the rest had 14 perforating (intra-extraoral) soft-tissue injuries and 5 soft-tissue defects (Graph 9).

6.4 Wound Treatment and Splinting in Preparation for Definitive Stabilization of the Fracture

6.4.1 Emergency Treatment

In the multiple traumatized patient admitted emergently with an open mandibular fracture, top priority is given to immediate life-saving measures. Once the patient's general condition has been stabilized, special diagnostic studies may be undertaken. Under no circumstances, however, should one remove the emergency dressing that was applied at the scene of the injury. Only about one-third of open fracture are contaminated on arrival at the hospital. For this reason a sterile mask and gloves should be worn during the clinical and radiographic evaluation.

6.4.2 Preoperative Preparation

The emergency dressing is not removed until the patient is in the preparation room and the wound can be inspected under reasonably aseptic conditions. With the aid of the postinjury radiographs, the surgeon evaluates the injury and plans the operation.

The area of operation is cleaned "from the inside out." The oral cavity and existing mucosal wounds are sprayed thoroughly with H_2O_2 solution, Betadine or Lavasept solution, and Ringer's solution in that sequence. Extraoral cleansing follows the same scheme, except that grossly contaminated parts of the wound and bone are scrubbed with a brush while irrigating them with Ringer's solution, or they are cleansed mechanically with Desogen spray. When the skin prep is completed, sterile drapes are applied to the head and neck, and the patient is taken to the operating room.

6.4.3 Intraoral Wound Care and Splinting

Treatment follows the "inside to outside" pattern used in cleansing the wound. Only the *oral* mucosal wounds (pharynx, tongue, floor of mouth) are closed with sutures; wounds in the *vestibular* mucosa are left open. This facilitates occlusal reduction and splinting and later makes it easier to close the rest of the mucosa. (Sutures preplaced in the vestibule can interfere with splinting and are easily torn out during manipulations.) Tailoring of the wound edges is seldom necessary.

After the bone fragments have been freed of broken and dislocated teeth, as required, and teeth in the fracture line have been removed, *splinting is carried out under sterile conditions.* For multiple or comminuted fractures we recommend applying divided splints over the individual fracture sites. When the occlusion has been established and intermaxillary fixation applied, the splints are interconnected using wire loops and self-curing resin. Once splinting is completed, the vestibular mucosal wounds may be closed with sutures.

6.4.4 Extraoral Wound Treatment and Debridement

First the operator makes a search for foreign matter and devitalized tissues in the wound. The devitalized tissue will appear cyanotic and will not show capillary bleeding. Contused and devitalized fat must be excised to eliminate a culture medium for bacteria. The skin is less frequently affected. Skin debridement is usually limited to the sharp tailoring of very ragged edges. In some cases the location or extent of the fracture may require extension of the traumatic wound. Thus, serious consideration must be given to the approach, the incision, and the most favorable site for the placement of a metal implant before the operation is begun (see p. 173ff.).

Dirty bone is freshened, and indriven foreign material is removed with a curet or ronguer. It is a good precaution to remove free cortical fragments or small, unpedicled fragments less than 1 cm in size; these are most commonly found at the basilar margin of the mandible. At the same time, it is unwise to leave large gaps at the fracture site unless dealing with a grossly contaminated area of comminution. That is the only situation in which primary bone grafting would be indicated. Avascular bone fragments corresponding to the size of a segment are reduced or replanted to ensure interfragmental contact. We maintain constant irrigation with warm Ringer's solution during and after the debridement. Then we redrape the area for the internal fixation that follows.

6.5 Internal Fixation of the Open Fracture

It is the experience of the ASIF that a functionally stable internal (or external) fixation following debridement constitutes the best prophylaxis against infection. Thus, definitive stabilization of the open fracture should be performed within 6-8 h of the injury if there is no general contraindication against it. In the mandible as elsewhere, vascularity forms the biologic basis, and stability the mechanical basis for uncomplicated fracture union. *The more the vascularity of the bone has been disrupted as a result of fragmentation and the paraosseous degloving of soft tissues, the greater the importance of stability* (see also pp. 33 and 70).

6.5.1 Indications for Bone Plating

Two basic requirements must be satisfied in the plating of fractures:

1) Application of the plate must not be associated with excessive mobilization of the soft tissues due to the potential for iatrogenic devitalization (see Fig. 22).
2) Careful preoperative planning is necessary in terms of selecting the appropriate type and length of plate.

Both requirements are based on the experience that faulty treatment planning, intraoperative tissue insult, careless handling of the soft tissues, and deficient fixation technique are the major causes of poor fracture healing.

Regarding requirement 1), the best way to avoid devitalization of the bone is by adhering to the principle of combined intra- and extraoral fracture treatment (see p. 169). The extraoral approach limits denudation to the lateral part of the mandibular base while the oral part remains intact. The strictly basoparietal exposure can then be extended distally or mesially as required. This bears upon the quality of the internal fixation, for it influences both the result of the reduction and the correct selection and adaptation of the plate.

Intraorally paramedian open comminuted fracture on the left side and subcondylar fracture on the right side (Fig. 270)

Fracture formula:	F_1 L_6/F_3 L_3 O_1
Clinical category:	F_3 S_1
Grade of severity:	IV A

Intraoral Procedure (Fig. 271)

Because of the marked instability and displacement of the fracture, divided splints are applied to the mandibular teeth. The occlusion is retained with the aid of an upper denture wired to the maxilla.

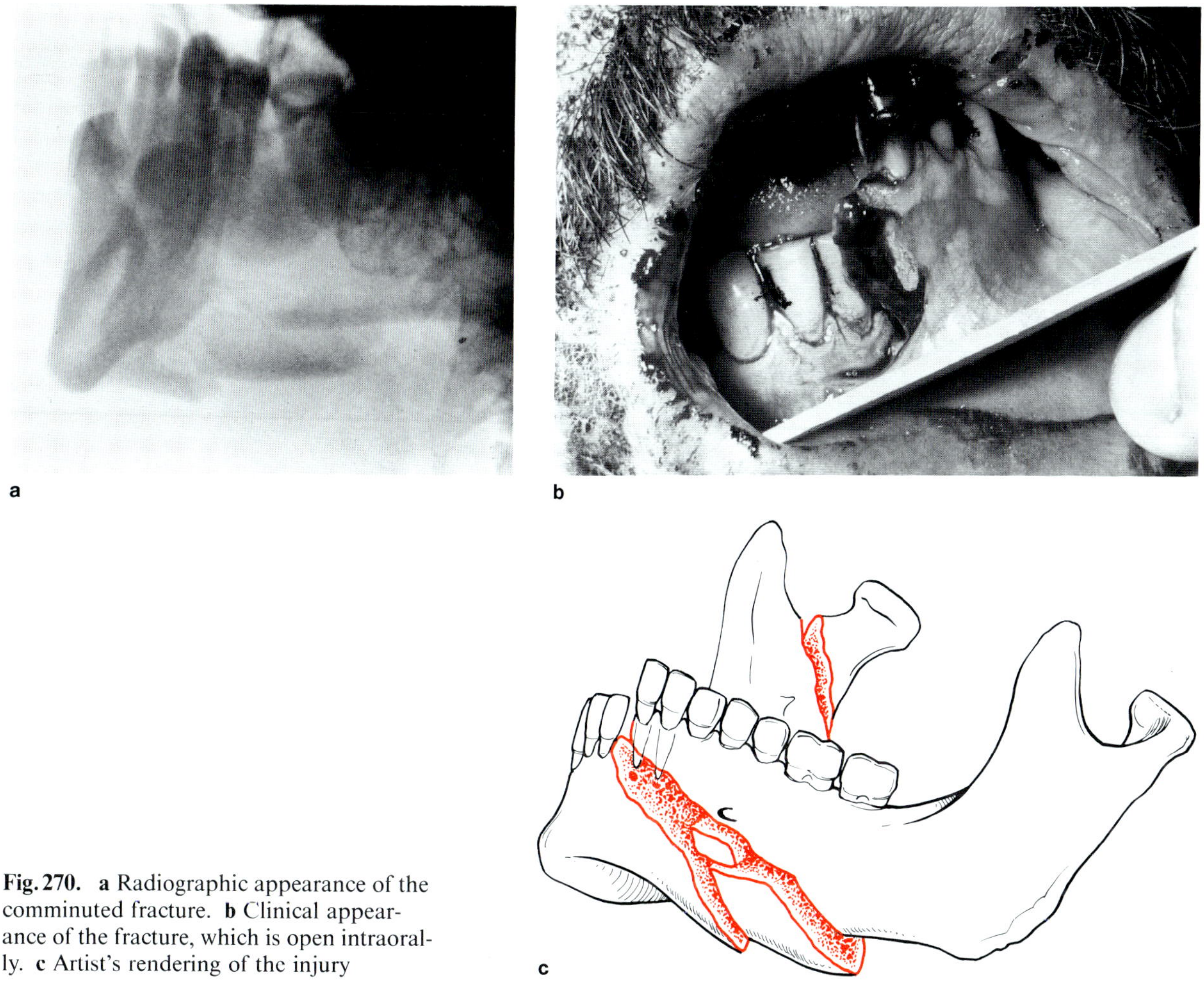

a b c

Fig. 270. **a** Radiographic appearance of the comminuted fracture. **b** Clinical appearance of the fracture, which is open intraorally. **c** Artist's rendering of the injury

Extraoral Procedure
The large intermediate fragment is fixed to the EDCP with a lag screw, which prevents slipping of the fragment while actively integrating is into the fixation system. Functional exercises were initiated after two weeks to rehabilitate the subcondylar fracture.

Figure 272 shows the status after removal of the fixation material.

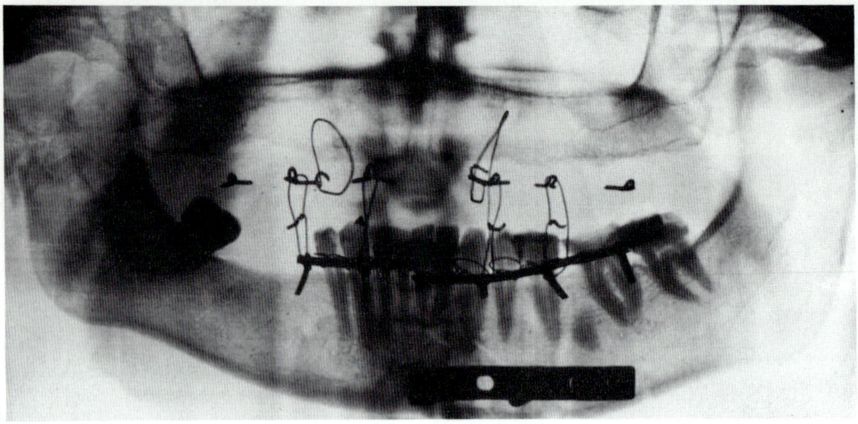

a

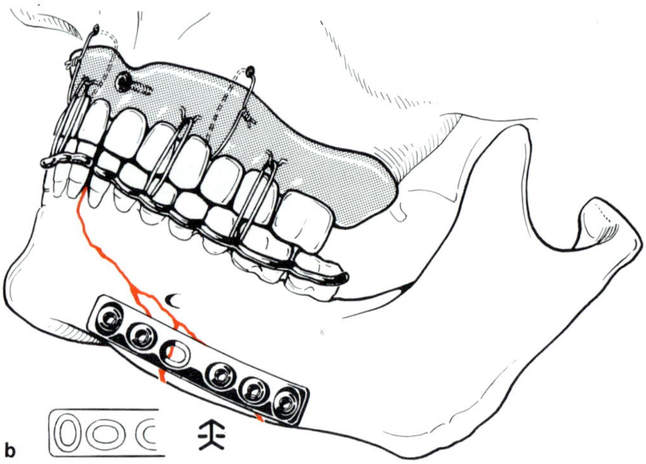

b

Fig. 271 a, b. General view of the fixation, showing the divided splint, six-hole EDCP, and peralveolar wires holding the maxillary denture (not visible in the radiograph) in position

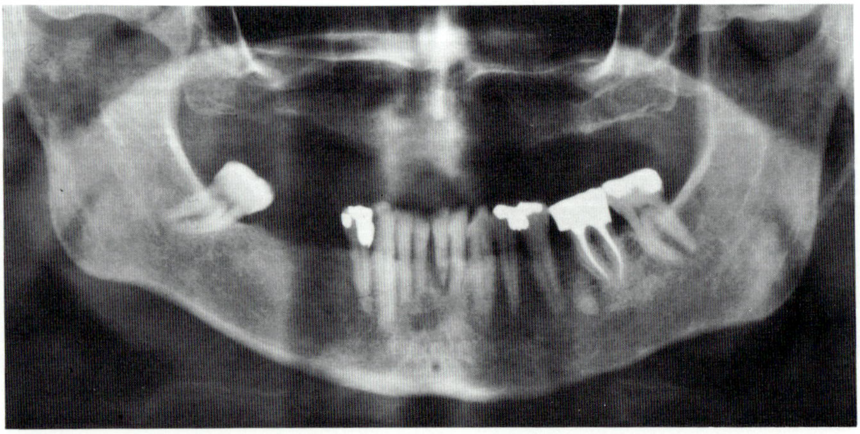

Fig. 272. Status after removal of the fixation material

Extraorally and intraorally open comminuted fractures of the right canine region and left postcanine region with a root fracture of the second premolar (Fig. 273)

Fracture formula:	$F_3\ L_2/F_3\ L_3$
Clinical category:	$F_3\ S_3$
Grade of severity:	IV B

Intraoral Procedure

The fractured left mandibular premolar is extracted. The fracture is manually reduced, and the whole dental arch is splinted to establish a tension band on each side. The occlusion is retained with Ernst ligatures.

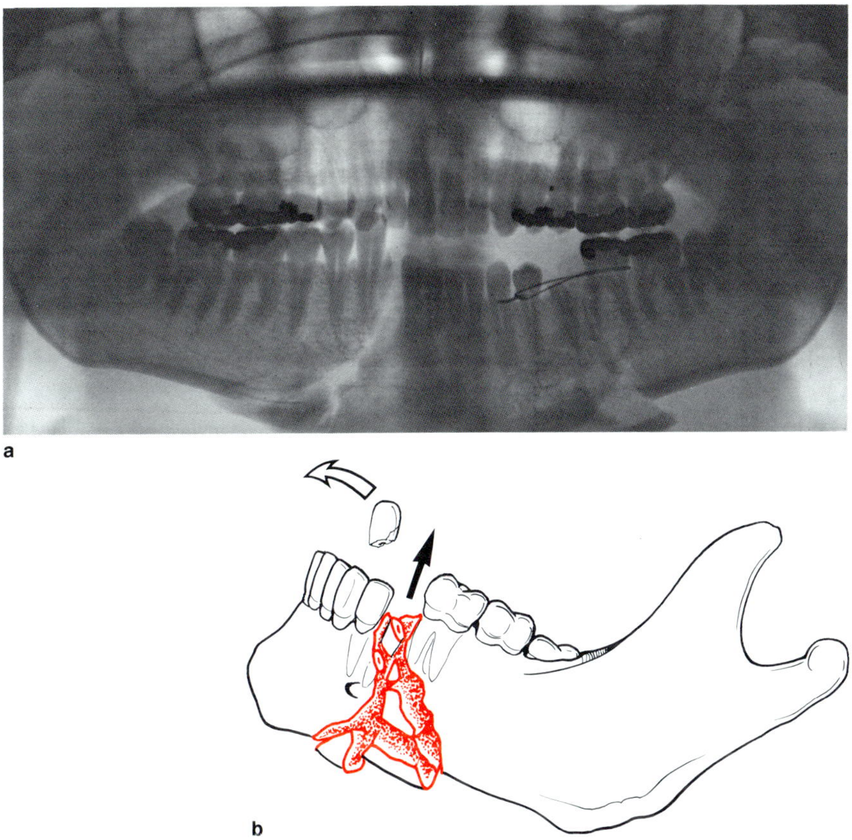

Fig. 273. **a** Comminuted fractures of the right canine and left postcanine regions. **b** Artist's rendering of the fracture on the left side

Extraoral Procedure (Fig. 274)
Right side:
An eight-hole DCP is applied as a buttress plate (compression is not attempted to avoid deformity from impaction of the fragments). A screw is driven into the largest of the three marginal fragments, thereby stabilizing an adjacent smaller fragment. The residual osseous defect is not large enough to warrant bone grafting.
Left side:
Smaller fragments and soft tissues are debrided from the fracture site, which is bridged with a ten-hole DCP applied as a buttress plate. The four central holes are left empty because of the extensive comminution of the underlying border. The large border fragment is left in place and attached to the plate with No. 0 Polytec.

Figure 275 shows the status after removal of the plates.

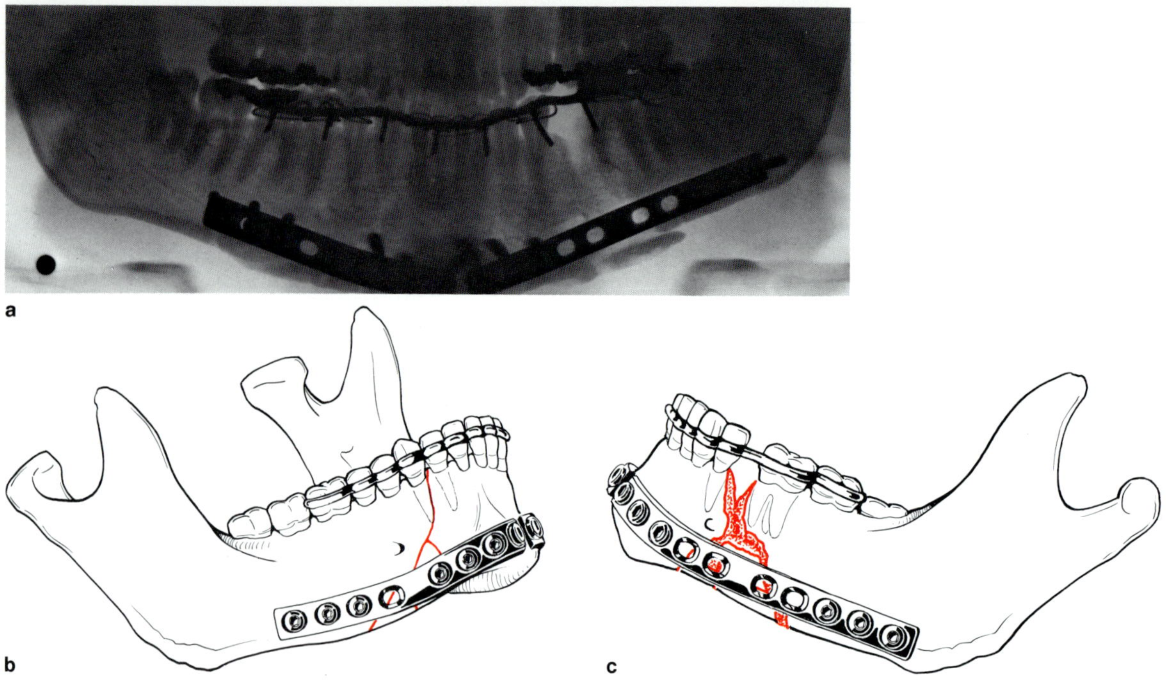

Fig. 274. **a** General view of the fixation, showing the tension-band splint, which also retains the reduced fragments, and the eight- and ten-hole plates used on the right and left sides, respectively. **b, c** Artist's renderings of the right and left sides

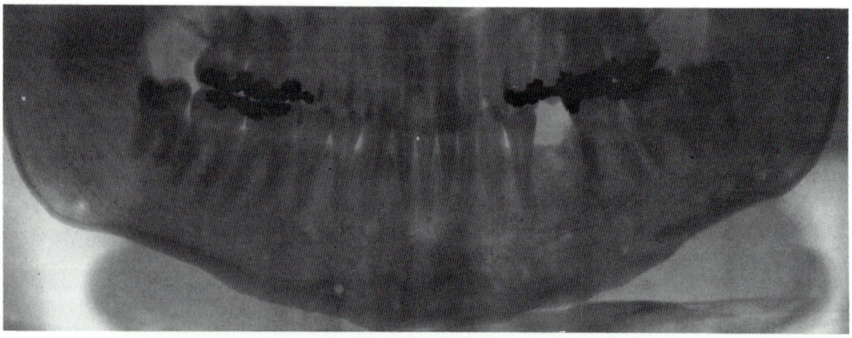

Fig. 275. Status after removal of the fixation material

Extraorally and intraorally open comminuted fracture of the left pre- and postcanine region and a preangular margin fracture of the right side with an associated subcondylar fracture (Fig. 276)

Fracture formula:	F_1 L_4 L_6/F_3 L_2 L_3
Clinical category:	F_3 S_3
Grade of severity:	IV B

Intraoral Procedure

The fractured teeth and the tooth in the line of fracture are removed. The dental arch is restored with a divided splint, carefully preserving the dentulous fragment. Intermaxillary fixation is then applied for eugnathic retention.

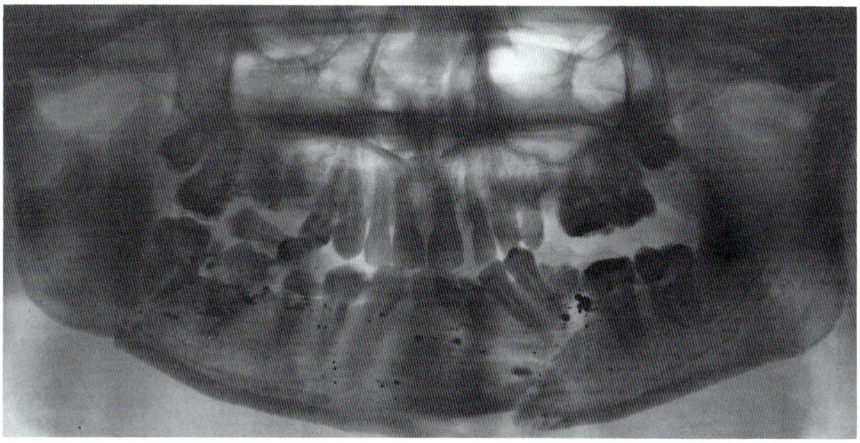

a

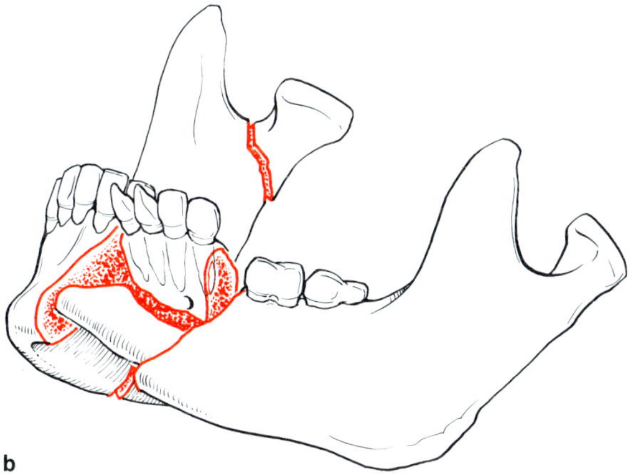

b

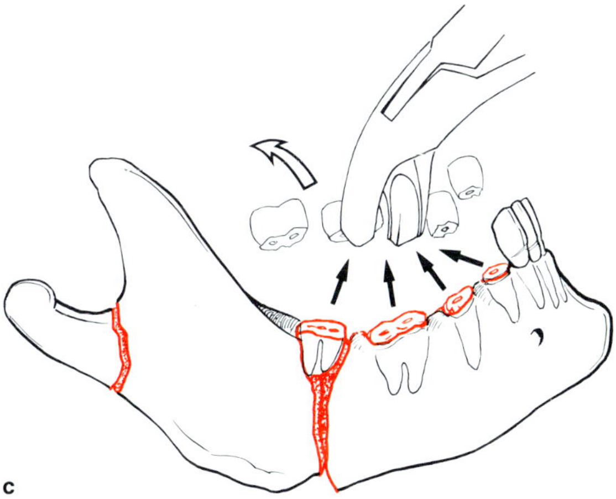

c

Fig. 276. a Comminuted fracture of the left precanine and postcanine region, right preangular margin fracture and subcondylar fracture. **b, c** Artist's rendering of the injury

Extraoral Procedure (Fig. 277)
Right side:
First the simpler, preangular margin fracture on the right side is fixed with a two-hole DCP applied as a tension band and a six-hole DCP applied as a stabilization plate. (Because of the inadequate mandibular height the tension band had to be removed.)
Left side:
The anterior comminuted area is bridged and buttressed with a 12-hole reconstruction plate attached with 4 screws in each of the main fragments (four screw rule); the 4 holes over the comminuted site are left empty. The smaller fragments that retain some periosteal coverage are left in place, eliminating the need for bone grafting. The general appearance of the fixation is shown in Fig. 277 c.

Figure 278 shows the status after removal of the plates (indriven bits of amalgam are visible on the right and left sides).

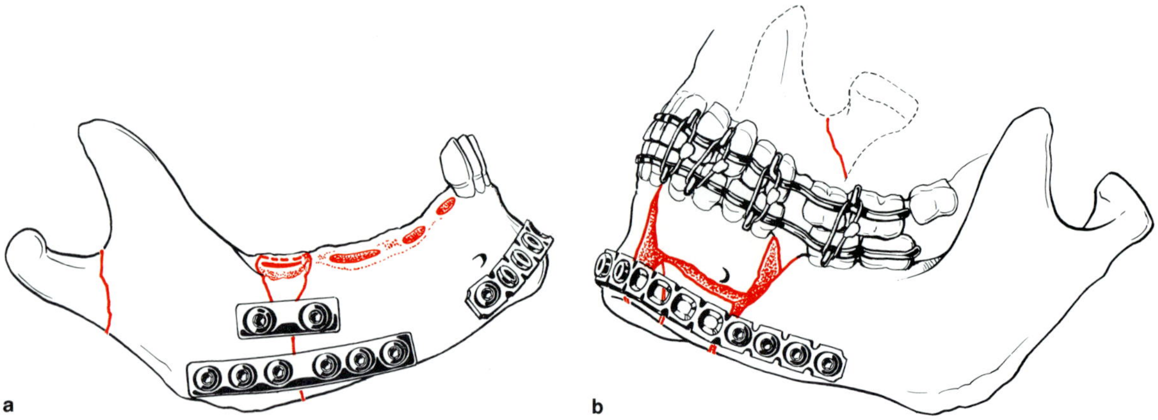

a b

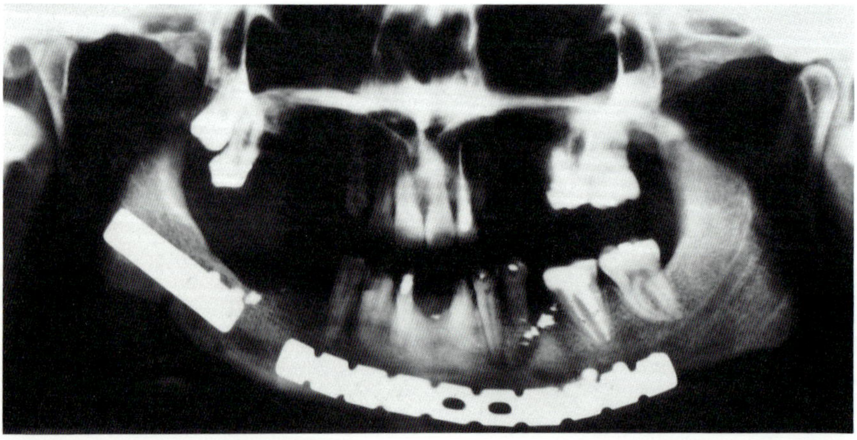

c

Fig. 277. **a** The single fracture is fixed first with a stabilization plate and tension band. (This plan of using a tension band was not realizable). **b** After intermaxillary fixation to retain the occlusion, the comminuted fracture is fixed with a long reconstruction plate. **c** Postoperative status

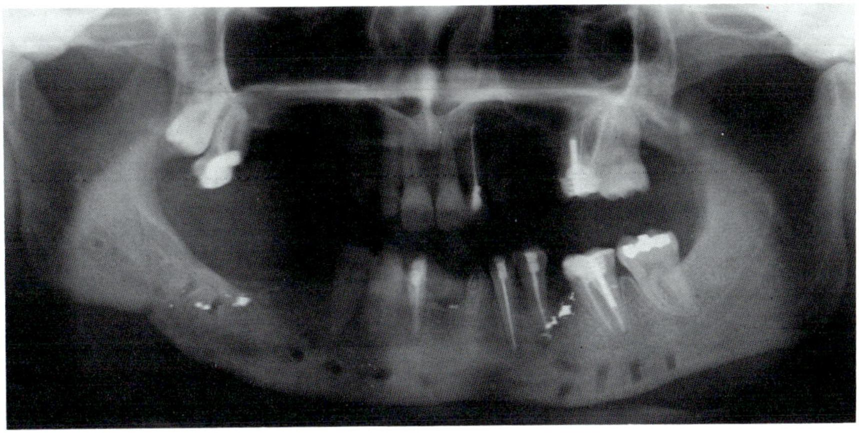

Fig. 278. Status after removal of the fixation material

Intraorally and extraorally open anterior comminuted fracture with loss of the alveolar process (Fig. 279)

Fracture formula:	F_4 L_1
Clinical category:	F_4 S_3
Grade of severity:	V A

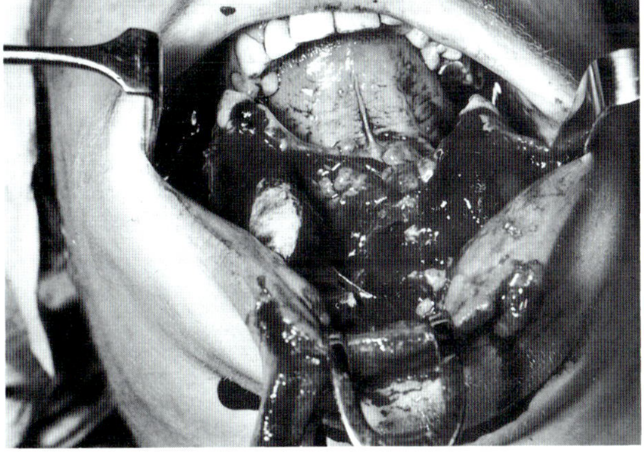

a

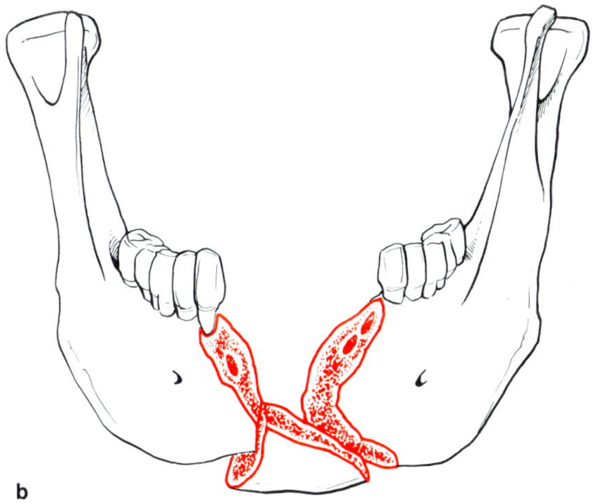

b

Fig. 279. **a** Comminuted fracture with bone loss, open intra- and extraorally. **b** Artist's rendering

Intraoral Procedure
The lateral mandibular stumps are fixed to the maxilla in normal occlusal relationship with Ernst ligatures.

Extraoral Procedure
Because the contused and lacerated wounds extend to the level of the molars in the lateral vestibular region, the internal fixation can be performed through the intraoral route without need for additional exposure. The remaining fragments of the alveolar process are prone to necrosis, infection, and sequestration and therefore are removed. The central symphyseal fragment, displaced lingually, is repositioned and fixed to the 14-hole reconstruction plate with 3 screws to help bridge the defect. The mucosal defect in the region of the alveolar process contraindicates primary cancellous bone grafting (Fig. 280).

Figure 281 shows the status after removal of the plate.

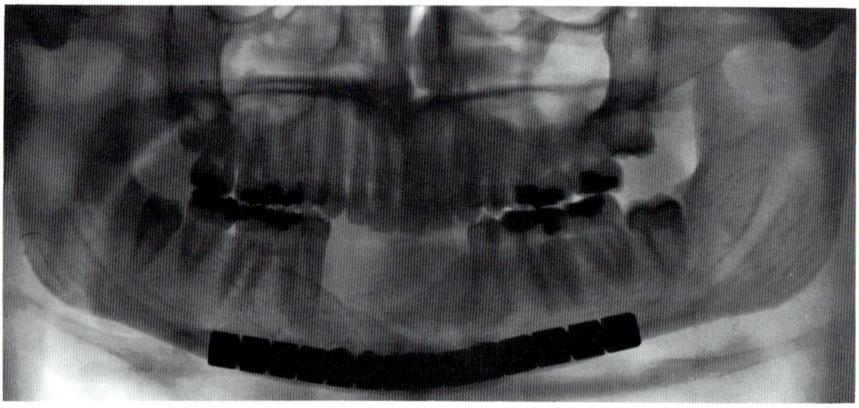
a

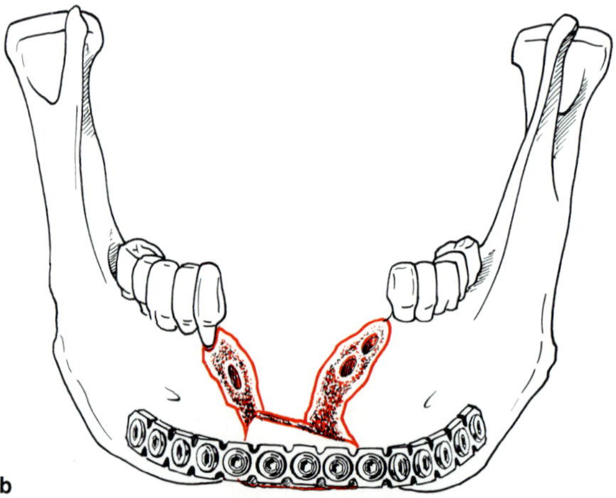
b

Fig. 280. **a** The fracture site and bone defect are stably bridged with a 14-hole reconstruction plate, obeying the 4 screw rule (see text). **b** Artist's rendering

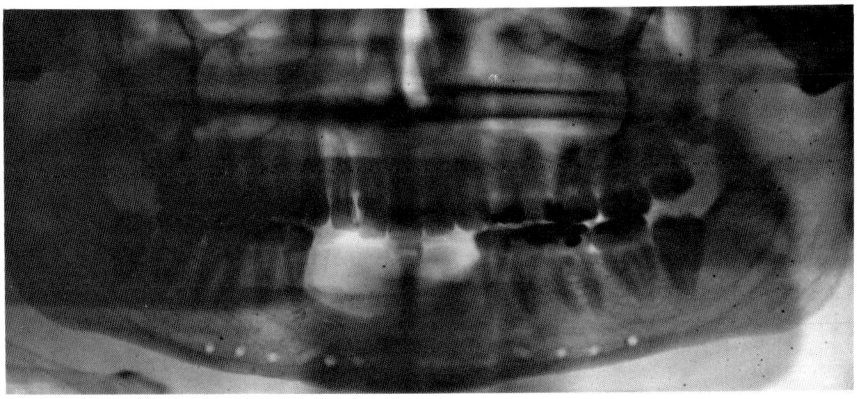

Fig. 281. Status after removal of the plate

Intraorally and extraorally open fracture of the anterior mandible with loss of the alveolar process (Fig. 282)

Fracture formula:	F_4 L_1
Clinical category:	F_4 S_3
Grade of severity:	V A

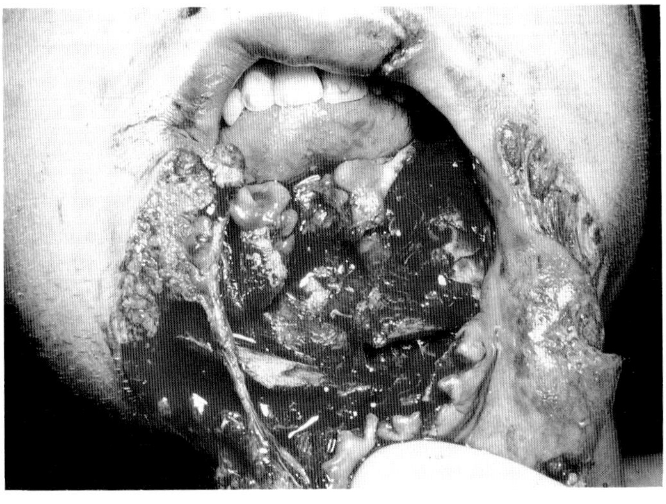

Fig. 282. Intra- and extraoral open fracture with a bone defect

Intraoral Procedure

Intermaxillary fixation of the mandibular stumps with Ernst ligatures applied to four remaining teeth on the right side and three on the left.

Extraoral Procedure

Option I (Fig. 283 a–c)

An eight-hole DCP is applied on the right side with its mesial end attached to the largest intermediate fragment; three plate holes over smaller fragments are left empty. On the right side, the large intermediate fragment is stabilized superiorly with a three-hole tension-band plate and interferiorly with a four-hole DCP.

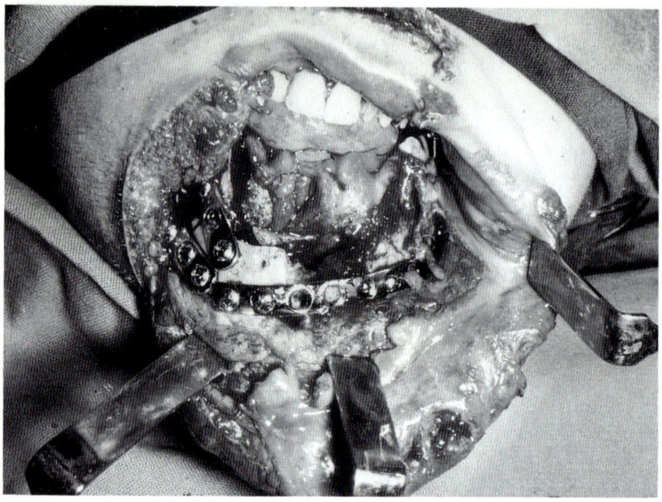

a

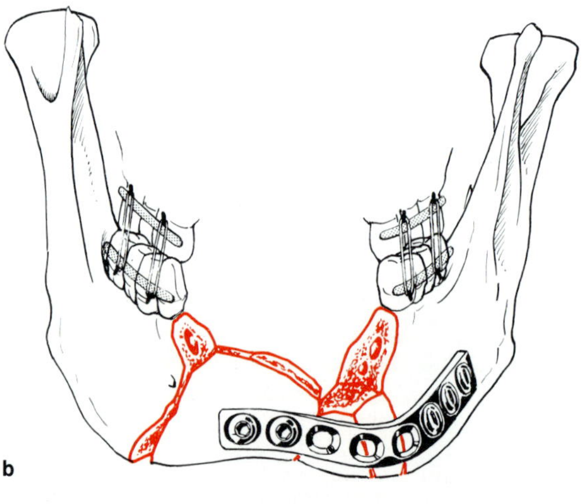

b

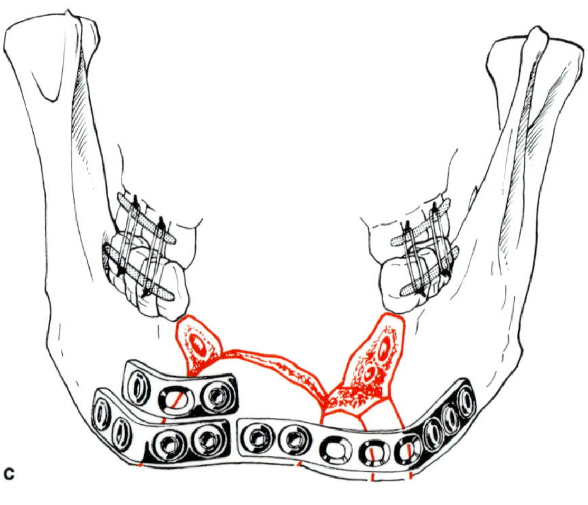

c

Fig. 283. **a** Option 1: internal fixation with three separate plates – a tension-band plate and stabilization plate on the right, a basal plate on the left. **b, c** Artist's renderings

Option II (Fig. 284)
A single 14-hole reconstruction plate is used to bridge the entire fracture site.

First corrective operation (Fig. 285)
Seven months later the plate is removed, and an autologous bone graft is inserted to reconstruct the alveolar process. The block is attached with an eight-hole DCP.

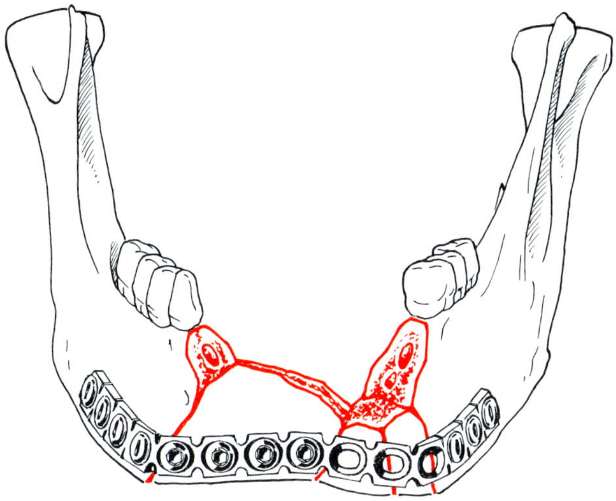

Fig. 284. Option 2: 14-hole reconstruction plate

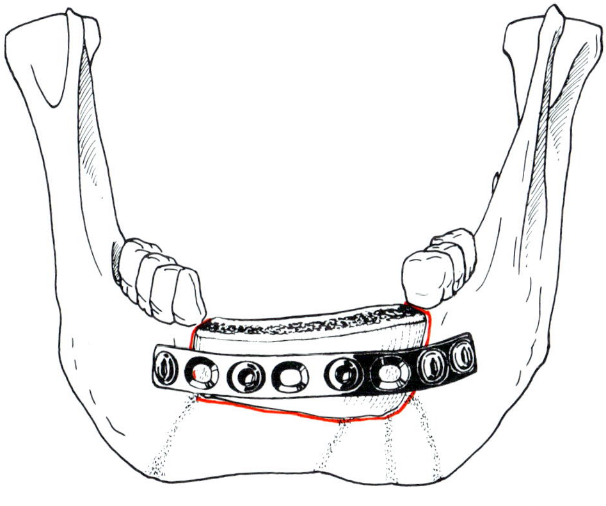

Fig. 285. First corrective operation: augmentation of the alveolar process

Second corrective operation (Fig. 286)
Eighteen months later the plate is removed. The healed graft now forms a base for the insertion of a DCI (dynamic compression implant) that will be used to support a partial denture.

The status nine years after implantation is shown in Fig. 287.

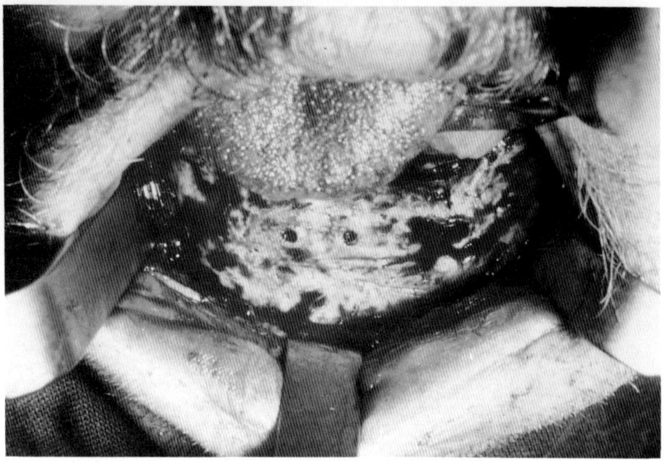

a

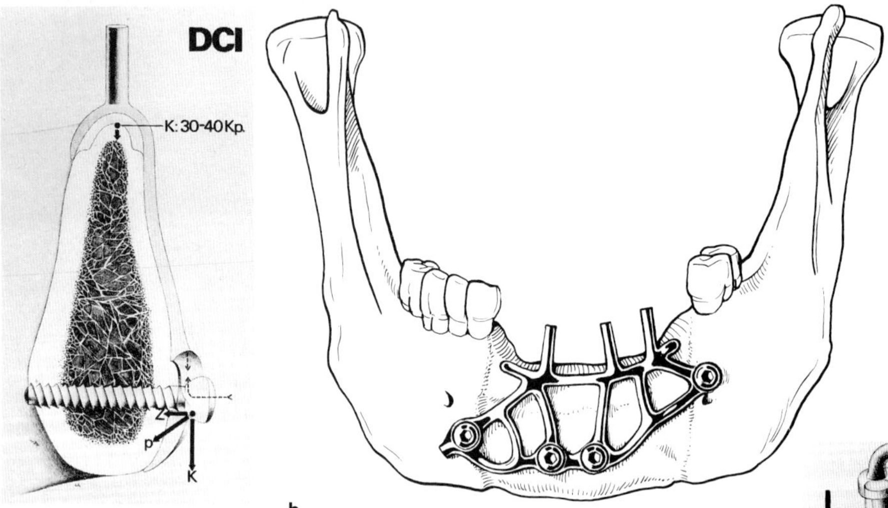

b

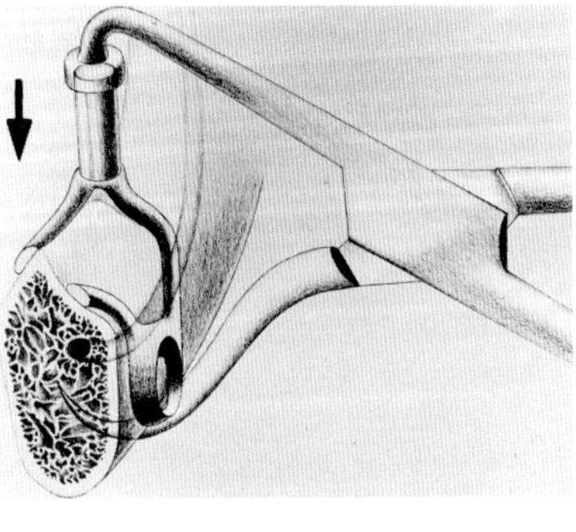

Fig. 286. a, b After healing of the bone graft, the plate is removed, and a dynamic compression implant (DCI) is attached by the spherical gliding principle (see p. 41). *Left:* Components of static compression in the vertical (K + P) and horizontal (Z) directions. *Right:* Manual precompression is applied before the eccentric 2.0-mm hole is drilled (see p. 98)

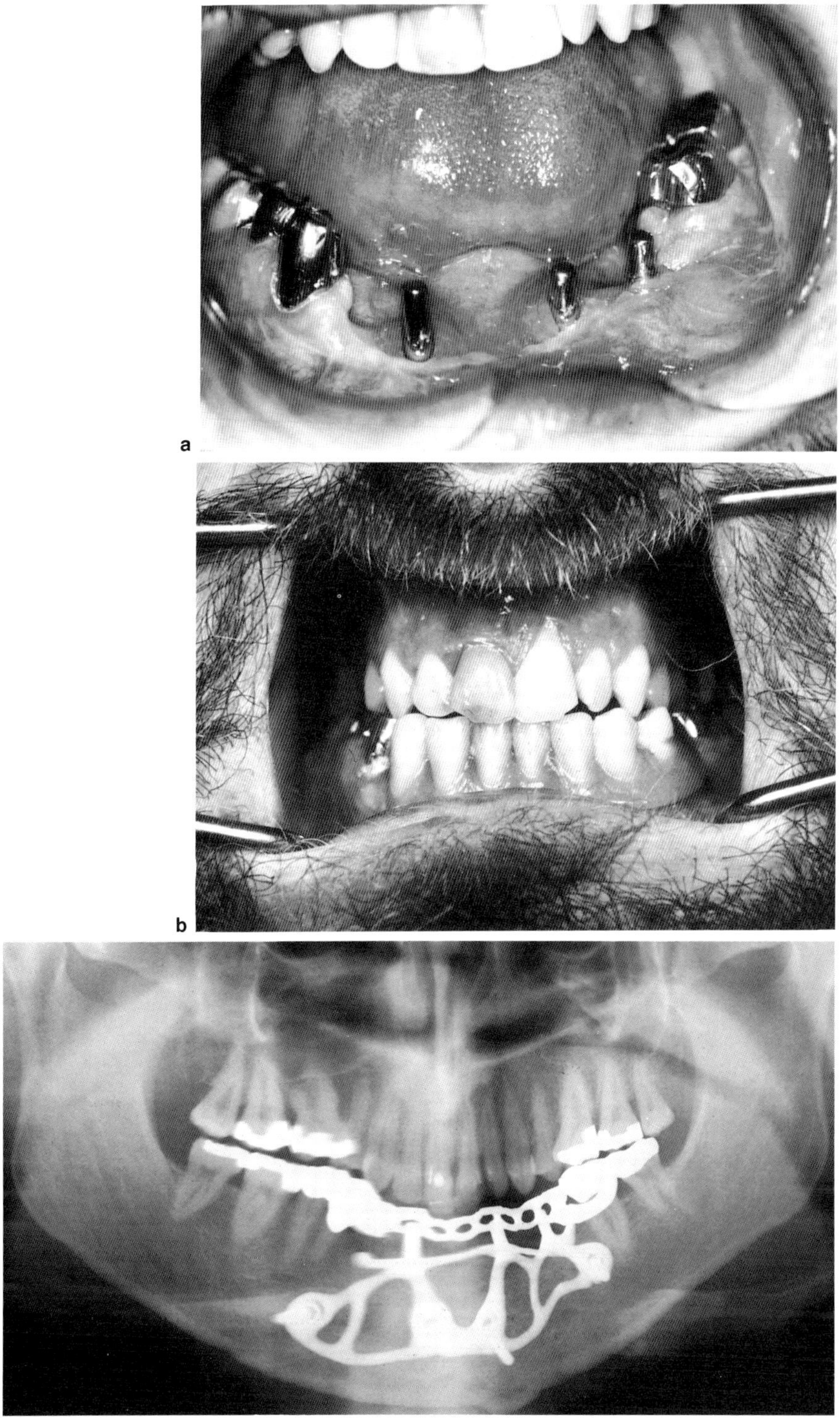

a

b

c

Fig. 287 a–c. Status nine years after implantation

6.8 Gunshot Fractures

These are injuries of category F_4 S_4 (severity V B) caused by a bullet or other missile in which a fracture with bone loss coexists with a soft-tissue defect.

The extent of facial bone loss in these injuries is exceedingly variable, especially in cases where the patient, while attempting suicide, places the muzzle of the firearm beneath the chin. When applied in this manner, the carbine rifle (a weapon commonly used in Switzerland) produces a typical pattern of injury involving extensive loss of substance from the midportion of the mandible and from the central or lateral midfacial region (Fig. 288). Frequently the orbital bone is bypassed as the missile, entering by a paramedian or anterior submandibular route, glances off the bone below the temporal fossa and exits at the temple. Trismus develops later as a result of damage to the masticatory muscles unless early, intensive mobilization is instituted under appropriate guidance.

There are two key aspects of initial treatment: bridging the bony defects with internal fixation appliances, and leaving the soft-tissue defect in its true extent. Simple coaptation of the wound edges would only promote soft-tissue contractures and secondary deformity of facial areas that are still morphologically intact.

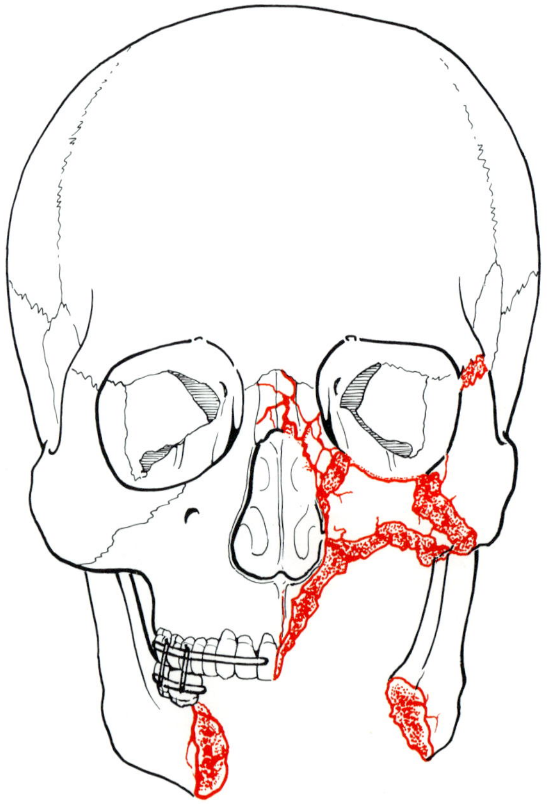

Fig. 288. The bullet in this patient entered submentally, causing loss of the mandibular body and portions of the maxilla, anterior orbit, and nasal bone (drawing made from radiographs of the patient in Fig. 289 a)

Bridging involves reestablishing the morphology of the mandibular arch, the intermaxillary relation, and the essential contours of the midfacial region (Fig. 289). Every tooth that is still present in the mandible and has a maxillary antagonist is a valuable aid to orthograde retention of the mandibular stumps. In the case in Fig. 289 b, a single retained molar was the key to shaping and attaching the bridge plate and to subsequent bone grafting (Fig. 290).

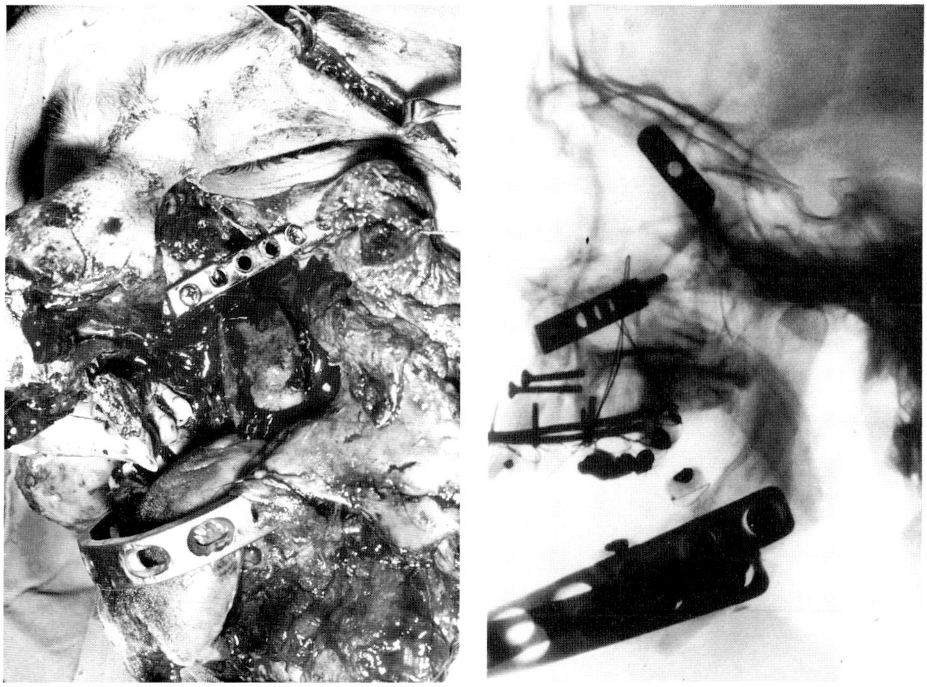

a b

Fig. 289. **a** Reconstruction of the mandibular arch using a contoured DCP (at that time, 1971, the reconstruction plate was still under development). Two DCPs are used to bridge the infraorbital defect and fix the residual zygoma to the frontal bone. **b** Status of skeletal fixation; the alveolar process is additionally fixed with two lag screws

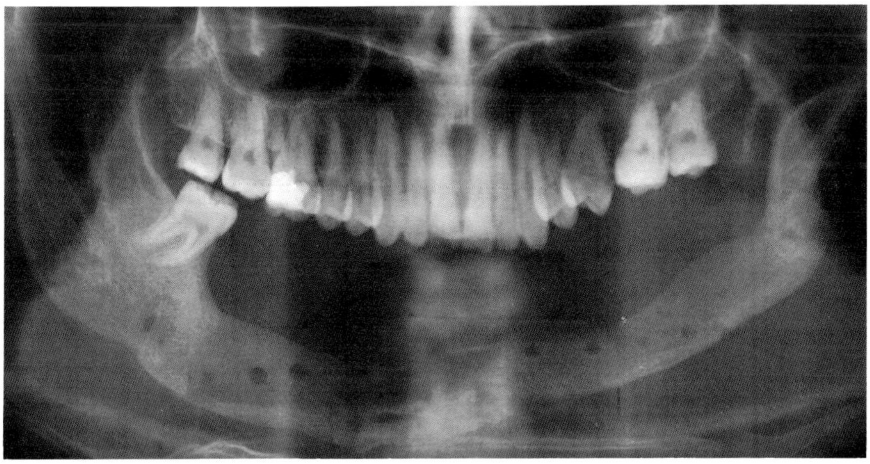

Fig. 290. The defect is bridged with an autologous bone graft

With total loss of the mandibular body, preformed reconstruction plates are used. They are available in three sizes (see Fig. 137 a–e).

Clearly, restoring the shape and continuity of the mandibular arch is a necessary prelude to a planned reconstruction of the walls of the oral cavity and the face. The baseline for all restorations is the portion of the face that remains. (Its deformation by primary coaptation of the wound edges would only hinder later reconstructive efforts.) Experience has demonstrated that primary bridging of the osseous defects with internal fixation material and the coverage of wound surfaces with mesh grafts constitute the best prophylaxis against soft-tissue contractures. The mandibular stumps, when stabilized with the reconstruction plate (applied with a minimum of four screws per side), may be left uncovered without danger of infection.

Depending on the local situation and the patient's psychological status, preparations for soft-tissue reconstruction can be made at an early stage. In the case shown in Fig. 289 a, for example, a round pedicled flap (Fig. 291 a) and visor flap (Fig. 291 b) were used to secure coverage of the residual defect (Fig. 292).

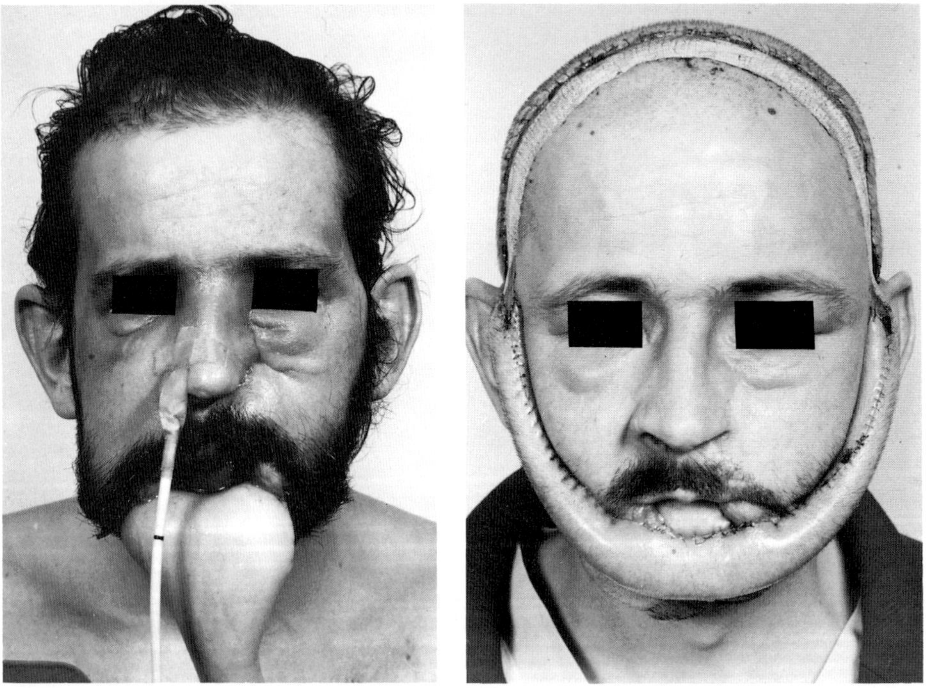

a b

291. **a** A round, pedicled flap is used to reline the oral cavity and reconstruct the lower lip. **b** A visor flap is utilized to reconstruct the chin

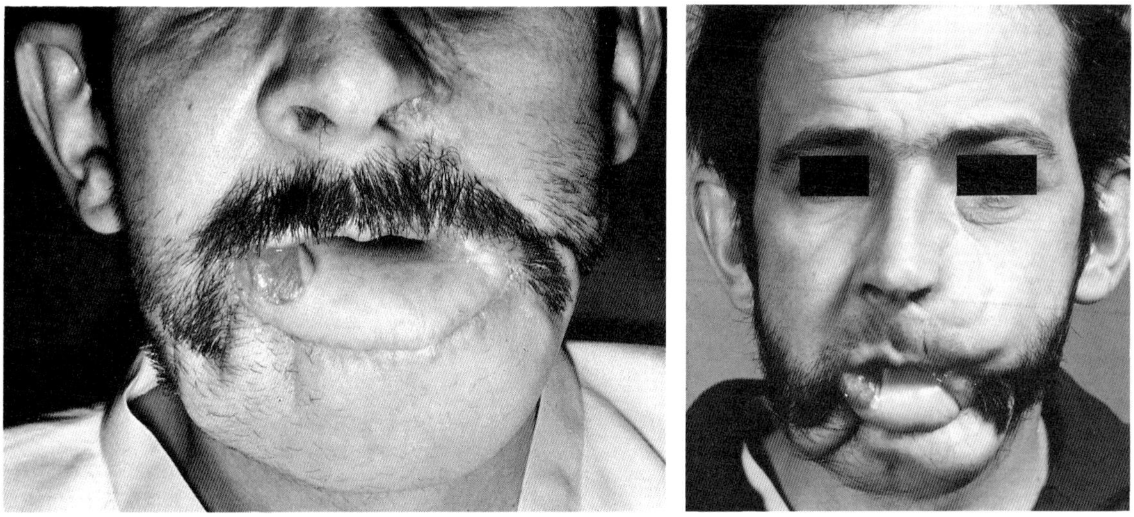

a b

Fig. 292. **a** Intermediate stage of the reconstruction. **b** Final stage of the reconstruction (patient declined further surgery)

7 Treatment of Mandibular Fractures in Children

Functionally stable internal fixation is contraindicated for fractures of the pediatric mandible. The fracture affects two substrates that are extremely sensitive to outside influences: the bone tissue and the tooth germs. Irreversible growth disturbances can result from damage to these structures.

The vulnerability of the germ tissue is offset by the tremendous regenerative capacity of the bone, which is inversely proportional to age. The pediatric fracture has the fastest rate of healing, and indeed it would take some effort on the part of the therapist to keep the fracture from consolidating. Nonunion is a virtual impossibility.

The guiding therapeutic principle, then, is "first do no harm." Conservative treatment is appropriate in the great majority of cases. A good rule to follow is to splint open or closed fractures that are undisplaced or minimally displaced. When the correct occlusion is established, minor degrees of axial malalignment, angulation, and displacements by the width of the mandible may be tolerated if a more accurate reduction cannot be obtained.

Only in older children and adolescents should one consider the open reduction and fixation of a closed fracture with an interosseous wire suture or a miniplate. This would be indicated, say, for a comminuted or severely displaced fracture that prevents manual restoration of the occlusion.

The open fracture lends itself to fixation with interosseous wires. The case illustrated involves an extraorally open, comminuted fracture of the angle and ramus with injury to the parotid gland and buccal facial nerve branches (Fig. 293 a).

Intraoral Procedure

The occlusion is retained by intermaxillary fixation with acrylated arch bars and wire ligatures.

Extraoral Procedure

The preauricular degloving injury gives direct access for interosseous wiring at the inferior border of the mandible, at the base of the condylar neck, and at the semilunar incisure (Fig. 293 b). Treatment of the nerve and soft-tissue injuries follows.

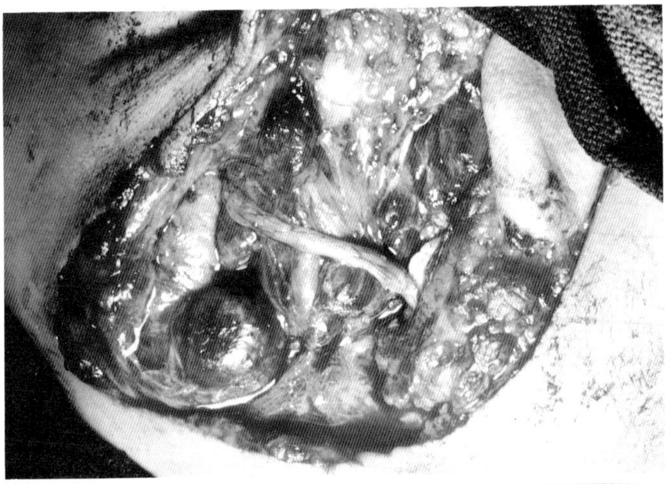

a

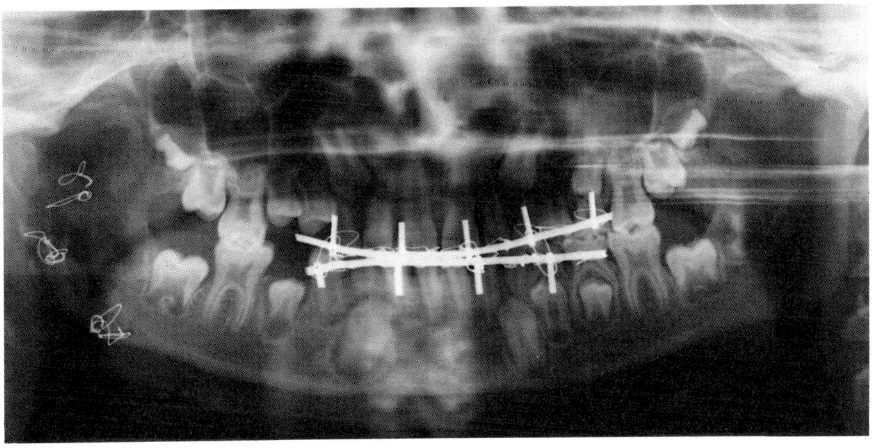

b

Fig. 293. **a** Degloving injury involving the parotid and angle region. (The superficial parotid flap is still attached to the skin; the severed facial nerve branch has been microsurgically repaired). **b** The fragments are approximated with interosseous wires. (The intermaxillary fixation may be released after three weeks by replacing the intermaxillary wires with loose elastic bands)

Part III

Reconstructive Surgery

1 Introduction

The goal of functionally stable internal fixation is the rapid restoration of form and function. That is why ASIF principles have applications not just in fracture management but also in the broad field of reconstructive surgery.

The main reconstructive application of ASIF principles is in the treatment if nonunion, defined as the local cessation of all reparative processes of bone healing. It is possible to reactivate these processes by applying interfragmental compression alone or in conjunction with autogenous bone grafting.

Another application is in the reconstruction of mandibular discontinuities caused by tumor resections. This basically involves the functionally stable bridging of segmental defects, which may be either a definitive treatment or a prelude to autogenous bone grafting. A major goal in these patients is the primary reduction of morbidity so that the immediate, functionally stable bridging of the defect can be integrated into the resective procedure.

Finally, the advantages of early mobilization and direct osseous union are of great benefit in orthognathic surgery. Experience has shown that stable internal fixation is as essential to a successful outcome as the corrective osteotomy itself.

2 Nonunion

Definition: We define a nonunion as *any fracture that has failed to unite by six months.* A varient of nonunion is pseudoarthrosis, in which there is a *true false joint with sealing of the medullary cavity,* formation of articular cartilage, and an articular pseudofovea. Pseudarthrosis is illustrated by the nearthrosis that is deliberately created by the functional therapy of a condylar neck fractures or fracture-dislocation of the temporomandibular joint.

"Delayed union" is present in a fracture that fails to consolidate within the sixth and twelfth postoperative week.

2.1 Causes

A number of factors contribute to the production of nonunion, the most common being instability and infection (see pp. 5 and 33). These are followed by inaccurate reduction, commonly seen in conservative fracture treatment (malalignment nonunion), and absence of contact between the bone ends (nonunion with a defect). A less important cause is soft-tissue interposition (interposition nonunion), which may result from laceration of the masticatory muscles over the fracture site.

2.2 Classification

We divide nonunions into two broad clinical groups: *noninfected* and *infected.* Within these groups we further recognize the reactive, *vascular* nonunion as opposed to the nonreactive, *avascular* nonunion.[11]

---

[11] An *avascular* or nonreactive state results from a failure of revascularization and the associated absence of cellular invasion. By contrast, *devitalized* fragments may still contain an osseoinductive matrix after cell death has occurred and therefore can be revascularized from surrounding tissues (e.g., larger exposed fragments in a comminuted area).

2.3 Clinical Aspects and Treatment of Noninfected Nonunions

Approximately 90% of nonunions that develop following a neglected or conservatively treated fracture are of the *vascular* (reactive) type. In some cases flared, elephant-foot-like bone ends may be seen on radiographs (Fig. 294a). This hypertrophy results from the rich blood supply to the ends of the fragments (Fig. 294b). Consequently, in this type of nonunion (see Fig. 294b) and in the delayed union it is unnecessary to resect the bone ends, and interfragmental compression is all that is needed for consolidation to occur (Fig. 295a–c). Once immobilized, the interposed connective tissue will rapidly mineralize and change to bone. Other examples of cases amenable to this form of treatment are presented below.

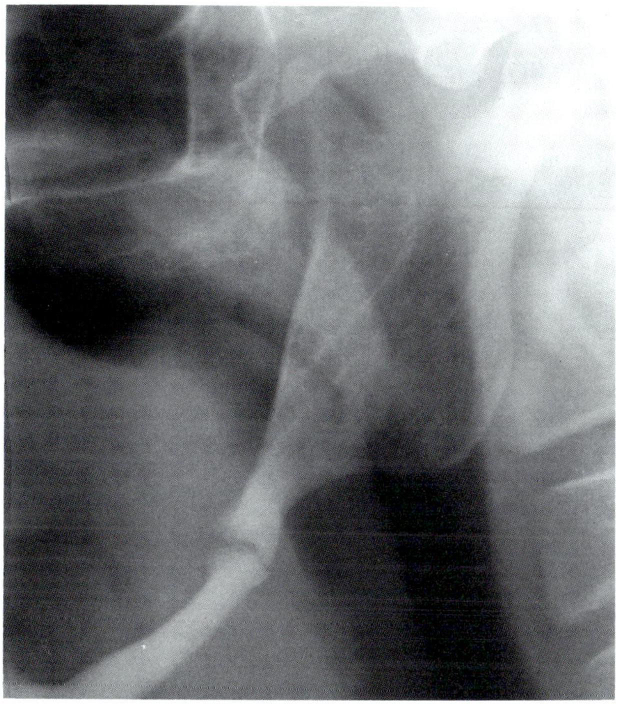

a

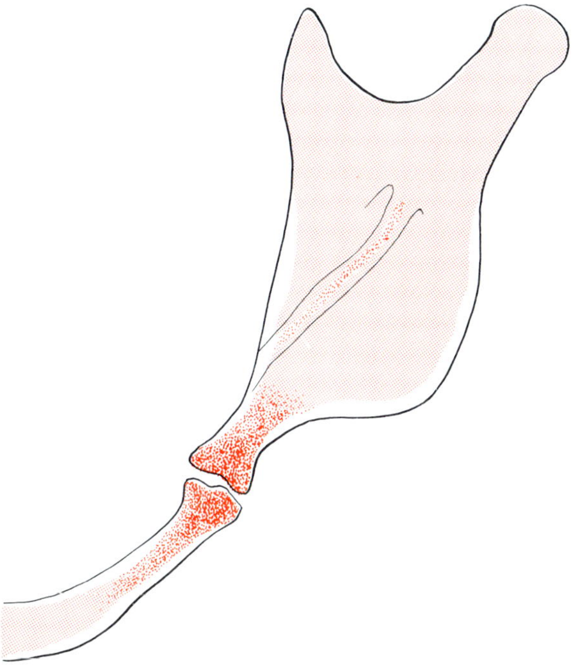

b

Fig. 294. **a** Vascular nonunion, recognized by the hypertrophic, "elephant-foot" flaring of the bone ends. (This hypertrophy is less obvious on films of the dentulous mandible.) **b** Artist's depiction of the blood supply to the bone ends

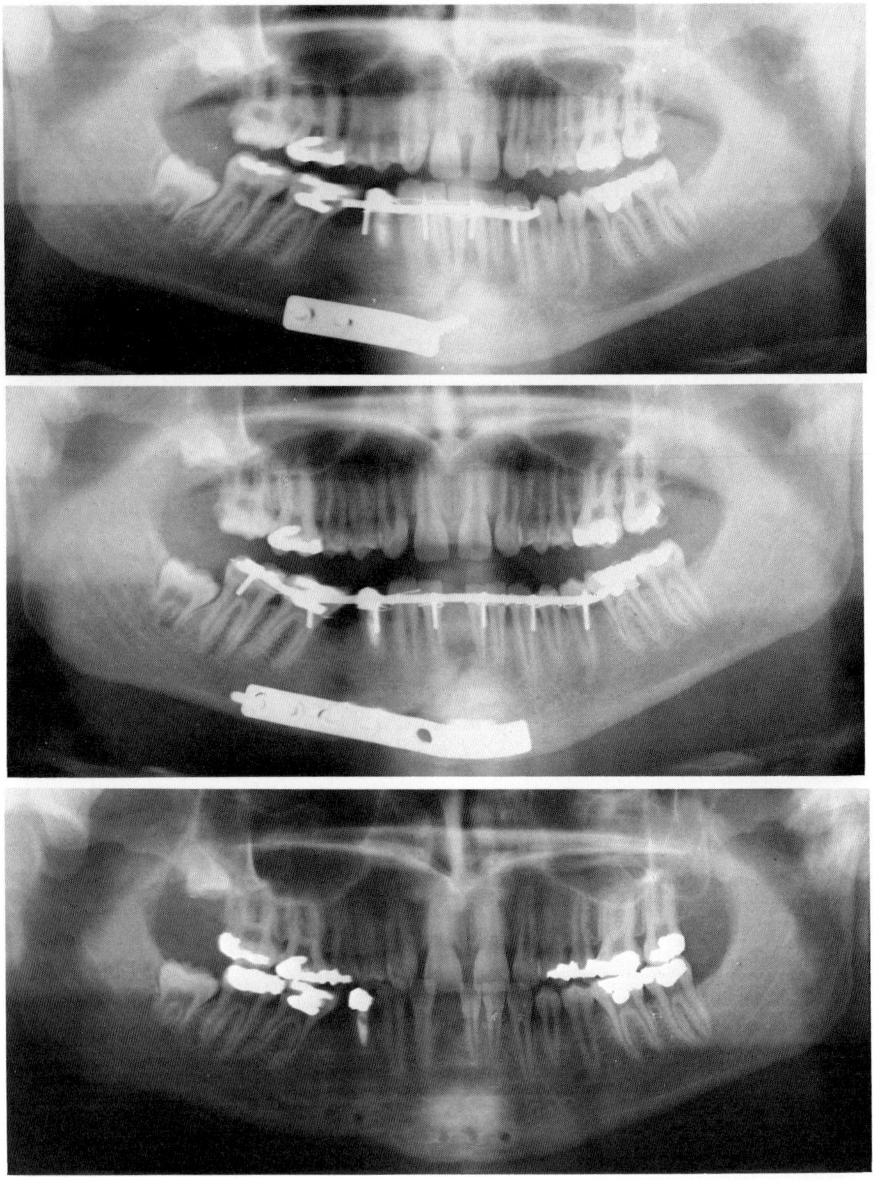
a
b
c

Fig. 295. **a** Vascular nonunion secondary to an inadequate internal fixation (a common error in fractures near the mental foramen due to underestimation of the anterior lever-arm forces). **b** Treatment consists of increasing the interfragmental pressure with a plate twice as long as the original. **c** Consolidation of the nonunion following the revision

Bilateral malalignment nonunion [six months after surgery (Fig. 296)]
This condition is treated by revising the internal fixation and applying adequate interfragmental compression (Fig. 297).
Right side:
Six-hole EDCP, as no teeth are available for a tension-band splint.
Left side:
Four-hole DCP combined with a tension-band splint.
Figure 298 shows the status after removal of the fixation material and restoration of the occlusion.

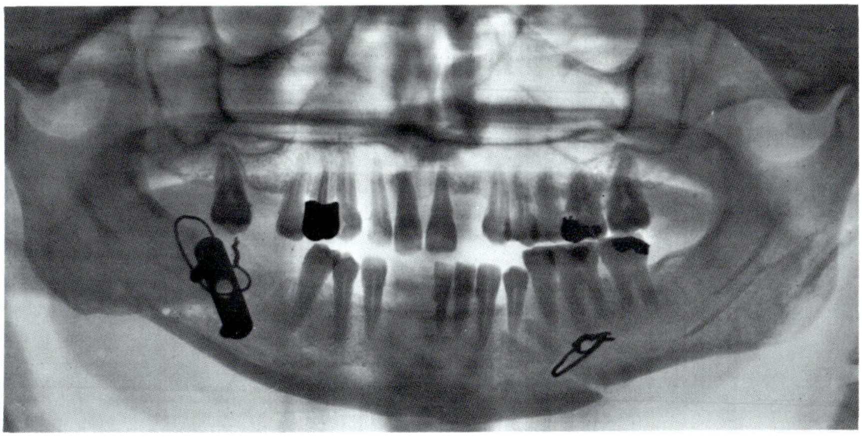
a

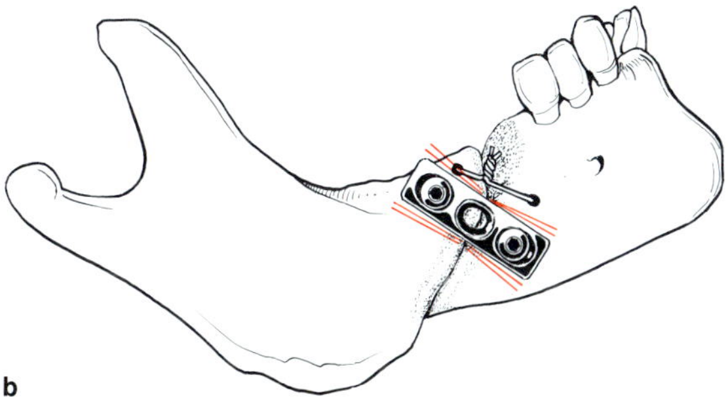
b

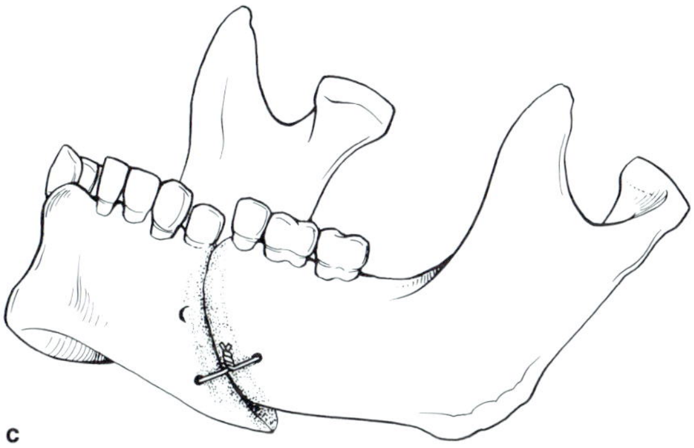
c

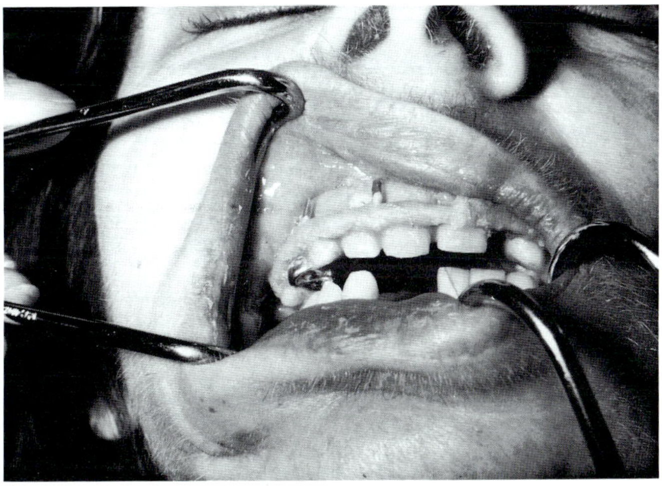
d

Fig. 296. **a** Bilateral nonunion secondary to an inadequate internal fixation performed elsewhere. **b, c** Artist's depictions. **d** Malocclusion resulting from the previous internal fixation

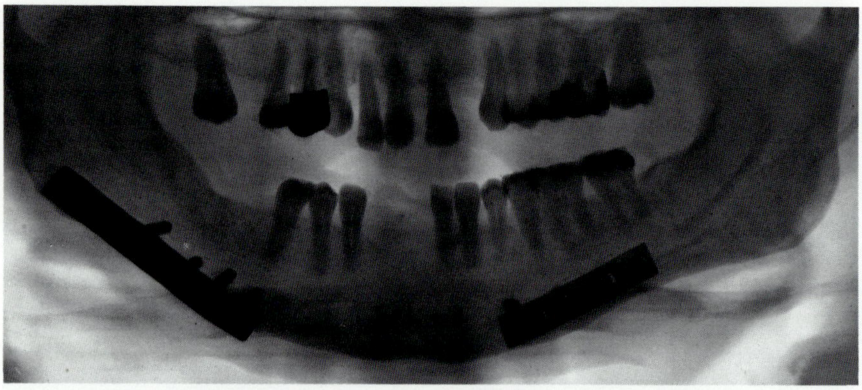

a

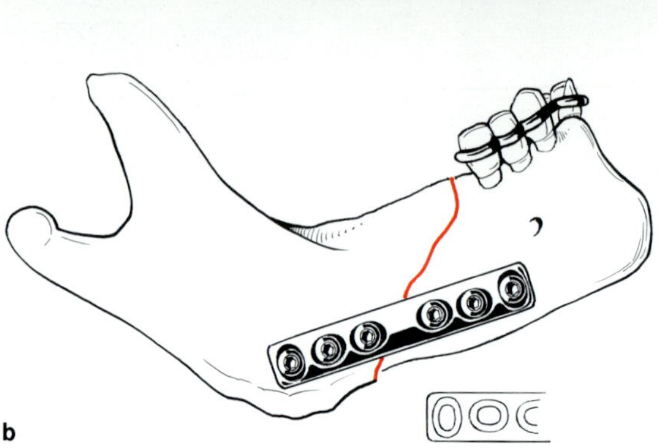

b

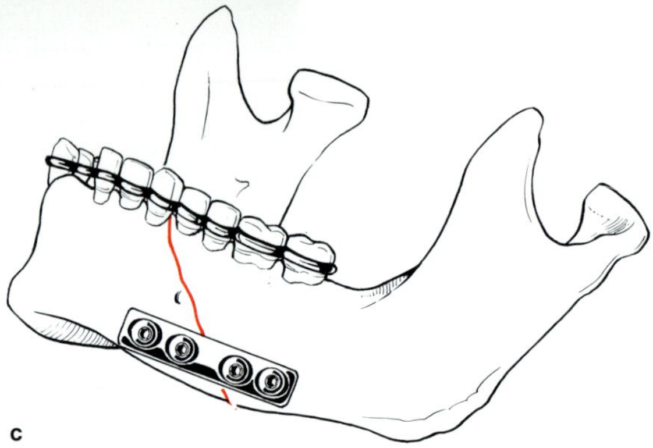

c

Fig. 297. **a** Panoramic view of the revisionary fixation. **b** The right side is fixed with an EDCP. **c** The left side is stabilized with a DCP and tension-band splint

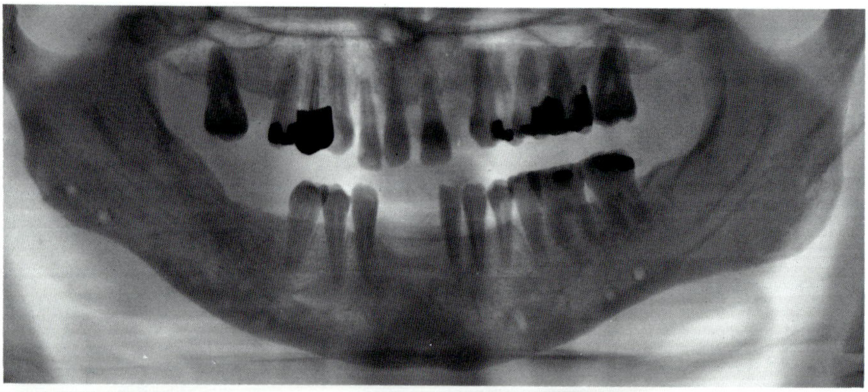

a

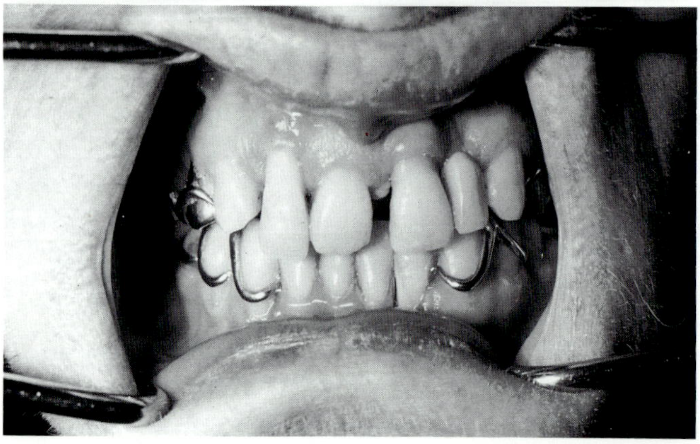

b

Fig. 298 a, b. Status following **a** removal of the fixation material and **b** restoration of the occlusion

Delayed union of an untreated low subcondylar fracture (sustained 8 weeks earlier) **coexisting with a consolidated angle margin fracture** (Fig. 299 a) The neglected subcondylar fracture has resulted in malocclusion and restriction of mandibular opening (Fig. 299 c).

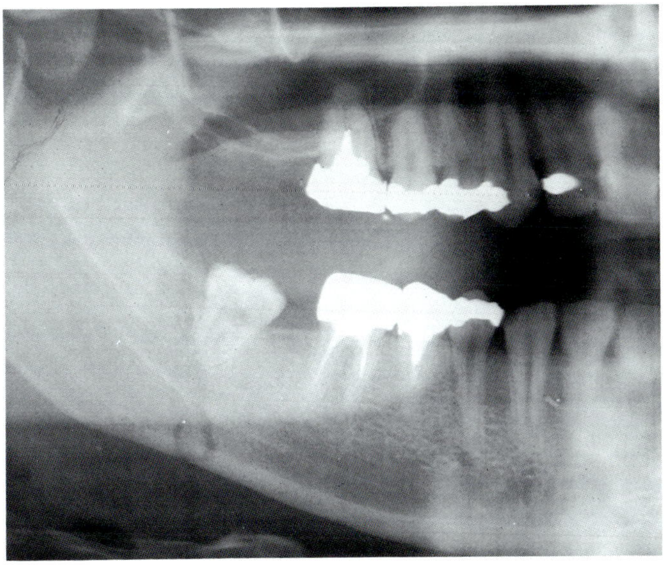

a

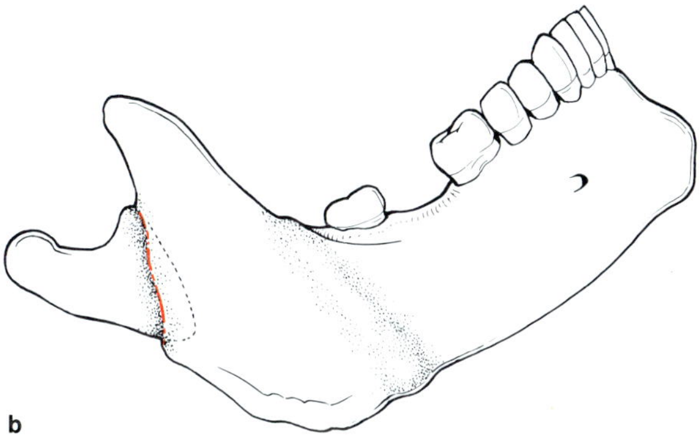

b

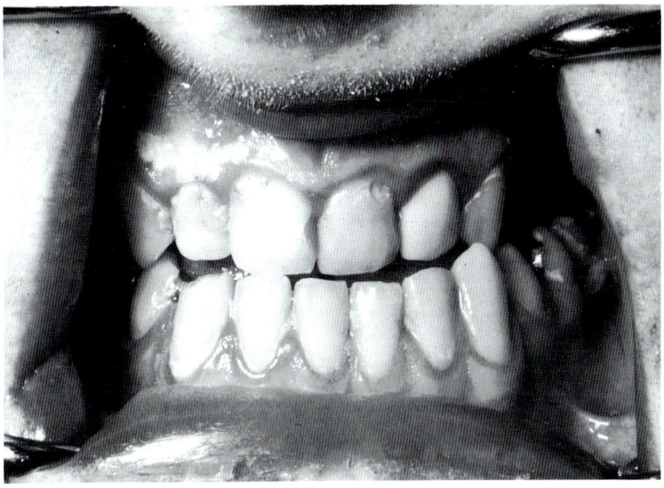

c

Fig. 299. **a** Delayed union of a subcondylar fracture with a consolidated angle fracture following conservative therapy. **b** Artist's depiction. **c** Nonocclusion resulting from the previous therapy

The delayed union is stabilized with a four-hole and a two-hole DCP (tension band plate) after the removal of interposed connective tissue and cartilage (Fig. 300a). First the normal occlusion is established and retained; this is aided by the newly gained mobility of the fragments. Because the vascularity of the bone ends cannot be assessed on X-ray films, so the vas-

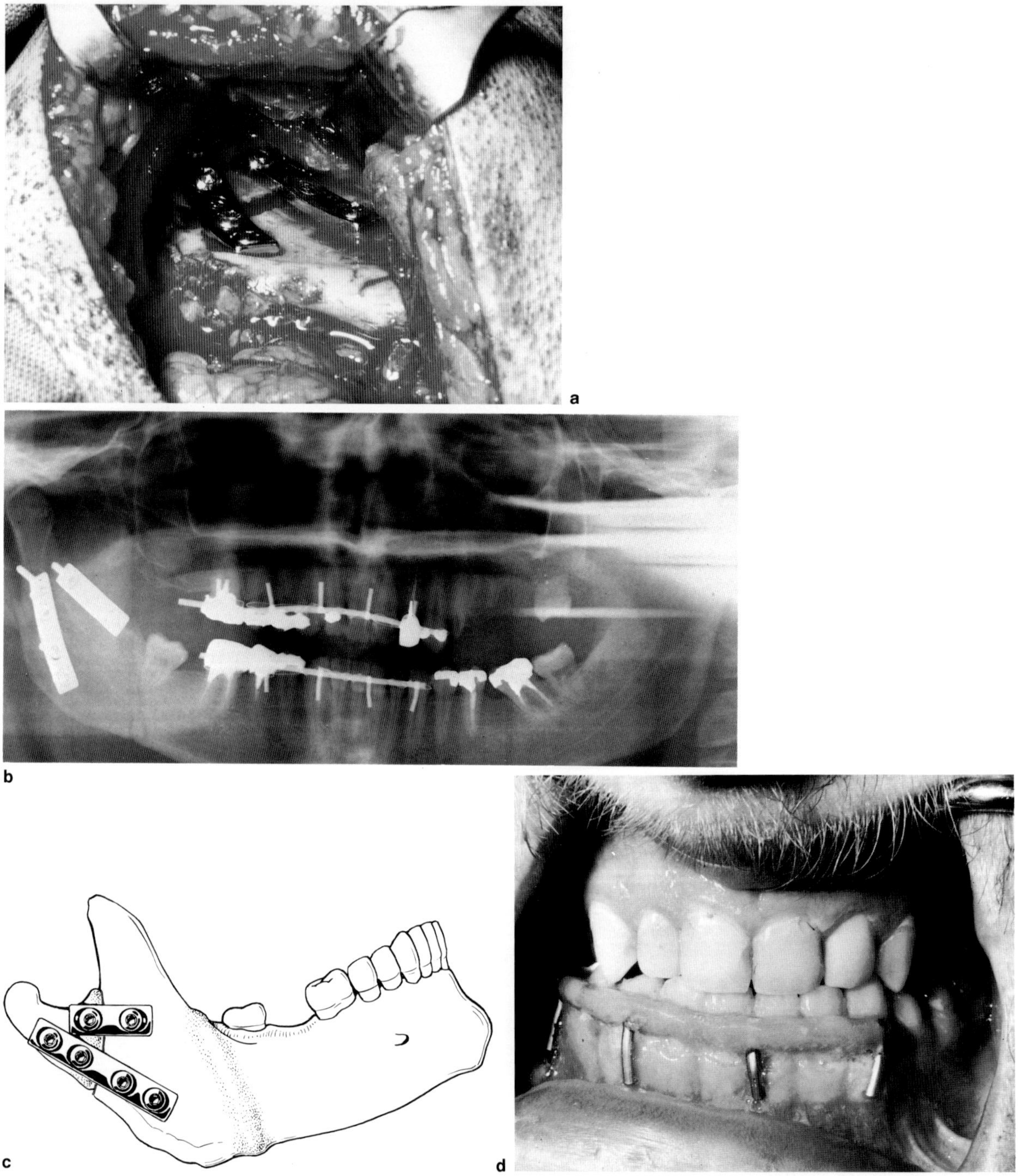

Fig. 300. **a** The delayed union is stabilized with a four-hole and a two-hole DCP. **b** Radiographic appearance. **c** Artist's depiction. **d** The restored occlusion

cular status cannot be determined until the site is surgically exposed and trial bur holes are made.

The radiographic appearance of the internal fixation is shown in Fig. 300b and an artist's depiction in Fig. 300c.

Figure 300d shows the restored occlusion and the auxiliary splint used for peroperative retention of the occlusion.

2.4 Clinical Aspects and Treatment of Nonreactive, Avascular Nonunions

The atrophic, nonreactive nonunion in the edentulous mandible presents unflared, avascular bone ends on radiographs (Fig. 301). This condition is prognostically and therapeutically equivalent to the osteoporotic, nonreactive, "oligotrophic" nonunion described by Weber and Cech (1973, 1976). Figure 302 shows a typical example: an avascular nonunion in a severely atrophic mandible diagnosed 9 months after the fixation of a double fracture by interosseous wiring and prosthetic splints. The patient, a 64-year-old woman, experienced significant physical and psychological deficits from the failed therapy relating to loss of masticatory function and post-traumatic trigeminal neuralgia. The osteoporotic state of the bone and the

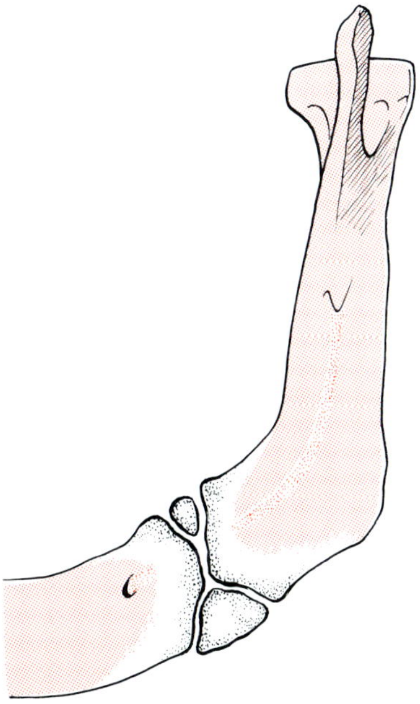

Fig. 301. Avascular, nonreactive nonunion with partial necrosis of the bone ends and necrotic intermediate fragments

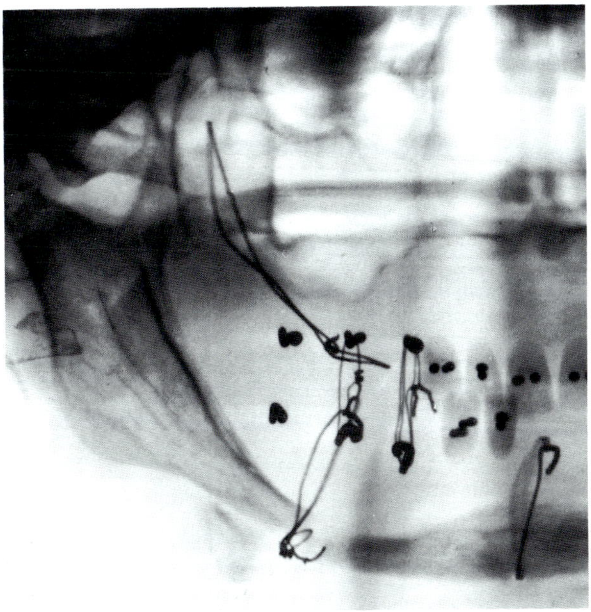

Fig. 302. Avascular nonunion

instability contributed to the production of a nonreactive, oligotrophic nonunion. Intermaxillary immobilization is contraindicated in this situation, as it promotes atrophy and removes functional stimulus from the hyporeactive bone ends.

When a functionally stable internal fixation is performed after removal of the a vascular bone ends (Fig. 303), the early mobilization and cyclic loading of the jaw create a situation in which the bone can regain its original strength. While the shielding action of the plate prolongs the consolidation process, much as in conservative therapy, it makes the posttreatment healing period far more acceptable to the patient.

The status after plate removal is shown in Fig. 304.

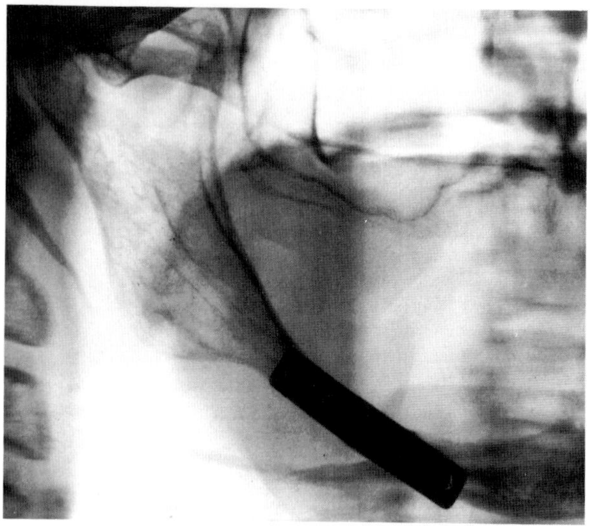

Fig. 303. Interfragmental compression with a six-hole plate after removal of the avascular bone ends

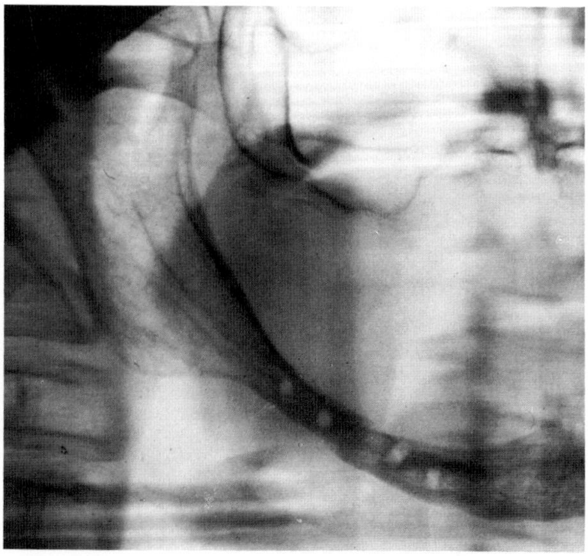

Fig. 304. Status following removal of the plate

2.5 Clinical Aspects and Treatment of Infected Nonunions

We recognize two categories of infected nonunion: the previously infected nonunion and the infected, draining nonunion.

2.5.1 Previously Infected Nonunion

The sequel to a resolved fracture-line osteitis may be a nonunion whose fragments are in contact or a nonunion with a bone defect.

The case in Fig. 305 is typical of a nonunion with a defect. It involves an infected, iatrogenic fracture caused by the surgical removal of an impacted premolar. The osteitis resolved with irrigation therapy, whereupon a six-hole DCP was applied to stabilize the fracture (Fig. 306a).

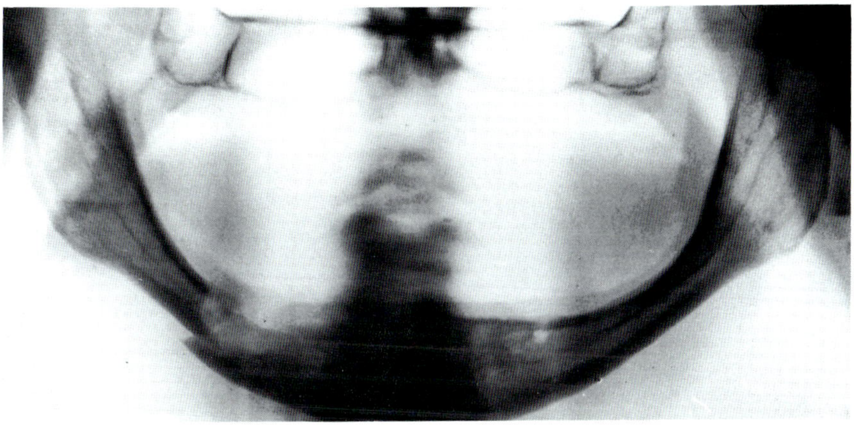

a

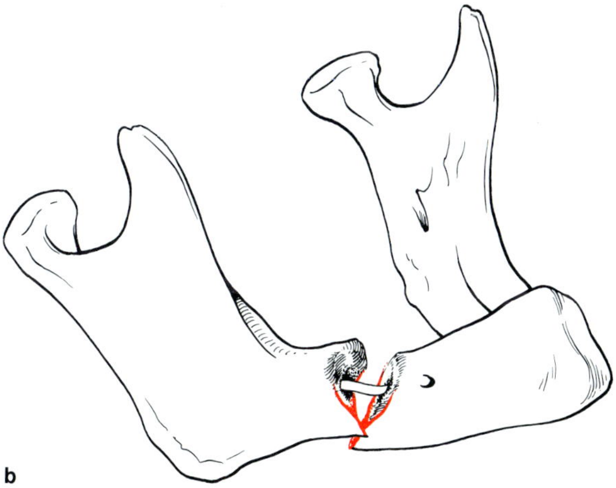

b

Fig. 305. **a** Infected iatrogenic fracture. **b** Artist's depiction

The result of the fixation is shown in Fig. 306b: an infected, draining nonunion caused by inadequate immobilization. It was wrong to attempt interfragmental compression with a DCP, for compression plating is not possible without an adequate bony buttress. Immediate removal of the plate is indicated.

It is clear that a nonunion caused by inadequate immobilization of the fracture should be treated by stable revisionary fixation. The associated infection will resolve quickly once the old implant has been removed. Compromises in the form of adjunctive intermaxillary fixation will only cause additional discomfort and further delay healing.

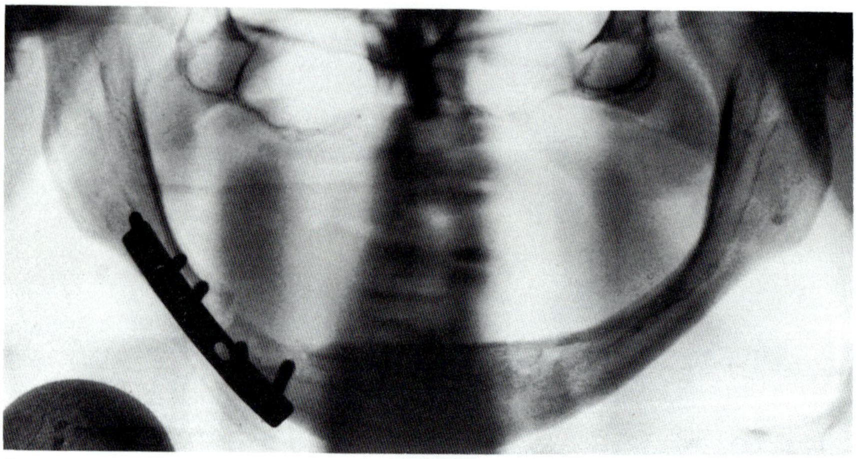

a

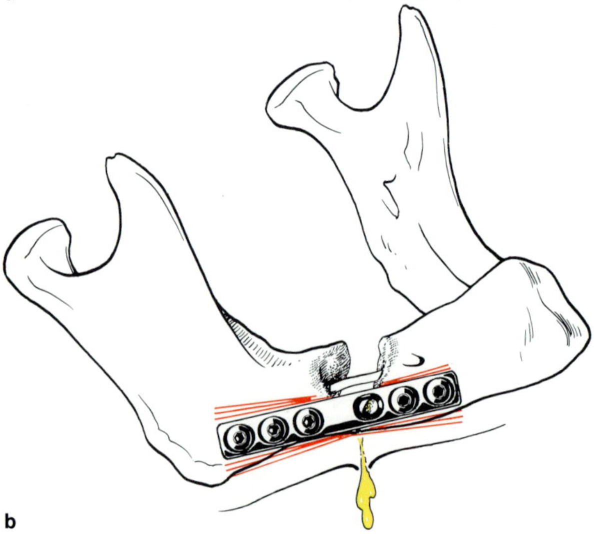

b

Fig. 306. **a** Status after initial fixation, which proved to be unstable. **b** Artist's depiction

Two problems must be addressed in this situation:

1) stabilization and
2) consolidation of the nonunion.

Our policy is to *stabilize the nonunion by revisionary fixation* with a reconstruction plate that buttresses the affected side of the mandible from the angle to the symphysis (Fig. 307 a). We combine this with *decortication and bone grafting* (Figs. 307 b and 308).

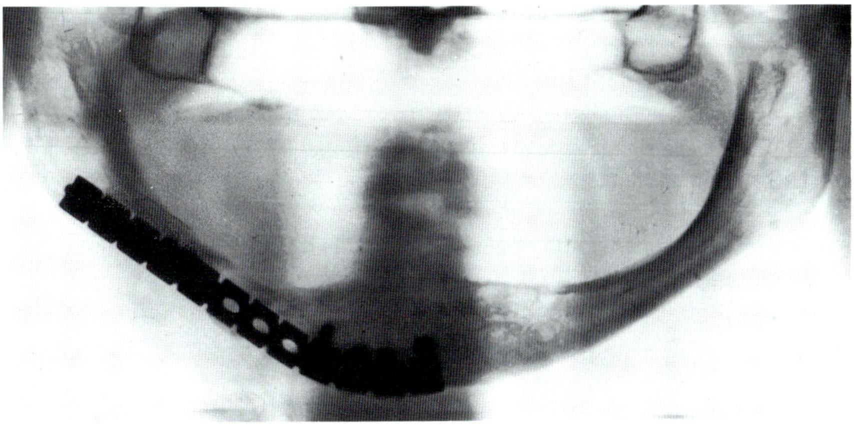

a

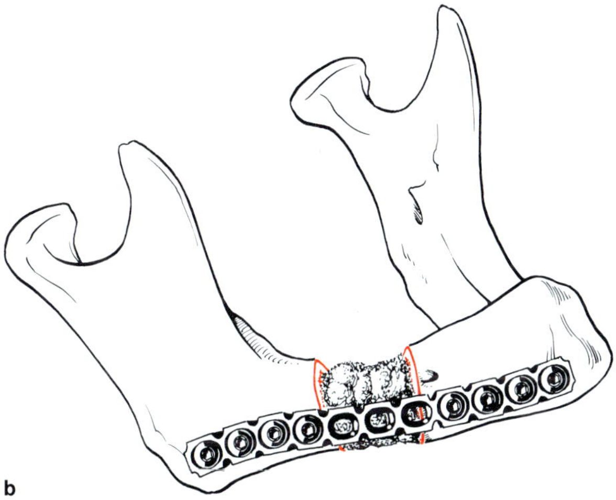

b

Fig. 307. **a** Previously infected nonunion with a bone defect. Therapeutic principle: stable buttressing with a reconstruction plate and autogenous bone grafting. **b** Drawing of the therapeutic principle applied in Fig. 307 a

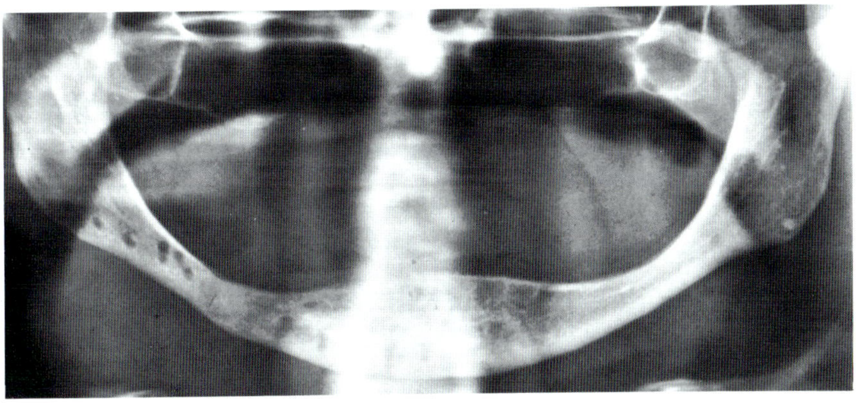

Fig. 308. Status after removal of the plate

2.5.2 Infected, Draining Nonunion

The most frequent cause of a permanent infectious focus is instability combined with the presence of the implanted material. Even one loose screw can sustain a chronic infection. Infection can also be perpetuated by a sequestrum or devitalized bone, and this should be suspected if the infection persists despite removal of the implant. These causes are eliminated by:

- immobilization of the fracture margins as a necessary prelude to consolidation of the nonunion, and
- eradication of the infection.

This therapeutic concept is illustrated by the following cases:

An indolent patient sustained a mandibular fracture followed 6 weeks later by a soft-tissue abscess that was treated with antibiotics by the woman's family physician. The infection did not respond, complaints persisted, and several months later the patient was referred to our care.

Infected, draining nonunion characterized radiographically by atrophic (avascular) bone ends and a sequestrum (Fig. 309)
Following removal of the infected granulation and scar tissue with a curet (Fig. 310 a), the avascular bone ends are removed and the ends freshened by making bur holes in the cortex (Fig. 310 b). The fragments are aligned and their position retained intraoperatively with extramaxillary clamps. Then the fistula is excised in preparation for the primary closure (Fig. 310 c).

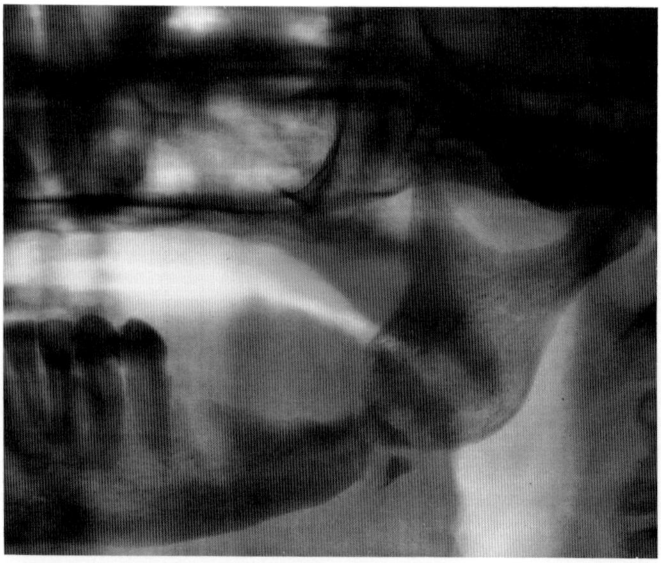

Fig. 309. Nonunion with atrophic (avascular) bone ends

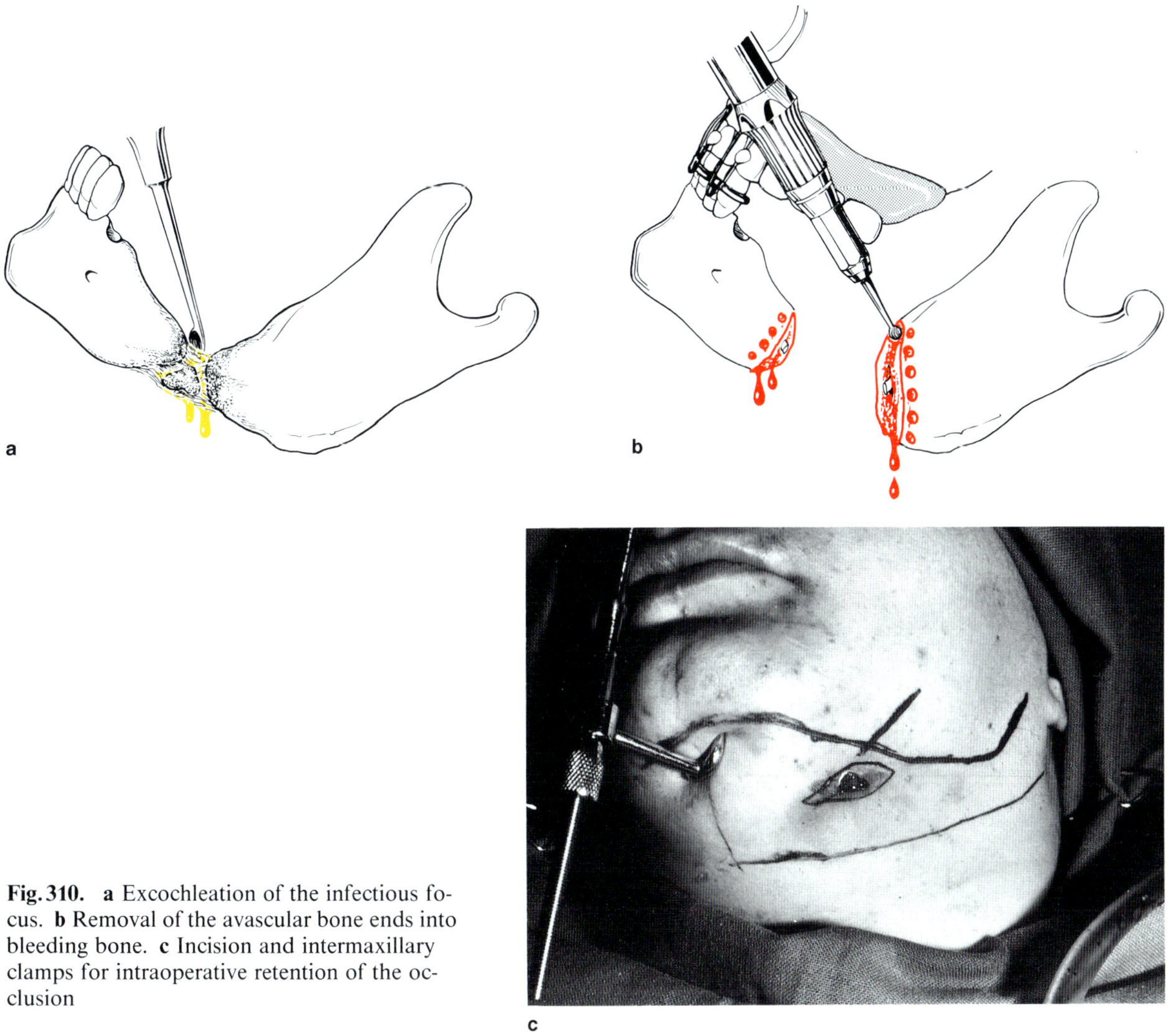

Fig. 310. **a** Excochleation of the infectious focus. **b** Removal of the avascular bone ends into bleeding bone. **c** Incision and intermaxillary clamps for intraoperative retention of the occlusion

The defect is bridged with a 12-hole reconstruction plate and then obliterated by the interposition of cancellous bone chips, which if necessary may be held in place with a piece of Vicryl mesh (Fig. 311). Finally primary wound closure is performed, which includes excision and closure of the fistulous tract.

Figure 312 shows the status after removal of the plate and primary healing. This outcome is anticipated in all cases where mechanical rest is provided as a precondition for revascularization of the grafted cancellous bone.

Note: Treatment of the infection is initiated 1–2 weeks preoperatively with antibacterial irrigations or the instillation of Neomycin and Bacitracin through the fistula. Parenteral antibiotic therapy is started 48 h before the operation in accordance with culture findings.

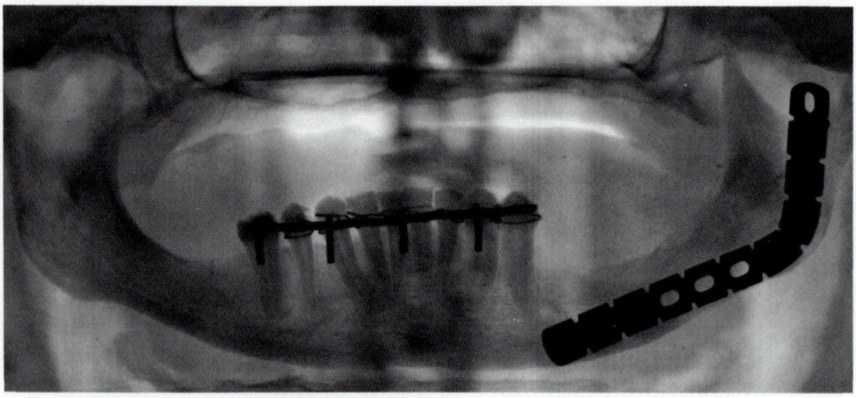

a

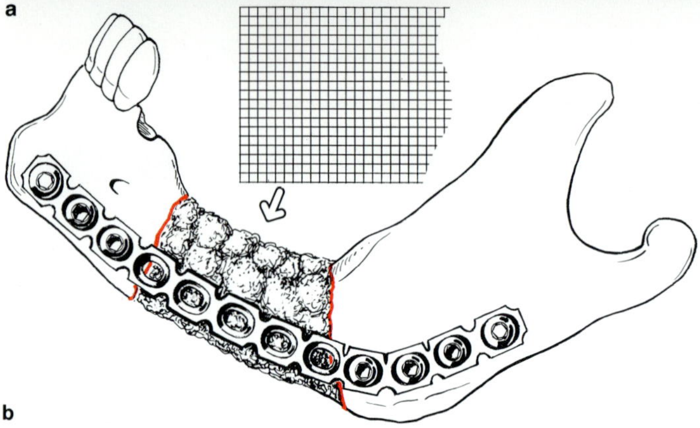

b

Fig. 311. **a** Bone graft protected with a reconstruction plate. **b** Artist's depiction

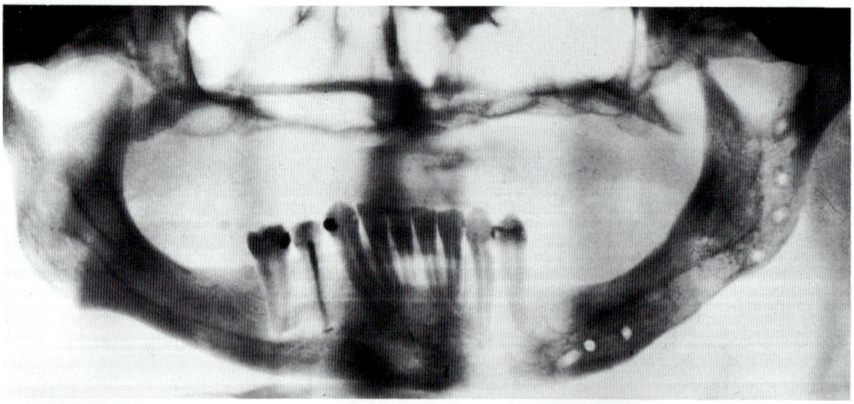

a

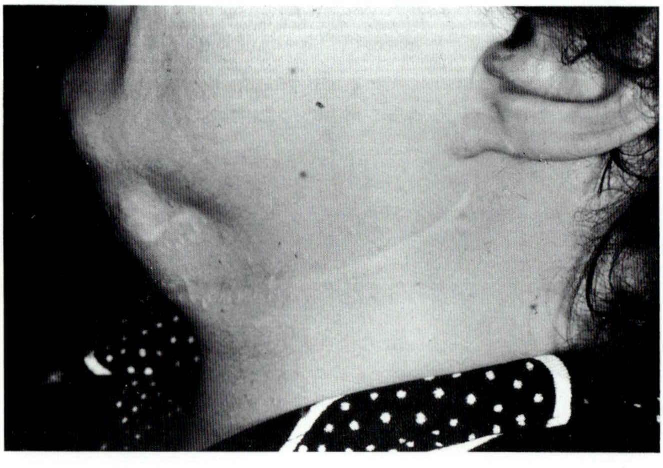

b

Fig. 312 a, b. Status following **a** removal of the plate and **b** primary closure of the fistula

Infected, draining nonunion with a defect

This resulted from the inadequate internal fixation of a severe comminuted fracture of the mandible (performed elsewhere) in which there was concomitant loss of the molar teeth. Within a few weeks a fracture-line osteomyelitis with sequestration developed and was perpetuated for months by the unstable fixation material (two loose screws in the distal fragment) (Fig. 313a, b).

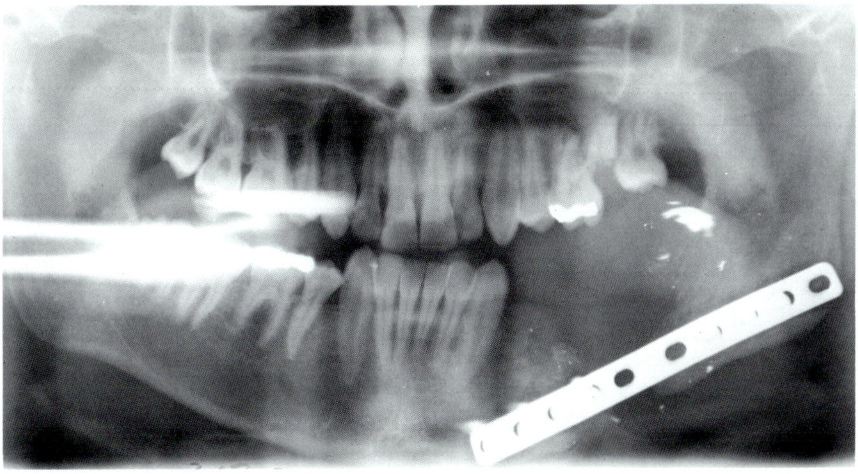

a

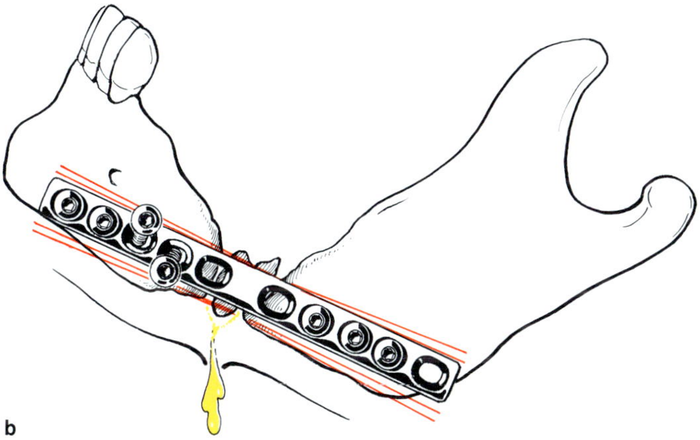

b

Fig. 313. **a** Radiographic appearance at referral. **b** Artist's depiction

The infected fibrous tissue is removed from the area of the defect with a curet, and the discontinuity is bridged with a 12-hole reconstruction plate and obliterated with cancellous bone grafts. Intermaxillary fixation is used for orthograde retention of the mandible during the operation (Fig. 314).

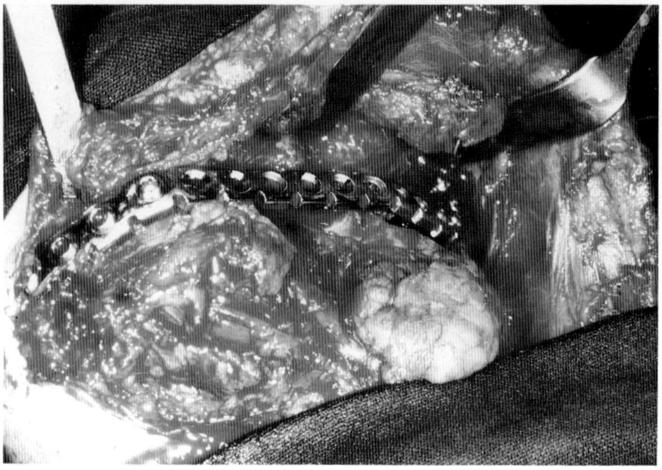

a

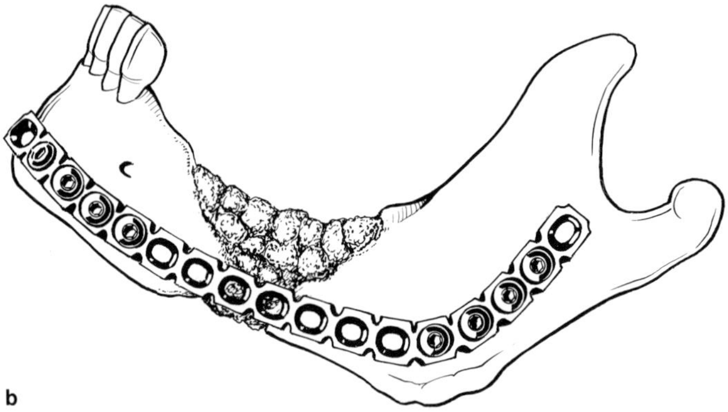

b

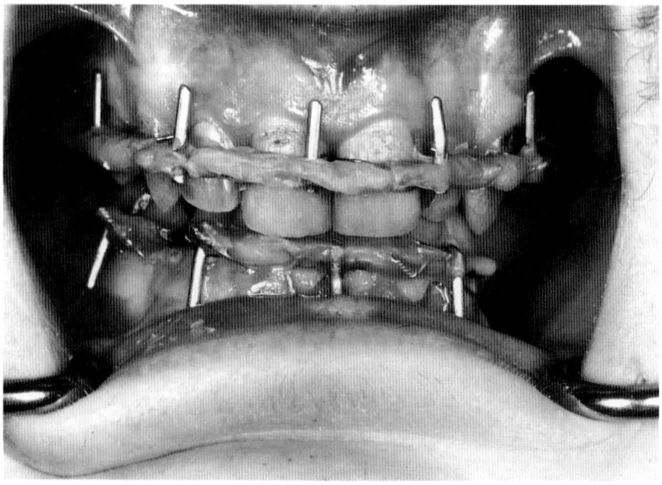

c

Fig. 314. **a** The freshened defect is bridged with a reconstruction plate, obeying the four-screw rule. **b** Artist's depiction of the concomitant bone graft. **c** Peroperative retention of the mandible with acrylated upper and lower arch splints

The radiograph after removal of the fixation material (Fig. 315) confirms the restoration of bony continuity. A second bone graft can be performed later to augment the deficient alveolar process.

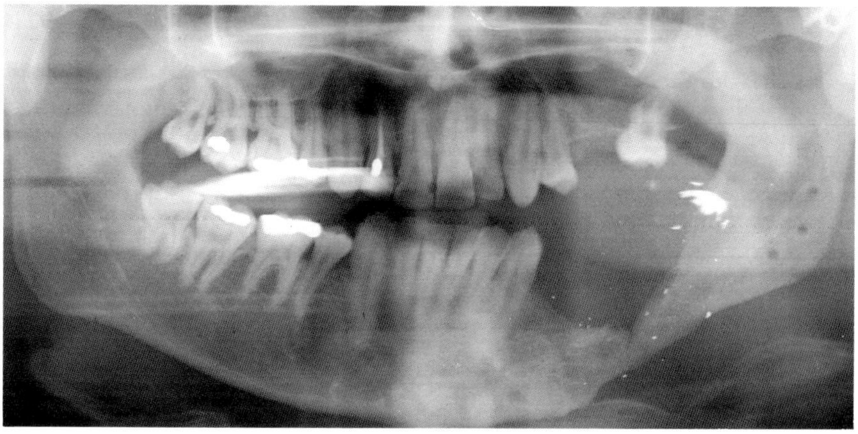

Fig. 315. Status after implant removal: the continuity of the jaw base is restored

3 Reconstruction of Segmental Defects in Tumor Surgery

3.1 Introduction to the Problem

The TNM system for tumor staging (UICC 1979, 1987) demonstrates the significance of transcortical invasion of the bone as a poor prognostic sign. Accordingly, bone involvement signifies a T4 lesion regardless of the surface area of the tumor. The problem of bone arises from the unique situation of the "mucosal bone" of the mandible to each of the three therapeutic modalities: surgery, radiation, and chemotherapy.

The main problem in surgical resection is one of limiting mutilation when there is occult infiltration in the area of T4 involvement. Because resections of the cranium are necessarily limited in their extent, a rationale exists for pre- and postoperative radiation therapy for patients with stage III and IV disease. Barring contraindications, radiation doses of 50 to 60 gyn are delivered. When administered *preoperatively,* this dose significantly increases morbidity (e.g., when tumorresection is performed as part of a multimodality therapy). To cite a representative study in this area, Flynn (1979) of Louisville University supplied data on 196 irradiated patients, 70% of whom underwent a hemimandibulectomy in addition to their radiotherapy. Most of these patients received 3000 rad of primary irradiation for 2 weeks or 5000 rad for 5 weeks. The outcome: 11% operative mortality, 50% local complications, and 30% systemic complications (mainly respiratory). The local complications included 6 carotid arterial ruptures, 4 cases of postoperative bleeding, 9 cases of significant wound necrosis, 6 wound infections, and 14 orocutaneous fistulas.

Although the complication rate is no longer this high owing to the increasing installation of linear accelerators and intensive care, morbidity continues to be the major problem of radiation therapy and surgical resection.

Adjuvant chemotherapy likewise has contributed little to solving the morbidity problem. It appears that toxicity can be reduced by the simultaneous administration of cis-platinum and radiation as a prelude to surgical resection (Slotman et al. 1986), but the remission achieved with this regimen does not reduce the necessary extent of radical surgery. A limited resection of the affected bone cannot be considered an adequate therapy at the present time. Consequently, the segmental defect that is produced by a mandibular resection remains a much-discussed problem of reconstructive surgery, and the question of immediate versus delayed reconstruction remains controversial.

Even today the decision for immediate or delayed reconstruction is influenced by the technical difficulty of primary reconstruction and its frequently dubious value. Many surgeons still prefer traditional immobilization (IMF) in the belief that it permits better wound healing and lowers the risk of infection.

This line of reasoning is apparent in the study of Lieberman et al. (1981), who studied the efficacy of immobilization (intermaxillary fixation) in 61 patients who underwent a mandibular resection or hemimandibulectomy. Forty of the patients received radiation therapy. In eight cases the mandibular defect was bridged with Kirschner wire as an adjunct to the intermaxillary fixation. Based on their analysis, the authors gave a positive assessment of the immobilization method despite the occurrence of severe postoperative complications, some with fatal outcomes. Seven patients died as a result of aspiration and pulmonary failure; acute glossoptosis developed in one case. The authors also reported five severe "pulmonary problems without a fatal outcome." Aside from four wound complications relating to the Kirschner wire, no other difficulties were reported. The operative mortality exceeded 10%, with respiratory insufficiency the leading cause despite routine tracheotomy. It is quite possible that this suspiciously high complication rate was not coincidental but related indirectly to the postoperative care difficulties caused by the intermaxillary fixation. The authors did not consider this possibility.

In a series 91 cases of TNM stage III and IV mandibular carcinomas treated in Basel, surgical resection was followed by immediate mobilization of the jaw, rather than intermaxillary fixation. The operative mortality in these cases was 0.5%. By facilitating postoperative care, we feel that routine, primary, stable bridging of the mandibulectomy defect is of significant value in reducing mortality and other complications. The capacity for immediate, pain-free mandibular opening after surgery carries major benefits: the ability to eat normally, the ability to raise secretions and keep the oropharynx clear, a shortened catabolic phase, avoidance of tracheotomy, and finally the psychosocial benefits of being able to speak in a normal manner.

The resulting limitation of morbidity makes functionally stable bridging of the defect an integral part of the mandibular resection.

3.2 Technical Principles

Segmental defects are bridged with the intent of restoring the continuity of the mandible in terms of its *function, form, and strength.*

Mandibular continuity is reestablished by a splinting device that attaches directly to the bone. The splint can exercise its load-bearing function if, when spanning a defect larger than 12 cm, it is sufficiently *rigid* under the action of deforming forces and is anchored to the mandibular stumps with sufficient *stability* (immobility).

The universal reconstruction plate has been tested in clinical use for more than 12 years (since 1973). Both steel and titanium plates are available (see p. 106), all are bendable in three dimensions, and all can be adapted to the contour of the mandible without significant loss of their biotechnical properties. This capability is crucial when one considers that long-term stability under functional loads depends largely on the response of the metal to the deformation that is imposed upon it during initial adaptation. If the material lacks sufficient strength and rigidity, eventual breakage is quite possible due to the very heavy stresses that result from the combination of the long "load arm" of the implant and the short "force arm" of the ascending ramus. The stresses take the form of alternating loads acting at points of contact between the metal and bone. To ensure long-term stability under these conditions, *a minimum of four screws should be used to attach the plate to each mandibular stump, and six to eight screws should be used in the free-end plate.*

If only the condylar neck is available for attachment of the plate, it can accommodate no more than three screws and probably only two. An "expandable screw head" system (THRP=Titanium Hollow Reconstruction Plate) is currently being developed for cases of this kind.[12]

The expandable screw head mechanism transforms the principle of the plate fixation screw into the principle of external pin fixation. It does this by permitting rigid fixation of the screw in the plate, producing a composite system so rigid that two screws can do the work of approximately four. This system also relieves stress on the underlying bone and does not impose transverse compression upon it like ordinary plate screws would do (Raveh et al. 1985).

3.2.1 Bridging Without an Autogenous Bone Graft

The simplest way to restore the basic shape of the mandible is by attaching an appropriately contoured reconstruction plate to the intact mandible before the resection is performed. The plate is fixed distal to the proposed lines of resection with two screws per side and then removed. The drill holes and corresponding plate holes will then provide reference points for bridging the defect and for restoring the basic contour of the jaw.

We have had excellent results with this technique for more than eight years. The case reports below illustrate the application of the technique both for *definitive reconstruction* and for *interim bridging* in preparation for future (secondary) autogenous bone grafting.

3.2.1.1 THRP or Reconstruction Plate for Definitive Reconstruction

The THRP system or the reconstruction plate offers an acceptable definitive solution for mandibular resection patients who have been previously treated for tumor, as illustrated by the ameloblastom case in Fig. 316. Multiple limited resections over a 12-year period had failed to check recurrences in this patient, who finally underwent a more radical resection (Fig. 317a), although she was considered unable to tolerate very extensive surgery (Fig. 317b). This titanium hollow screw and reconstruction plate system (THRP) developed by Raveh et al. in 1985 makes it possible to perform a stable free-end fixation with only four expanding-head screws. Bony in-

[12] Additional information is available upon request from SYNTHES AG, CH-4436, Waldenburg, Switzerland.

growth into the hollow, perforated screw shanks further stabilizes the fixation. The curative, functional, and aesthetic result in this patient (Fig. 319) has been constant since the last surgical procedure 5 years ago.

The more widely used alternative at present is the universal reconstruction plate, shown in Fig. 318 attached by the necessary 7 or 8 fixation screws.

3.2.1.2 Bridging as Definitive Treatment for Mandibular Metastases

Bridging can be the only definitive treatment recommended following a palliative resection for metastatic carcinoma of the mandible. A pathologic fracture is usually present as a result of hematogenous spread and may be unrecognized initially due to a lack of symptoms. Even when the patient complains of numbness or trigeminal nerve pain, the physician may not suspect metastatic carcinoma of the jaw even when the primary disease is known. Brack (1980) points to the breast (8 cases), lung (5 cases), and liver (3 cases) as the most common sites of origination.

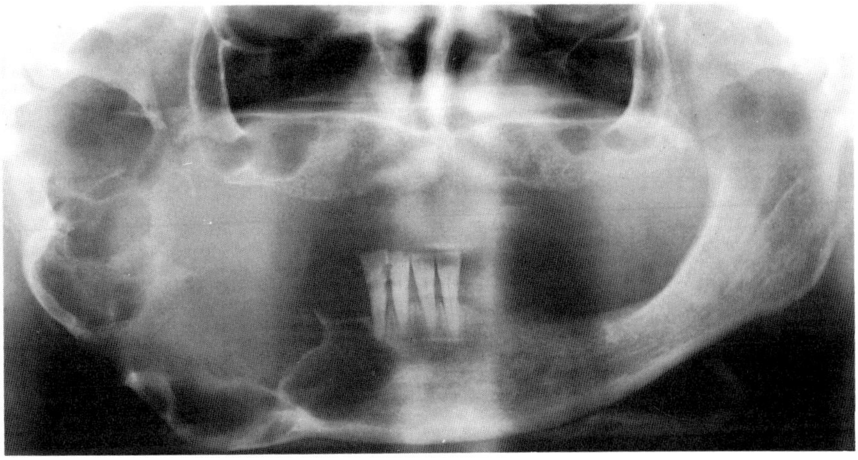

Fig. 316. Multiply recurrent ameloblastoma

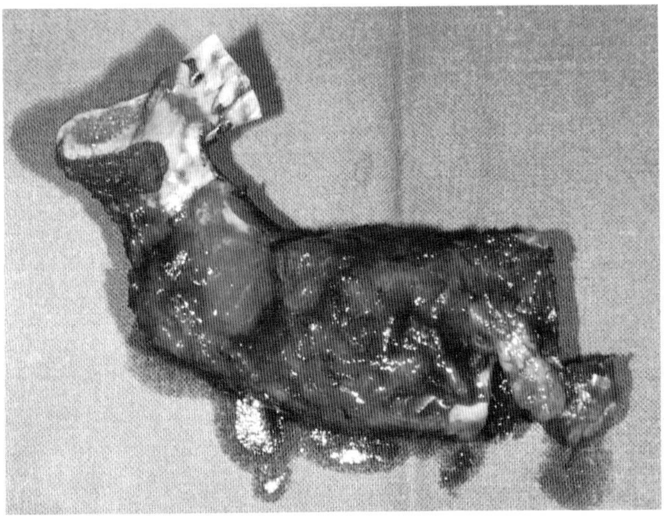

Fig. 317. a Exarticulated specimen.

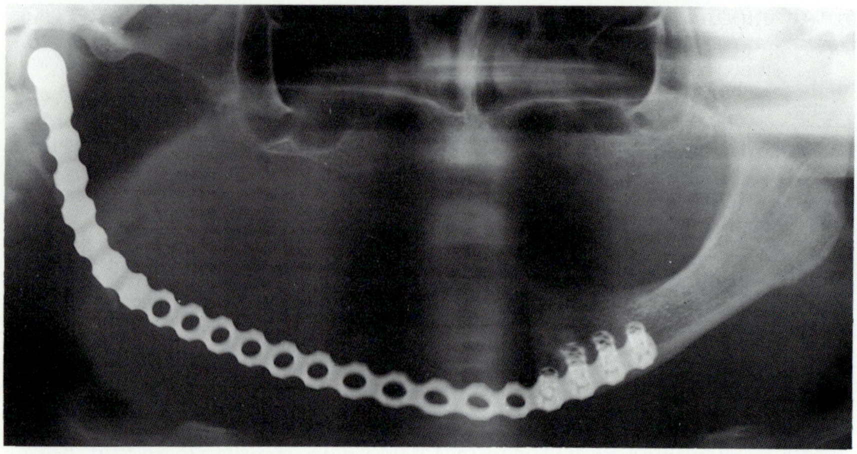

Fig. 317. b Primary, definitive reconstruction of the hemimandible is accomplished with a free-end resection plate. In the THPR system used here, four hollow screws are sufficient to give permanent bone-plate stability (THRP, titanium hollow screw and reconstruction plate)

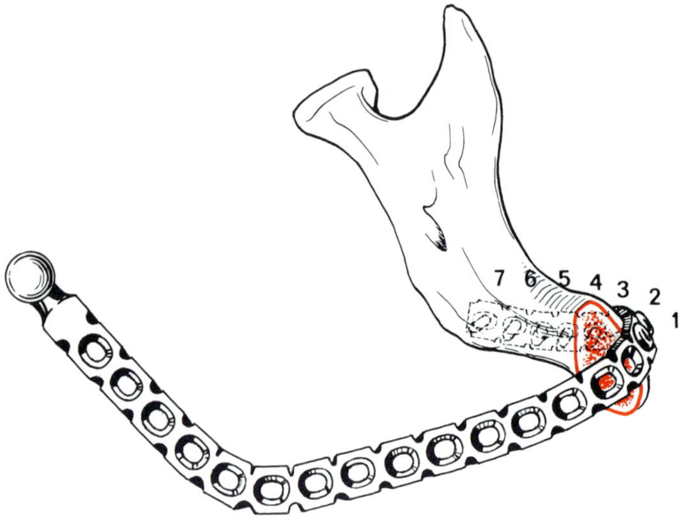

Fig. 318. Alternative to the THRP system: the universal reconstruction plate attached with 7 or 8 screws

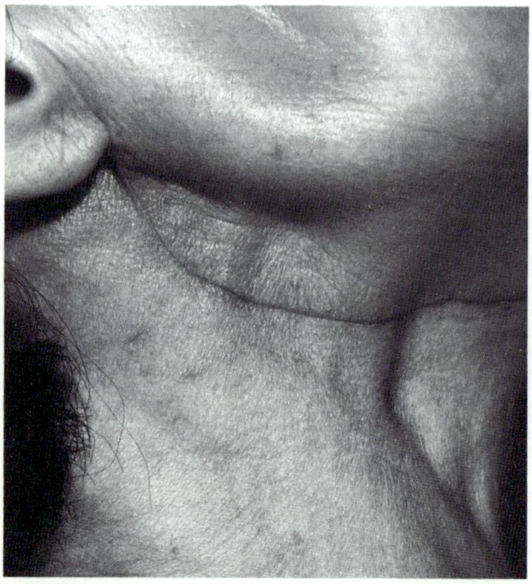

Fig. 319. Aesthetic result of definitive hemimandibular replacement with a titanium hollow screw and reconstruction plate (THRP)

If the metastasis is located distal to the apophyseal and articular portion of the mandible and is reasonably well circumscribed, its removal by segmental resection is indicated. As a result of modern organ-conserving therapeutic regimens, the patient's general condition remains relatively constant and his survival time is prolonged. The increasing use of the Karnofsky index[13] reflects ongoing efforts to mitigate the consumptive terminal stage of cancer through appropriate preventive measures.

The criteria defined are a valuable decision-making aid in difficult cases of patient selection, as in the present case of a hypernephroma (Fig. 320). The patient's general condition rated a Karnofsky index of 2, while the metastasis in the left mandibular angle and ramus caused acute discomfort only during mastication. The growth had already infiltrated the submucosa of the alveolar process, and ulceration was imminent along with a rapid decline in quality of life. The case was managed by resection and primary reconstruction (Fig. 321), which has proved to be a truly palliative, well tolerated surgical procedure.

[13] Karnofsky index:
0 = Normal activity with no disability
1 = Normal activity with minimal disability
2 = Unfit for work but capable of self-care
3 = Unfit for work, requires occasional help
4 = Unfit for work, requires support, not bed-confined
5 = Requires nursing care, bed-confined
6 = Severely debilitated, hospitalization required
7 = Active treatment is necessary to preserve life
8 = Moribund
9 = Not known

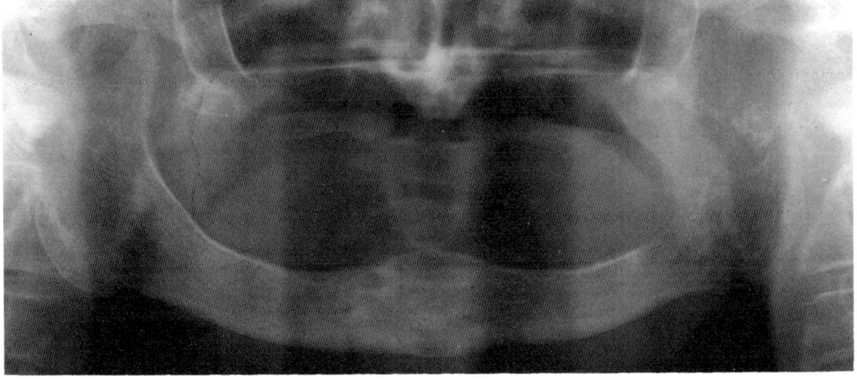

Fig. 320. Central osteolytic tumor of the left ascending ramus with reactive bone formation, presumably metastatic from a hypernephroma that had been removed several years earlier

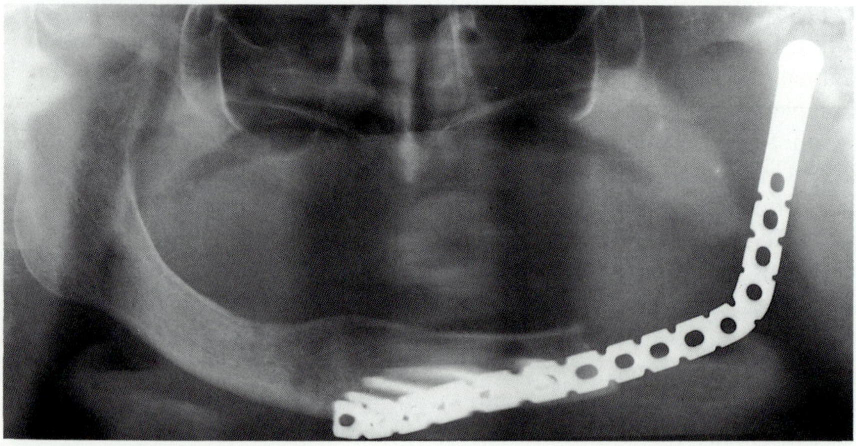

Fig. 321. Reconstruction plate with condylar head for definitive replacement of the exarticulated mandibular segment

3.2.1.3 Reconstruction Plate for Interim Bridging

Interim bridging facilitates

- radical surgical resection,
- follow-up of the operated area,
- autogenous bone grafting (generally done after a disease-free interval of 1-2 years).

A typical case of interim bridging is illustrated in Fig. 322. Owing to the capability for preliminary, functionally stable bridging of the defect, we did not hesitate to resect the lesion with wide margins (Fig. 323 a). Postoperative appearance and function were excellent (Fig. 323 b), so the 1- to 2-year waiting period before bone grafting imposed no hardship whatsoever. At that time the defect was reconstructed with a corticocancellous graft placed between the previously stabilized mandibular stumps (Fig. 324 a, b).

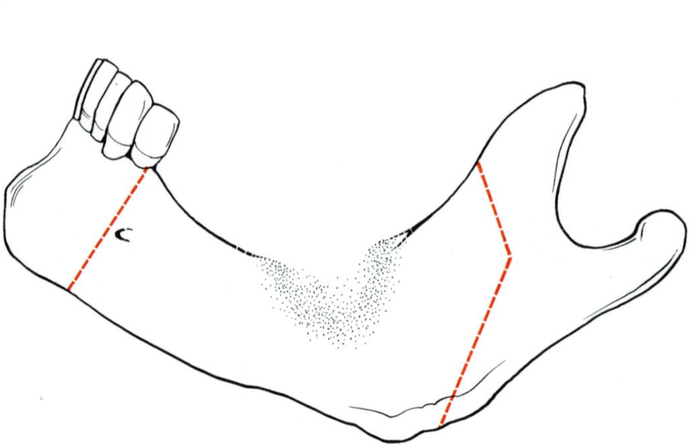

Fig. 322. Osteolytic focus of an alveolar-process carcinoma. The lines of resection are indicated

The *danger of plate fracture* should be noted in cases where the patient comes to regard the interim bridging as an acceptable permanent solution. The repeated deferral of bone grafting from year to year or the outright refusal of bone grafting can ultimately lead to breakage of the implant. From a biomechanical standpoint, bridging the defect with a plate alone is unfavorable due to the *absence of a bony buttress.* The metal is subjected to al-

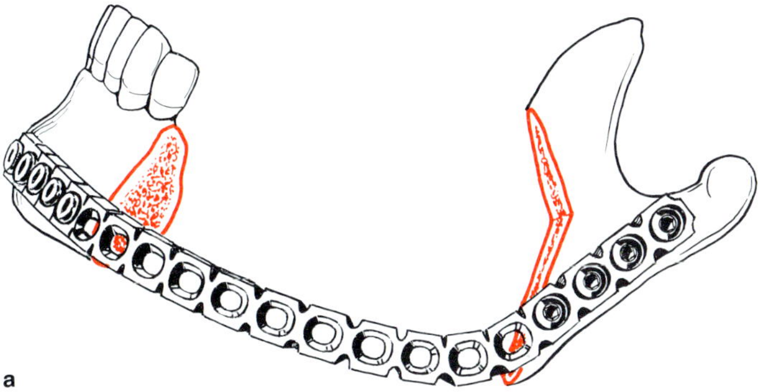

a

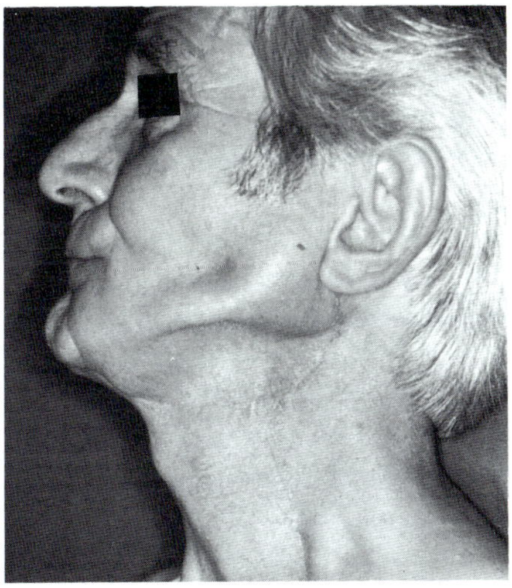

b

Fig. 323. **a** Reconstruction plate for interim bridging (note adherence to the four-screw-minimum rule for plate fixation). **b** The interim bridging produces a typical mandibular contour and intact basic function

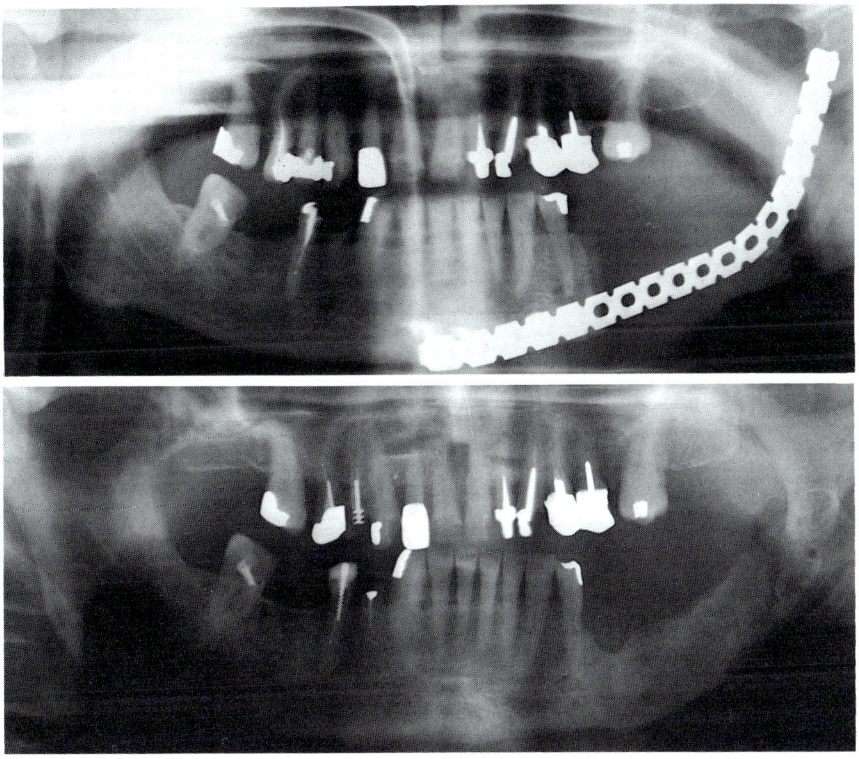

a

b

Fig. 324. **a** After 1.5 years' interim bridging, there is no evidence of instability at the screw sites. **b** The excised segment is replaced with autogenous bone under the protection of the reconstruction plate (interim bridging). Radiograph taken 3 months after plate removal (Figs. 322 and 323 a are artist's depictions of this case) ternating bending loads that will eventually cause it to fail after a given number of cycles, depending on the thickness of the plate (see p. 133 ff.).

We have observed five such cases of fatigue fracture. The failure occurs after a period of five to six years, as it did in the case of an alveolar-process carcinoma that necessitated a segmental resection beyond the midline (Fig. 325). The plate was contoured most heavily in the midline area, creating a site of predilection for fracture (Fig. 326).

The effects of the plate fracture finally convinced the patient of the need for a second operation, in which a corticocancellous bone graft was

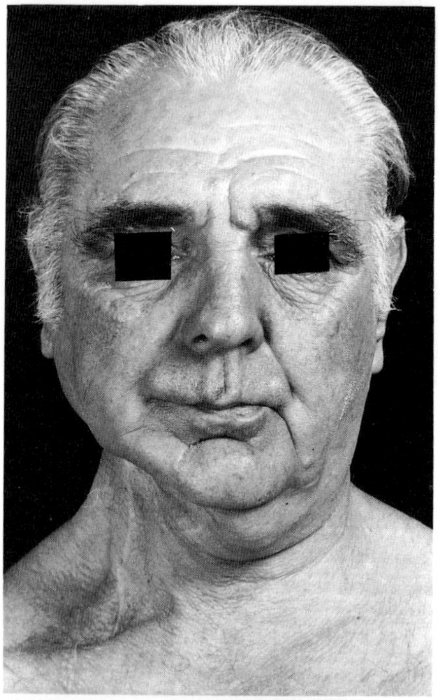

a

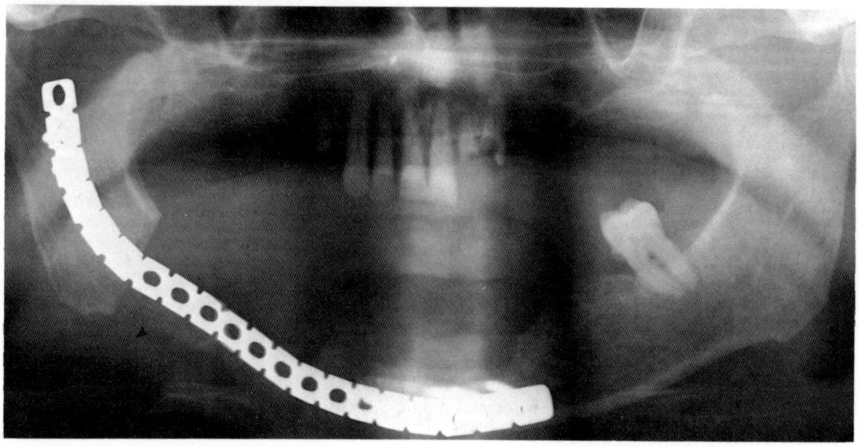

b

Fig. 325. **a** Part of the mandible presents an angular contour after more than 5 years' "interim" bridging with a reconstruction plate. **b** Corresponding orthopantomogram

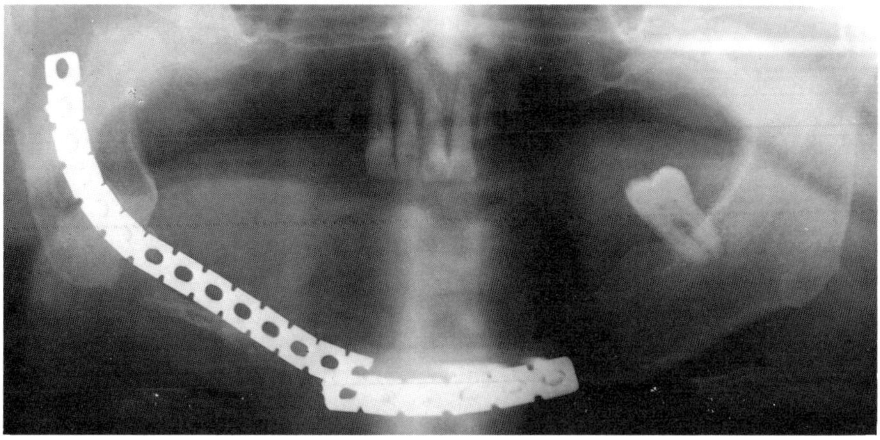

Fig. 326. Eventually the plate fractured at the point where it was bent to follow the chin contour

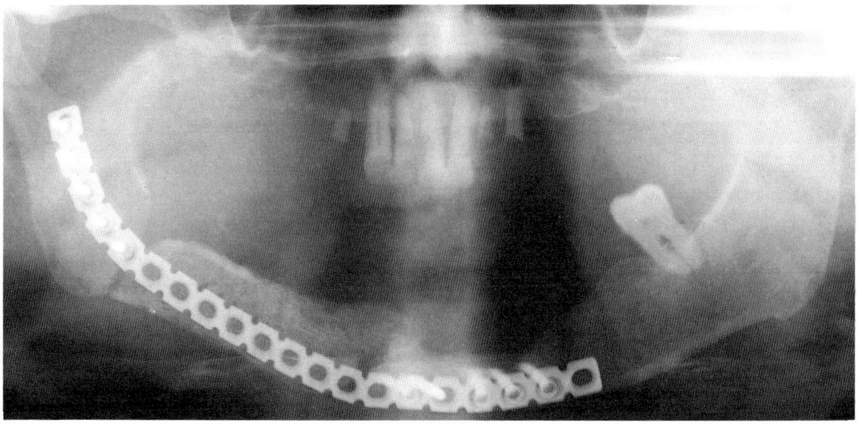

Fig. 327. The defect is reconstructed with a bone graft, and a new plate is applied

interposed under the protection of a new plate (Fig. 327). There are plans to make the titanium reconstruction plate slightly thicker with the object of eliminating fatigue fractures of this kind (we know of no plate fractures that have occurred in the internal fixation of fractures). Fatigue bending tests indicate that the greater plate thickness increases the bending stiffness of the implant several-fold.[14]

[14] These plates have to fulfill the function of a prosthesis for extended periods of time. The new available titanium plate is therefore thicker (3.1 mm compared with the universal type 2.7 mm; see p. 110) and has larger holes and notches on the side facing the bone.

3.2.1.4 Covering Soft-Tissue Defects and Bridging Segmental Defects

The use of musculocutaneous flaps (Aryan 1979) greatly facilitates the coverage of defects and contributes to the success of bone grafts. While the deltopectoral flap (Bakamjian 1965) has been a mainstay of reconstructive surgery for many years and still has its indications, the myocutaneous flap offers significantly greater advantages owing to its excellent vascularity. This makes it especially valuable for cases that require bone grafting and for repairing defects produced by the radical removal of residual tumor or a postradiation recurrence.

The pectoralis flap has proved to be the most useful flap by far for reconstructing defects in the mandibular region. It makes a good island flap for intra- and extraoral transfers owing to its excellent mobility. In thin patients it is ideal for resurfacing the interior of the oral cavity. On the other hand, a thick fat layer between the skin and muscle not only makes the flap too bulky but also renders it susceptible to necrosis.

The free forearm flap offers an alternative in such cases, especially for the closure of large, bilateral, full-thickness defects. Its thinness and size (25 × 15 cm) and the length of its vascular pedicle make it excellent for intraoral use, while the pectoralis flap is appropriate for exterior coverage. The disadvantages of the forearm flap include its proneness to postoperative edema, which is difficult to treat in the oral cavity and may lead to induration of the flap. Thus, as many venous anastomoses as possible should be established to ensure maximum venous drainage of the flap. Another disadvantage is that the donor site is in a conspicuous location.[15]

Another alternative is the dorsalis pedis flap, a free fasciocutaneous flap that is favorable in terms of its size, thickness, and pedicle length.

We have no personal experience to relate concerning the use of transplanted intestinal mucosa.

All of the flap procedures can be used in conjunction with a reconstruction plate for definitive reconstruction or interim bridging. A primary bone graft is contraindicated due to the palliative nature of the majority of these operations, the extended length of the operation, and the danger of infection in the recipient bed. The timing of a secondary bone graft is guided by the follow-up findings and prognosis.

[15] We are grateful to Dr. Helali, Clinic for Plastic and Reconstructive Surgery, Aarau, for his cooperation in the application of the forearm flap and to Dr. Brennwald, Microsurgery Section, Department of Surgery, Basel, for his cooperation in the use of the dorsalis pedis flap.

3.2.2 Bridging With an Autogenous Bone Graft

Two main problems are involved in the replacement of an excised mandibular segment by autogenous bone: *revascularization* and *heterotopia*.

3.2.2.1 Revascularization

The revascularization of a bone graft depends directly on the *mechanical stability* that exists between the graft and mandibular stump and also on *immunogenicity*.

Importance of Stability
Stability is essential so that undisturbed revascularization can take place under conditions of constant rest. This condition must exist

- between the graft and mandibular stump to increase the rate of "interface healing" and
- between the graft and tissue bed to hasten "creeping" substitution of the transferred bone.

Creating the necessary stability is a practical problem that can be satisfactorily solved by establishing close contact between the graft, mandibular stump, and tissue bed over a maximum area and also by *securing the graft-recipient junction through stable bridging of the defect.*

Thus, it is important that a compact graft such as a corticocancellous graft or orthotopic allograft be fitted precisely into the space between the mandibular stumps. In addition, the reconstruction plate used to bridge the defect must have adequate stiffness, even when spanning defects longer than 12 cm, and must be attached very securely to the mandibular stumps ("four screw rule" as a minimum demand).

Double plating of the bone graft, i.e., applying one or two short plates at each end of the graft, does not offer the same long-term mechanical protection for undisturbed substitution of the transplanted bone as a single, long reconstruction plate. This clinical experience has been confirmed experimentally (Habel et al. 1980).

Importance of Immunogenicity
Immunogenetics is a more difficult problem that is encountered in the grafting of homologous materials. Immunogenic processes lead to the formation of transplant antigens which destroy the cell groups responsible for osteoblastic bone formation and hamper or prevent revascularization, depending on tissue compatibility.

Experimental studies on the use of immunosuppression are in progress (Aebi et al. 1984) and should yield results that will benefit transplantation surgery. Until then, *freshly harvested autogenous bone is superior to any other material in terms of its capacity for revascularization.* Of course many problems remain to be solved in autogenous bone grafting as well, including 1) the risk of infection posed by facultative pathogens in the oral cavity and 2) poor revascularization at the graft-recipient junction caused by the small cross-sectional area of the mandible and the absence of a closed muscular envelope to provide a well-perfused recipient bed and an environment conducive to the inductive effect of the grafted bone on the undifferentiated mesenchymal cells ("intrinsic osteogenic inductor"). Another problem is the potential failure of osteoinduction in a radiation-damaged tissue bed.

3.2.2.2 Heterotopia[16]

Lack of congruity between the donor and recipient sites presents a problem in autogenous reconstructions of the mandible. No part of the skeleton is as highly differentiated structurally as the mandible. The most difficult parts of the mandible to reconstruct, aside from its apophyseal and articular portions, are the anterior symphyseal segment and the angle.

Despite the problems mentioned, the following requirements are satisfied for a successful *secondary* interposition bone graft:

- mechanical rest of the recipient bed, which is present after 1 to 2 years of uncomplicated interim bridging;
- a relatively intact tissue bed and an implant bed that does not communicate with the oral cavity (requires atraumatic preparation of the recipient bed).

3.2.2.3 Secondary Interpositional Corticocancellous Bone Graft

3.2.2.3.1 Obtaining the Graft

The iliac wing is the donor site best suited for the replacement of excised mandibular segments. The corticocancellous graft should be taken from the medial aspect of the ilium if at all possible. The curvature of the *right* iliac crest approximates the curve of the *right* half of the mandibular body and vice versa (Fig. 328a). The *left* iliac crest is better suited for replacing the right ramus and angle, and the anterior iliac spine makes a satisfactory condylar substitute (Fig. 328).

It is most difficult to find a one-piece replacement for the anterior arch of the mandible. An acceptable substitute is either the midportion of the iliac crest (at the level of the tuberosity), which has the greatest curvature medially (Fig. 329a), or the outer part of the anterior curve of the iliac wing, one fingerwidth below the outer lip of the iliac crest at the site where it terminates in the anterior spine (Fig. 329b). The block graft is sawed from the iliac wing in one piece. The skin incision extends to the groin and requires that the subcutaneous tissue be separated from the gluteal fascia and the iliotibial tract of the fascia lata (Fig. 329b) in order to preserve the cutaneous nerves (branch of cutaneous iliohypogastric nerve and lateral cutaneous femoral nerve). The hip is flexed and medially rotated in preparation for the incision. At the outer lip of the iliac crest, the fascia at the attachment of the obliquus externus abdominalis and gluteus medius muscles is divided to the bone so that the lateral aspect of the anterior superior iliac spine is visualized. Aided by a template, the surgeon excises the full-

[16] The problem of heterotopia could be largely solved by appropriate suppression of the immune response. This would make practical the grafting of banked segmental mandibular homografts obtained from cadavers.

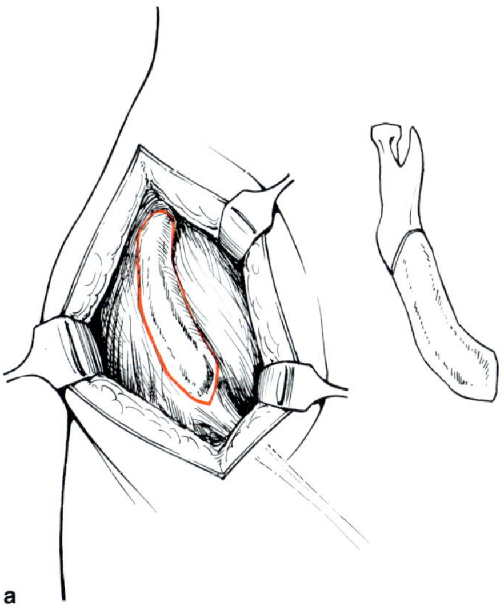

a

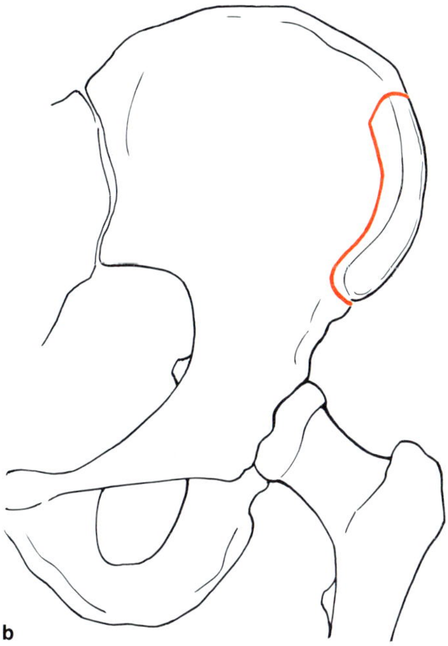

b

Fig. 328. **a** The iliac crest graft most closely approximates the shape, length, and thickness of the horizontal ramus of the mandible. **b** The iliac crest with the anterior iliac spine for replacement of the ascending ramus and condyle

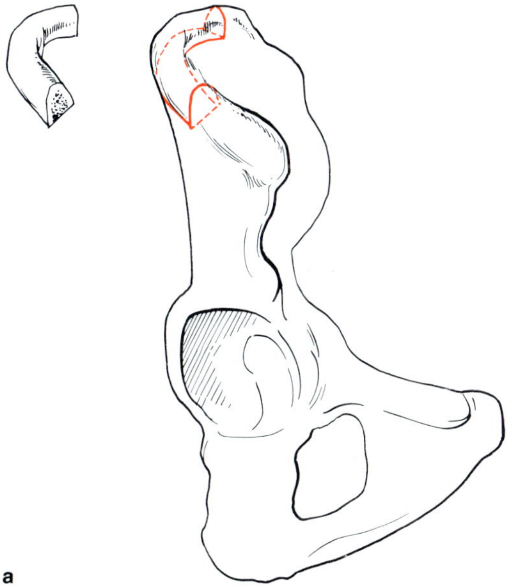

a

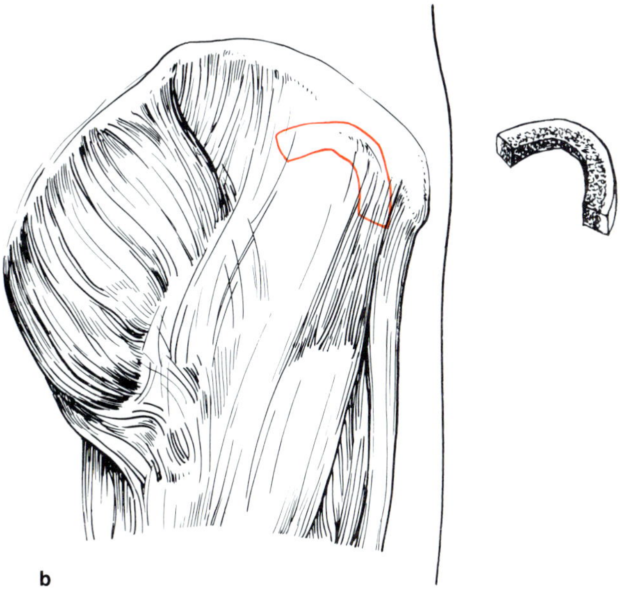

b

Fig. 329. **a** The midportion of the iliac crest with the iliac tuberosity at its center is an acceptable substitute for the anterior jaw base. **b** A graft of appropriate size and shape is drawn on the lateral aspect of the iliac wing and excised with an oscillating saw thickness graft with the large oscillating ASIF bone saw. The graft will have a fairly uniform thickness of 7.5–10 mm. An artificial posterior mental spine is helpful as it will permit two or three bur holes to be placed for attachment of the oral floor muscles.

Several factors favor taking the graft from the inner table of the pelvis. The soft tissues in that area can be mobilized and retracted more widely and less traumatically than on the lateral side, where the removal of larger grafts necessitates a wide release of the gluteal muscles. The postoperative sequel to this trauma is a characteristic trailing of the leg ("gluteus gait"), whose duration depends on associated damage to the fascia lata and fascial tensors.

Another reason to obtain the graft on the medial side is to ensure *contact of the cancellous bone surface with a "better" (more richly vascularized) tissue bed*. The mandibulectomy involved in the removal of malignant tumors frequently necessitates a neck dissection which leaves a sizable soft-tissue defect in the ipsilateral floor of the mouth. In such cases the buccal soft tissues adjacent to the bony contact surfaces provide the sole basis for graft revascularization. Clearly this process will be aided by having an open cancellous bone surface in apposition to the soft tissues around the graft.

3.2.2.3.2 Hazards of Obtaining an Iliac Crest Graft

During exposure of the inner table of the ilium, the lateral femoral cutaneous nerve coursing in the iliac fascia is vulnerable to damage by retractor tension. This is avoided by elevating the soft tissue from the inner table with a Hohmann retractor as far posteriorly as possible (Fig. 330). In addition, the surgeon should keep strictly on the subperiosteal plane to avoid injury to functionally important structures like the iliacus muscle, the deep circumflex iliac artery, and the femoral nerve (Fig. 331).

3.2.2.3.3 Fixation of the Graft

Absolute immobilization of the interposed bone graft is essential for undisturbed revascularization. It might be supposed that the graft should be rigidly attached to the reconstruction plate with screws, but clinical experience indicates otherwise: screws used to attach the graft to the plate tend to loosen within a few months, usually accompanied by infection. This loosening results from the vascularization and demineralization that take place in the first six months after operation. The bone resorption that accompanies these processes seriously weakens the hold of screws. It is preferable, then, to secure the bone graft without screws by wedging the graft firmly between the mandibular stumps. Bridging the operative defect with the reconstruction plate (Fig. 332a) makes it possible to determine the exact length of the discontinuity, and this measurement is transferred to a template. The template is then used to tailor the bone graft to the appropriate size so that it will fit the defect precisely, with its cancellous surface facing toward the soft tissues that have the best blood flow – in our case the buccal side (Fig. 332b). Revascularization is further aided by placing multiple bur holes in the opposite cortex. In the present case, removal of the implant at one year showed evidence of disturbed remodeling of the graft directly adjacent to the plate: remnants of granulation tissue and lacunar voids in the newly formed osseous surface (Fig. 333a). However, these changes re-

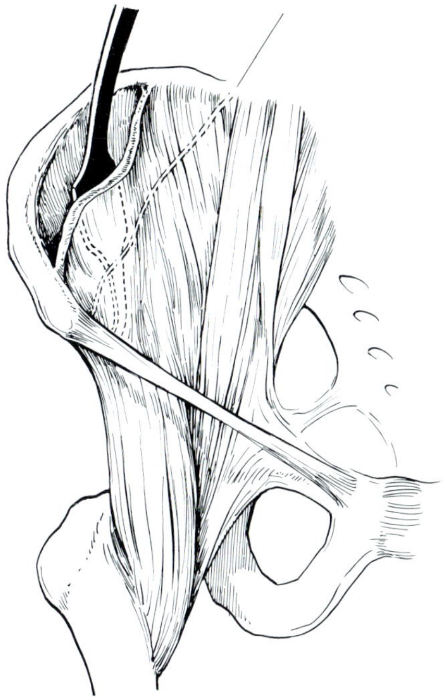

Fig. 330. The Hohmann retractor is inserted posteriorly to preserve the lateral femoral cutaneous nerve. Deep, anterior palcement of the instrument would jeopardize the nerve, which is relatively immobile in this area

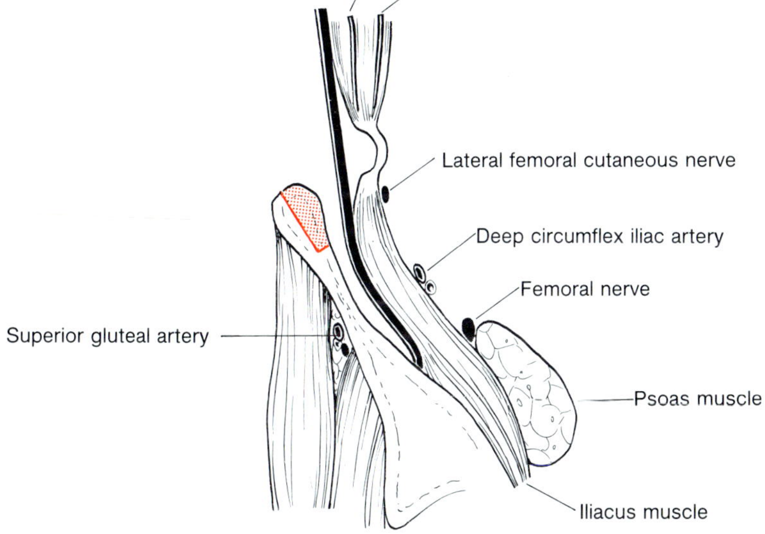

Fig. 331. Anatomy of bone graft removal from the inner table of the ilium. The incision and fascial mobilization are initiated at the outer lip of the iliac crest. The inner table is exposed strictly on the subperiosteal plane so that the iliacus muscle with the lateral femoral cutaneous nerve, deep circumflex iliac artery, and femoral nerve can be retracted atraumatically and far enough medially to permit harvesting of the graft

gress very quickly after plate removal as the graft undergoes remodeling in response to functional stresses (Fig. 333b) (Roux's law).

The interposed bone graft may be tied to the plate with absorbable threads if desired (Fig. 334), but this additional fixation is not crucial. The success of the reconstruction relies on an immobile bed between the mandibular stumps and the reconstruction plate. Screw fixation of the graft is necessary only if the graft is not long enough to span the defect completely. In that case a pair of emergency screws may be placed at each end of the graft, or one screw may be placed at its center.

A different fixation technique is needed in cases where the defect is not stably bridged with a plate, e.g., when a tumor patient consents to the secondary bone graft only on condition that the reconstruction plate be permanently removed. In such cases the bone graft functions both as the bridging device and as the bony buttress. The cortical surface of the graft faces outward, which prolongs revascularization but lessens the danger of premature screw loosening (Fig. 335). Excellent stability is obtained using a minimum of fixation material: three lag screws and two interosseous wires (see p. 119). Even in the initial osteoblastic phase, the pressure at the graft-recipient junction "welds" the graft to the recipient bone and promotes ear-

a

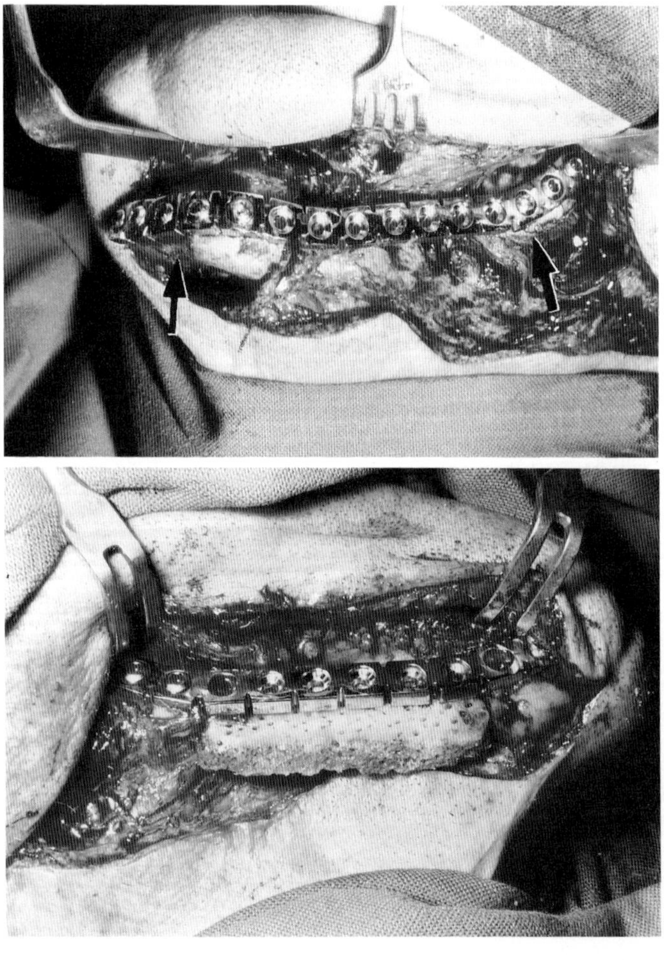

b

Fig. 332. a The defect is stably bridged according to the four-screw rule *(see black arrows)* as a prelude to accurate size determination and interposition of the graft. **b** The cancellous surface of the graft faces the well-perfused buccal tissue bed to enhance revascularization

Fig. 333. **a** At implant removal, granulation residues adjacent to the plate site indicate impairment of early revascularization by the plate itself. (Analogous findings would be seen around the screw holes if the graft had been fixed with screws. These screws would have become loose and would almost certainly have led to infection and failure of the graft. Biomechanical integration of the interposed graft is obtained by omitting screw fixation of the graft and instead wedging it firmly between the bone ends. **b** Functional remodeling of the healed graft is apparent several years after plate removal

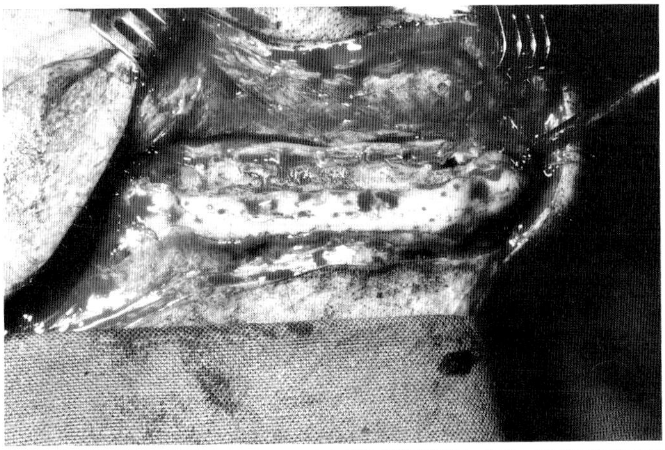

a

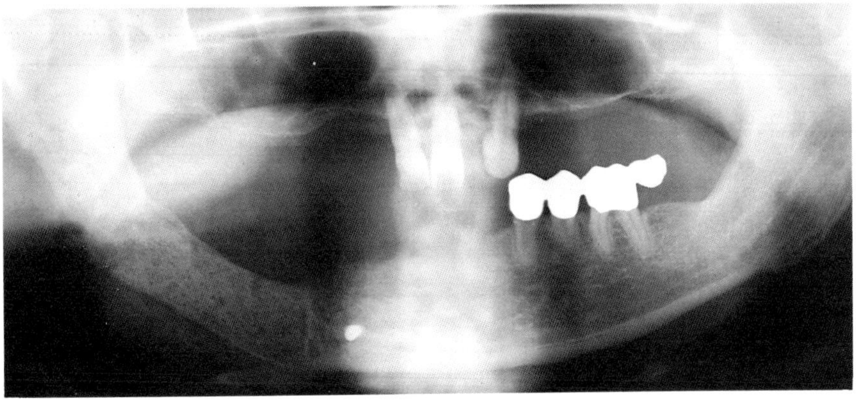

b

ly revascularization. At least a six-week period of rigid intermaxillary fixation (with maxillary and mandibular splints, Fig. 335 c) is recommended to allow for the concomitant processes of bone resorption and new bone formation (substitution). This is followed by fixation with elastics to assist remodeling; by six months, continuity is reestablished by lamellar bone (Fig. 336).

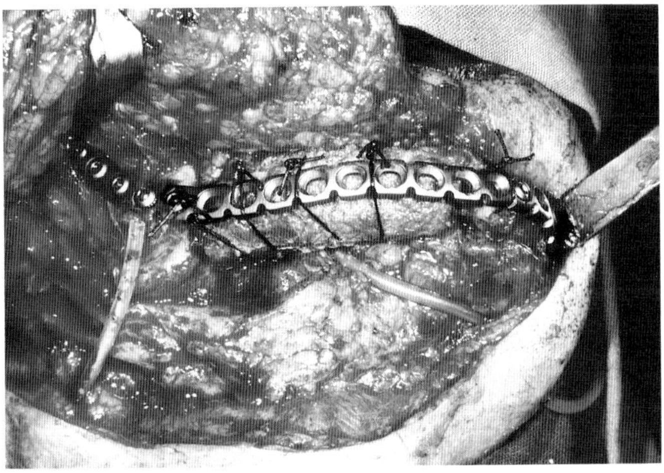

Fig. 334. Interpositional graft tied to the reconstruction plate with absorbable sutures

3.2.2.4 Primary Interpositional Autogenous Bone Graft

3.2.2.4.1 Indications

Two circumstances limit the use of primary bone grafting: the increased risk of infection and the potential for loss of the bone graft and of any local or distant flap transfers in the event of a tumor recurrence.

Even the best grafting technique cannot fully compensate for intraoperative contamination of the recipient bed by intraoral flora. What is more, a primary bone graft is not appropriate when pre- and postoperative radiation is given as an adjuvant to surgical resection. This does not apply to recurrences that were irradiated some time before, in which case the radiation-damaged tissue bed can be reconstructed with myocutaneous flaps that will provide for good graft vascularization and osteoinduction.

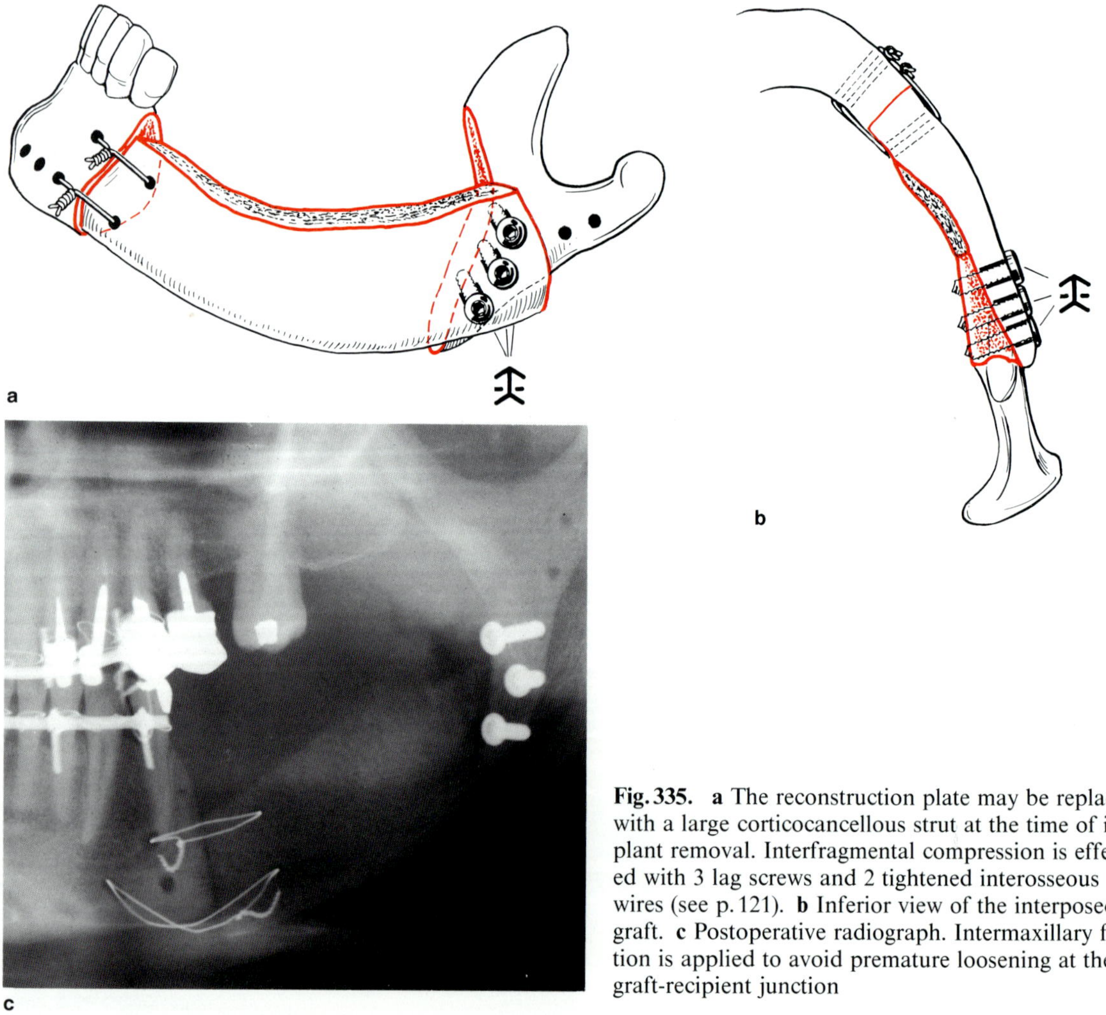

Fig. 335. **a** The reconstruction plate may be replaced with a large corticocancellous strut at the time of implant removal. Interfragmental compression is effected with 3 lag screws and 2 tightened interosseous wires (see p. 121). **b** Inferior view of the interposed graft. **c** Postoperative radiograph. Intermaxillary fixation is applied to avoid premature loosening at the graft-recipient junction

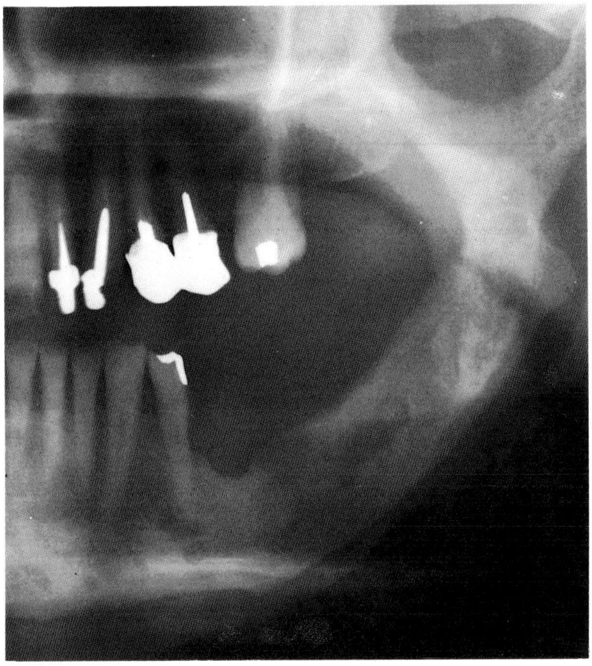

Fig. 336. Status following implant removal

Thus, primary bone grafting after a malignant tumor resection should be limited to highly selected cases. These would include T4 N0 carcinomas of the alveolar process in which the lymph nodes are clear and there is only circumscribed involvement of the bone.

A primary bone graft may also be considered in older patients with T4 osseous involvement and palpable lymph node involvement (N1). Not infrequently, these patients will categorically refuse an en bloc resection and will consent only to radiotherapy. But the side-effects associated with the delivery of a certain focal radiation dose will prompt the patient to discontinue treatment and agree to the recommended surgery. A one-stage resection and recontruction is justified in these exceptional cases to reduce morbidity. We would also advise using a cancellous bone graft so that risk factors are minimized.

A primary bone graft is less problematic in patients with semimalignant tumors. Many are ideal candidates for primary reconstruction with a *cancellous* or *block bone graft*.

3.2.2.4.2 Compressed Autogenous Cancellous Bone Chips

Principle of the Cancellous Bone Graft

Recent clinical and experimental experience confirms the earlier assertion (Mattis 1929, 1932) that autogenous cancellous bone can be transplanted with a far lower risk than any other nonmicrovascular autograft or allograft material. A great many live bone cells can be transferred with the freshly harvested cancellous bone and can survive as a result of diffusion and early revascularization (Decker et al. 1976). When present in sufficient numbers, these cells can make a significant contribution to new bone formation. This ability, known as osteogenic potential (cell-specific osteogenesis), and the osteoinductive potential are mutually supportive in their effect. The inductive differentiation of mesenchymal cells in the tissue bed apparently plays the greater role. The inductive effect depends on an unaltered bone matrix (Schweiberer 1970) and is believed to be mediated by a "bone morphogenetic protein" and inhibitor (Urist et al. 1970).

The essential point is that new bone formation in a cancellous graft depends upon the *quantity* of unaltered matrix that is transplanted with the graft. This underlies the rationale for using *compressed* cancellous bone, whose osteoinductive effect increases in proportion to the amount of matrix that is present in the graft per unit volume.

Removal of the Graft

An excellent donor site for cancellous bone is the anterior iliac crest (Fig. 337 a), which can provide sufficient material to reconstruct a mandibular defect 5–6 cm long. A wide osteotome is used to raise a bone flap on a medial hinge of periosteum (Fig. 337 b, c). Exposure of the outermost rim of the iliac crest terminates anteriorly three fingerwidths behind the superior spine to perserve the cutaneous iliohypogastric and lateral cutaneous femoral nerve branches. The reflected bone flap is replaced and fixed in place with a periosteal-fascial suture to restore the contour of the iliac crest and prevent hematoma formation.

If the ilium cannot serve as a donor site, the necessary quantity of cancellous bone can be harvested from the greater trochanter (Fig. 338). As on the ilium, a cortical cap is raised on a periosteal hinge (Fig. 339), taking care to preserve the calcar so as to avoid the risk of fracture. The skin incision is made over the right greater tuberosity (Fig. 340). The tensor fascia is incised longitudinally, simultaneously separating the fibers of gluteus medius and maximus down to the bone.

The posterior portions of the iliac wings are a good cancellous bone source for grafting defects more than 6 cm long. Starting a handswidth cranial to the posterior iliac spine, a pair of incisions are made three fingerwidths from the midline on each side and are carried to the lumbodorsal fascia. Placed in this fashion, the incisions will not sever the main branches of the superior cluteal nerves (Fig. 341, left). The site for creation of the bone flap and the harvesting technique are shown in the right half of Fig. 341.

Production and Use of Compressed Cancellous Bone Grafts

To produce compressed cancellous bone grafts, we use a pneumatic press consisting of a plunger, upper die, and lower die which compress the cancellous bone chips into sections that match the shape of the three principal

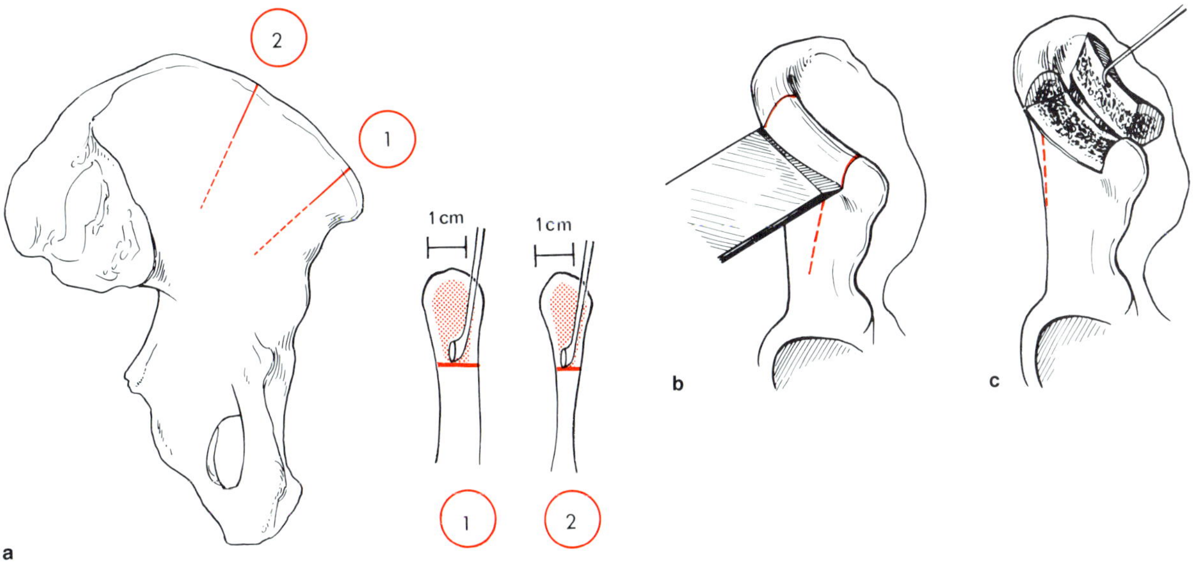

Fig. 337. **a** The iliac wing as a source of cancellous bone. *1* Cross-section of the drawing in Fig. 337b. The anterior part of the iliac creast contains a large cancellous bone reservoir extending almost to the acetabulum. *2* Cross-section of the drawing in Fig. 337c. The cancellous bone reservoir narrows in the direction of the acetabulum. **b** An osteoperiosteal flap is raised from the anterior iliac crest with a broad chisel, leaving an intact medial hinge of periosteum. **c** The flap is elevated on its periosteal hinge for harvesting of the cancellous bone

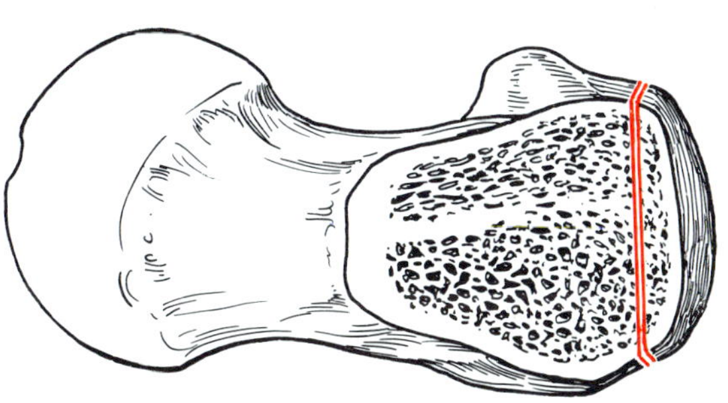

Fig. 338. Cross-section through the proximal portion of the greater trochanter. The calcar should be left intact during cancellous bone removal so that the proximal femur is not weakened

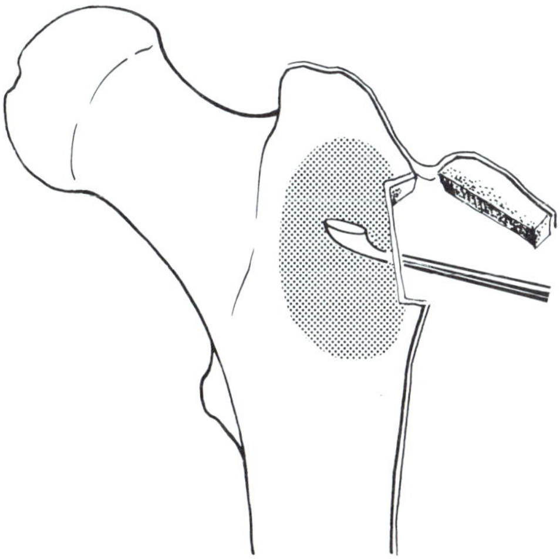

Fig. 339. The bony cap is elevated on a periosteal hinge

segments of the mandibular body[17] (Figs. 342 and 343). The compressed central (chin) or lateral segment is interposed between the ends of the fragments.

Because of the viscoelasticity of cancellous bone, the graft will swell shortly after removal from the lower die, increasing its volume by approximately 20%. It should be placed into the mandibular defect without delay, therefore. One advantage of this swelling effect is that it enhances the inductive effect on the tissue bed. Overcompaction of the cancellous bone should be avoided, as it will delay revascularization. The pressure should

[17] Manufacturer: Synthes AG, G. Hug, D-7801 Umkirch bei Freiburg, West Germany.

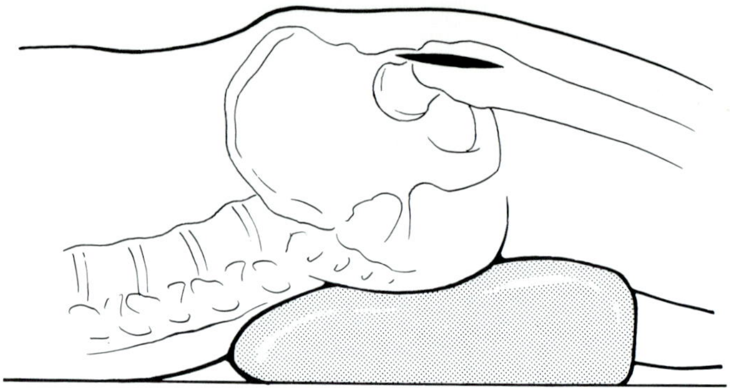

Fig. 340. Position for obtaining cancellous bone from the greater trochanter: left lateral positioning with the right buttock elevated on a pad

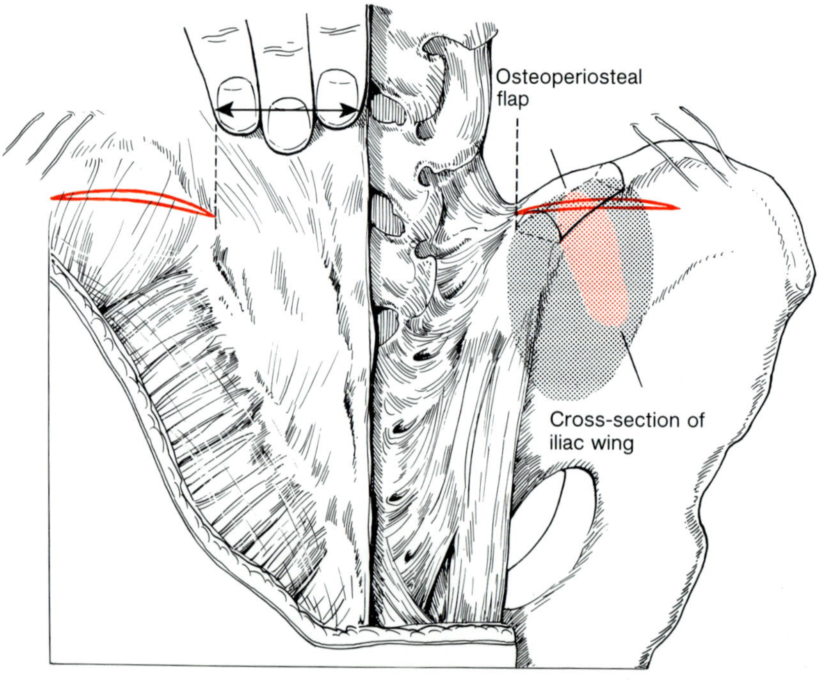

Fig. 341. *Left:* Approach for removing cancellous bone from the posterior iliac wing while sparing the cutaneous branches of the superior clunial nerves. Starting 3 fingerwidths from the midline, the skin is incised to the lumbodorsal fascia on each side at a level one handwidth above the posterior iliac spine. *Right:* Topography of the donor site on the posterior iliac wing showing the cross-section of the wing and the contours of the osteoperiosteal flap

not exceed a maximum of 90 kg and should be increased gradually (over about a 10-min period) so that the graft does not become overcompacted and biologically inferior to unaltered cancellous bone chips despite its greater osteogenic potency. Because osteoinductive potential is also diminished by prolonged exposure to air – a 50% decrease in 90 min (Puranen 1966) – the cancellous bone should be transferred to the recipient site as soon after harvesting as possible. If delay is unavoidable, the graft should be stored in Ringer's solution.

To prevent secondary flaking, the tissue around the bone graft should form a closed bed, as in Fig. 346b where the lingual muscles form one con-

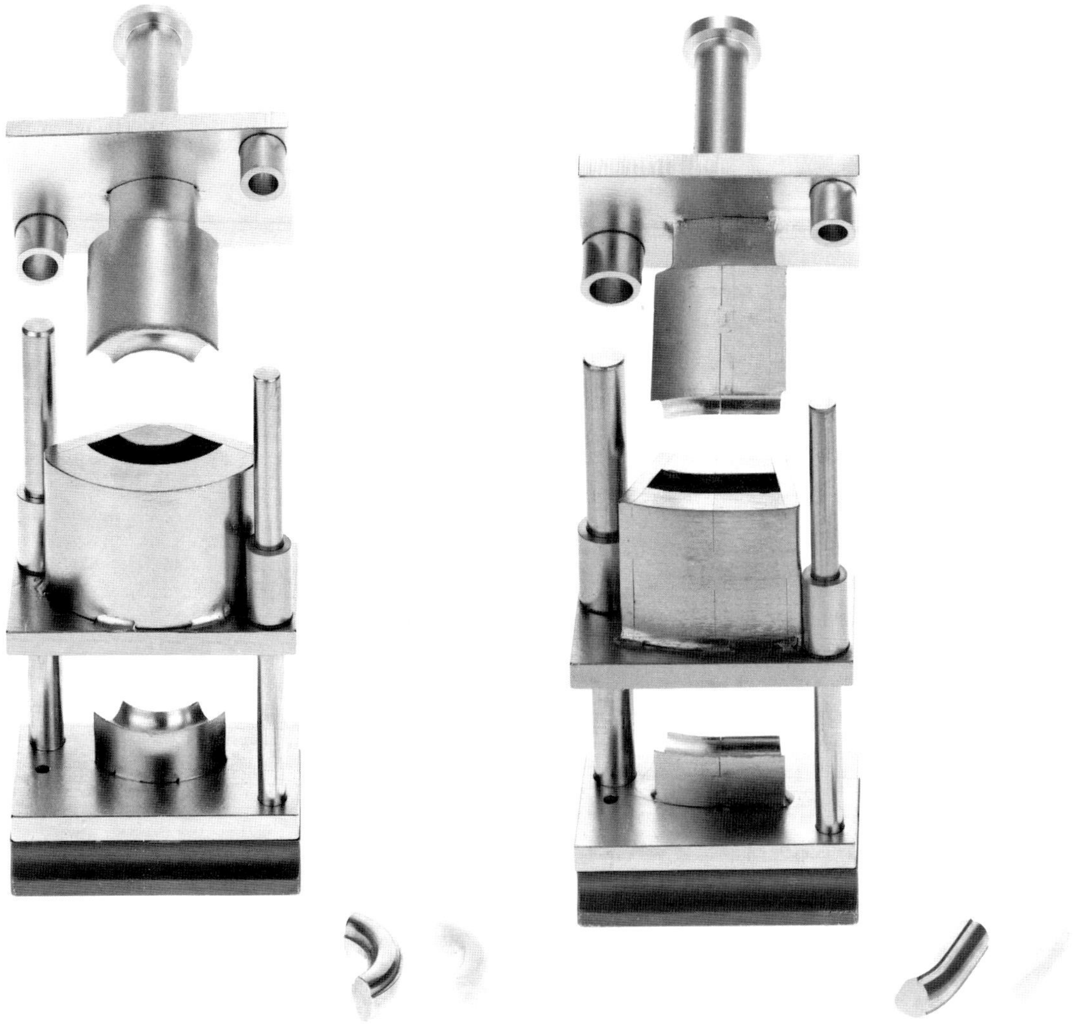

Fig. 342. Upper and lower dies of the cancellous bone press. *Left:* For production of the central (chin) segment. *Right:* For production of a lateral segment

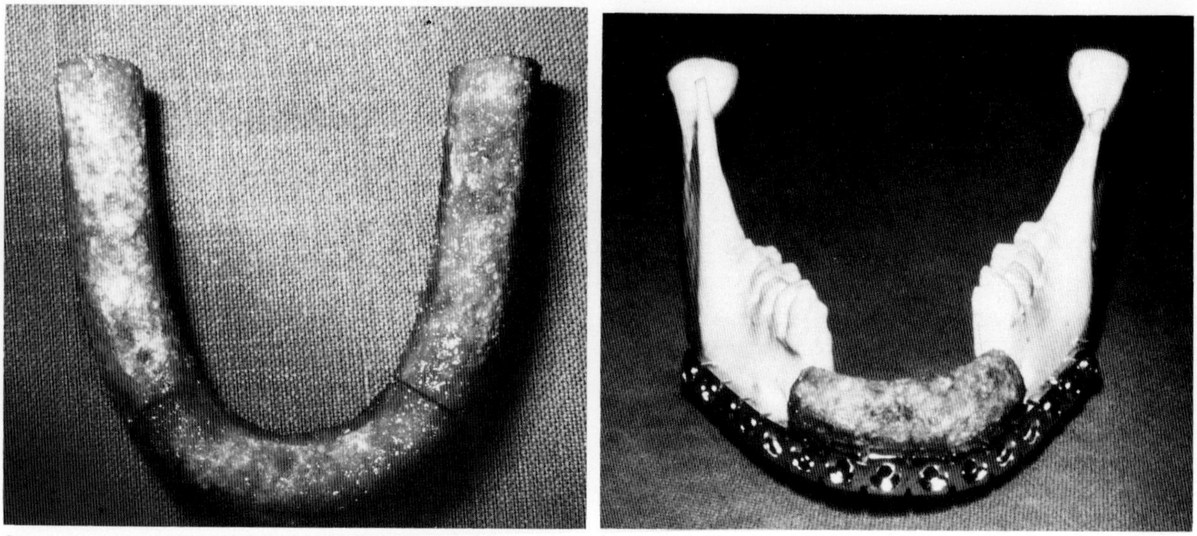

a b

Fig. 343. **a** Compressed cancellous bone graft segments assembled for replacement of the mandibular body. **b** Model of a functionally stable reconstruction consisting of a reconstruction plate and an interposed cancellous bone block pressed into the desired shape

taining wall and the cheek flap the other. If the graft is not well contained by local tissues, a Vicryl mesh implant can be used. As in any primary bone grafting of the mandible, a special technique is used to close the oral wall of the bed. Because the oral mucosa does not have a muscular coat or an adventitia or serosa, it generally is closed in a single layer, especially in the area of the alveolar process. Consequently, suture line dehiscence at this site is the most frequent cause of postoperative infection of the graft bed. This can be avoided by reinforcing the mucosal suture with a second, submucosal suture. Due to the absence of a muscular coat, the second suture should encompass adjacent muscle if at all possible (e.g., the intrinsic and extrinsic muscles of the tongue or the skeletal muscle of the floor of the mouth. The submucosal stitch (that adjacent to the graft) is placed first, using simple interrupted threads of absorbable material that broadly approximate the edges of that layer. Then the epithelial layer on the oral side is sutured with a nonabsorbable, material such as Supramid 4-0, preferably using continuous technique. Finally it is recommended that both suture lines be reinforced with a third row of all-layer sutures. The reinforcing sutures may be applied in stages *before* closing the individual layers (e.g., 3 Supramid sutures spaced 1 cm apart), or the all-layer interrupted sutures may be placed after the wound has been closed in layers (Fig. 344).

The following case reports are offered in place of a summary:

T4 N1 Carcinoma in a 75-year-old woman (Fig. 345)
(The side-effects following the delivery of 40 gyn of radiation to a residual tumor motivated the patient to consent to the operation originally planned.)

Figure 346 shows the extent of the resection and the preliminary attachment of a reconstruction plate with two screws each in the proximal and distal stumps. Following the segmental resection and the definitive fixation of the mandibular stumps according to the "four-screw-minimum" rule, a compressed cancellous bone graft is interposed.

The postoperative radiographs demonstrate the screw placement and the compressed cancellous bone graft interposed without additional fixation material (Fig. 347).

Thc radiograph after plate removal clearly shows the formation of new cortical bone on the graft (Fig. 348 a). Figure 348 b shows the intraoral appearance of the closed recipient bed.

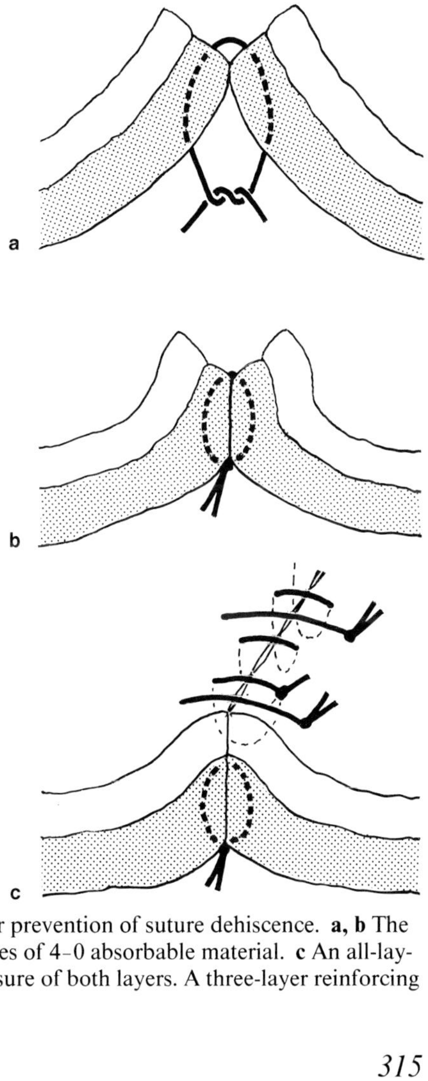

Fig. 344 a–c. Two-layer closure technique for prevention of suture dehiscence. **a, b** The first row consists of simple submucosal sutures of 4–0 absorbable material. **c** An all-layer reinforcing suture is applied following closure of both layers. A three-layer reinforcing stitch is used if skeletal muscle is present

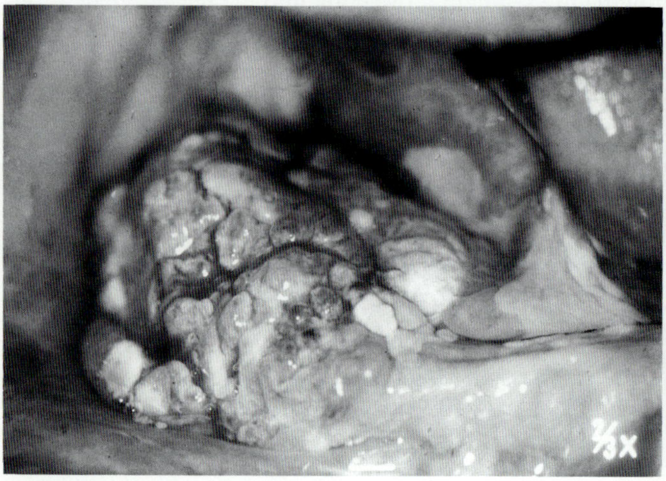

a

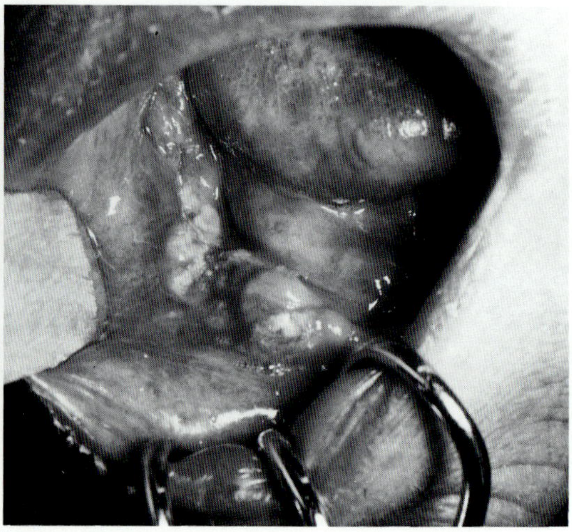

b

Fig. 345. **a** Exophytic carcinoma of the right alveolar process. **b** Residual tumor after discontinuation of radiotherapy

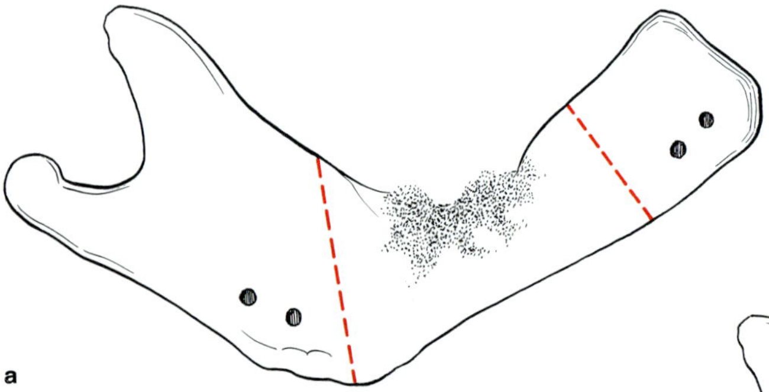

a

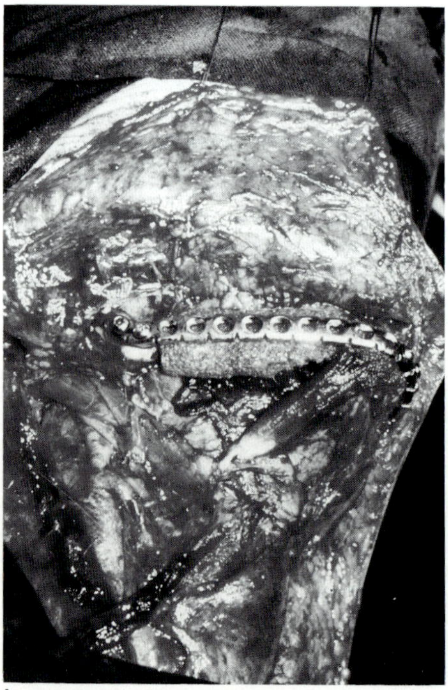

b

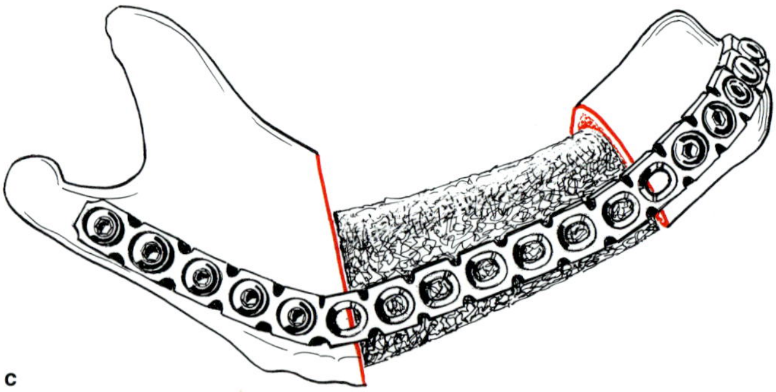

c

Fig. 346. **a** Lines of resection and preliminary drill holes for subsequent bridging of the defect with a suitably contoured reconstruction plate. **b** Stably bridged defect with interposed compressed cancellous block. **c** Artist's depiction

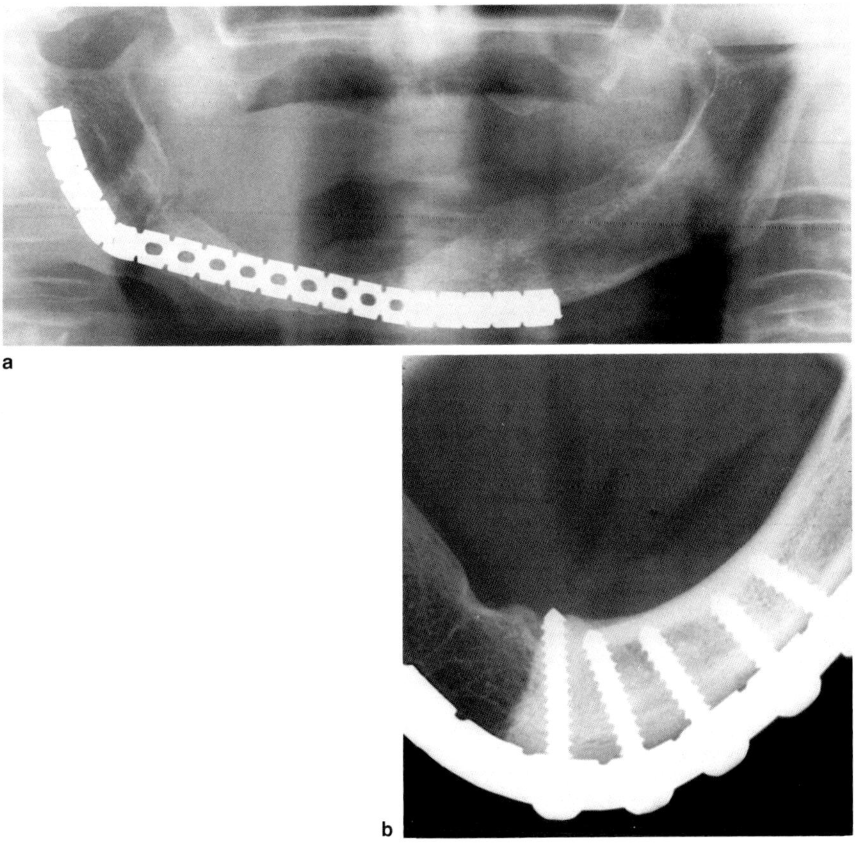

a

b

Fig. 347. **a** Postoperative radiograph. **b** Application of the four-screw rule is well documented

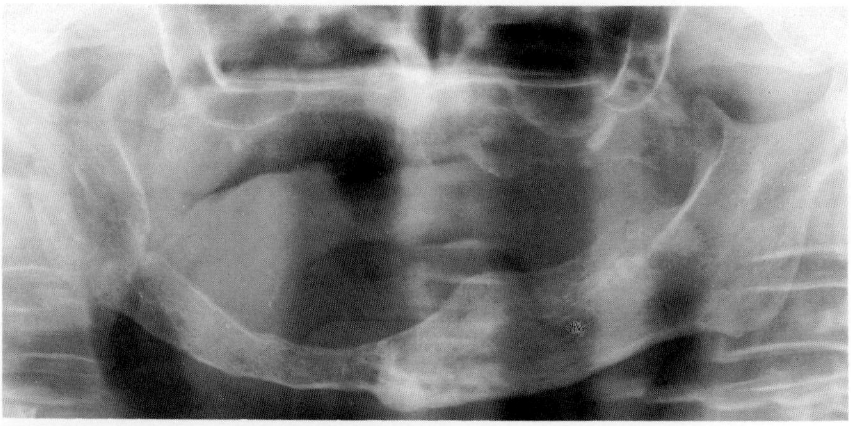

a

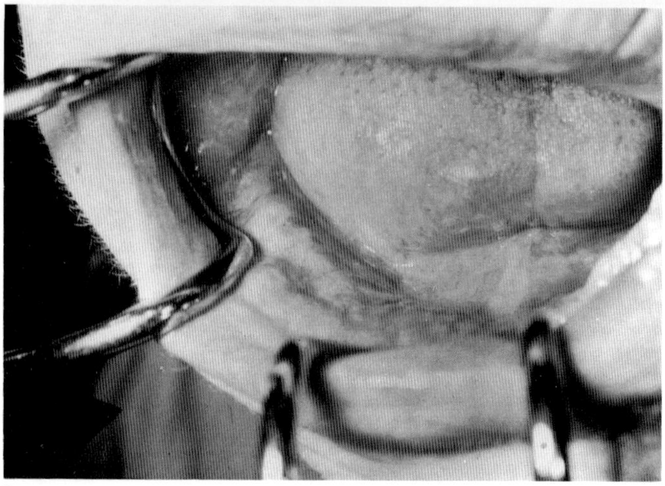

b

Fig. 348. **a** Status after plate removal. **b** Intraoral appearance at 4 years

3.2.2.4.3 Autogenous Block Bone Graft

It is clear that preliminary stabilization greatly facilitates a radical mandibular resection and the interposition of a block graft. This technique has emerged as the dominant therapy for adamantinoma. This semimalignant tumor most commonly affects the mandible, and multiply recurrent growths can assume a malignant character through local or intracanalicular spread. Even today the rate of recurrence is relatively high.[18] This has led to recommendations for a standardized, radical surgical therapy for these tumors, as the following case illustrates:

[18] In 1986 the German-language UICC Multicentric Study, started in 1977, reviewed data from 526 patients with osteosarcoma, fibrosarcoma, Ewing's sarcoma, malignant lymphoma and ameloblastoma. Approximately half (258) the tumors were ameloblastomas, of which 25 (about 6%) recurred; 2 patients developed distant metastases.

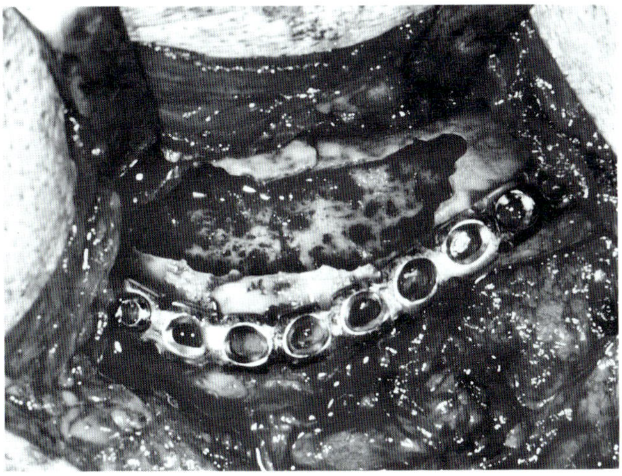

a

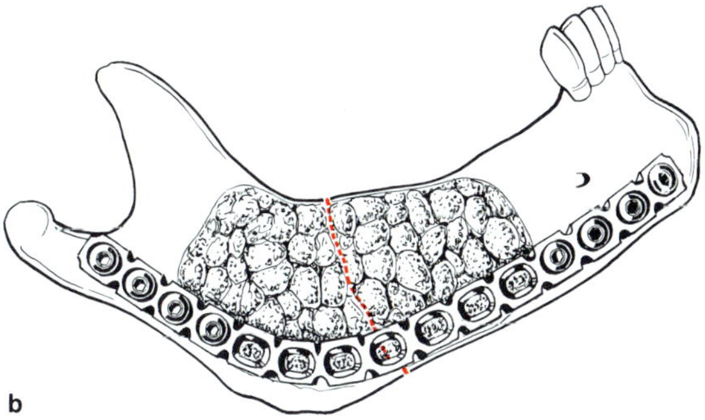

b

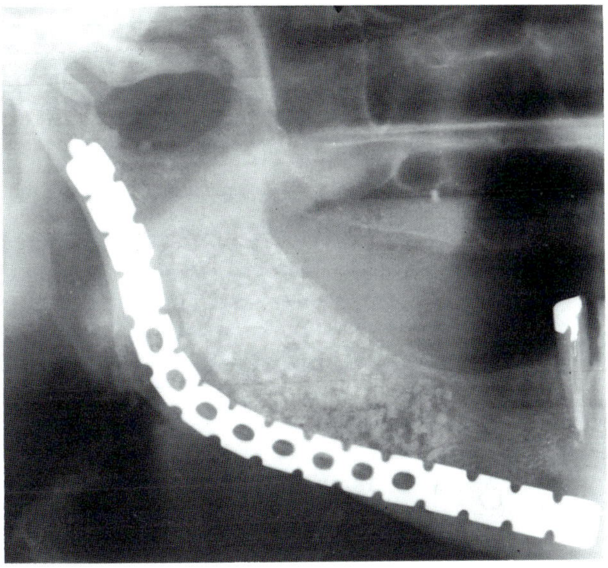

c

Fig. 353. **a** Multiple erosions through the bone are apparent on the lingual side of the cyst. **b** The defect is obliterated, and a neutralization plate is applied. **c** Postoperative radiograph

periosteal sheath is preserved on the lingual and marginal aspects and a protective neutralization plate is applied (see Fig. 353 a), there is no longer any danger of fragment displacement.

A large cystic cavity can be obliterated with a mixture of autogenous cancellous bone chips and Ceros 80 (hydroxylapatite)[19] (Fig. 353 b, c).

[19] Highly porous, polycrystalline hydroxylapatite granules. R. Mathys & Co, CH-2544 Bettlach.

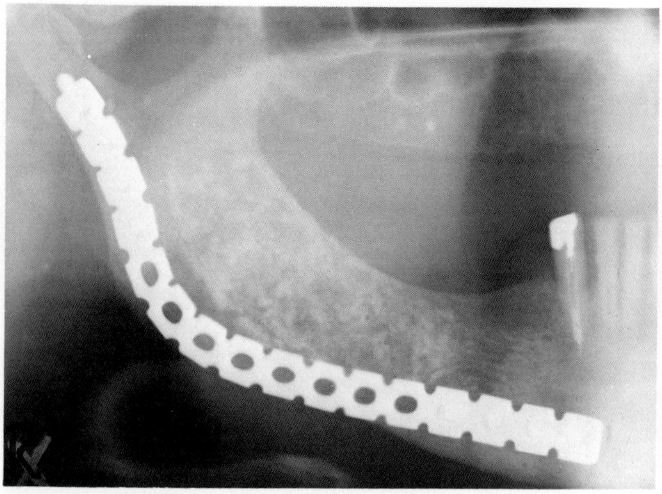

Fig. 354. Radiograph at 5 years. The hydroxylapatite is integrated into the bone but has not been fully absorbed

Figure 354 shows the status at 5 years after surgery. The hydroxylapatite is absorbed slowly but shows satisfactory osseous integration. So far the patient has declined to have the plate removed.

4.2 Plating for the Removal of an Impacted Wisdom Tooth

The neutralization plate is occasionally indicated for the removal of an impacted third molar from an atrophic mandible (Fig. 355). Although this requires a more extensive operation, it is justified by the risk of iatrogenic fracture with a bone defect and the danger of subsequent osteitis (see Fig. 305).

The neutralization plate is removed at once after autogenous cancellous bone grafting is completed (Fig. 356 a).

Figure 356 b shows the status at 2 months.

6 Osteotomies

Definition
Mandibular osteotomies are planned surgical divisions of bone for the purpose of shortening or lengthening the mandible or increasing or decreasing its size.

The success of the corrective osteotomy depends on how well the osteotomy site is stabilized against skeletal displacement and relapse during the healing period. That is why stable internal fixation has become a valuable adjunct to surgical orthopedics. Examples are the lag screw fixation of the sagittal split osteotomy of the ascending ramus and the plate fixation of sliding osteotomies and ostectomies of the mandibular body.

6.1 Sagittal Split Osteotomy of the Ascending Ramus (Laminotomy)

Definition
The sagittal split ramus osteotomy involves the separation of the outer cortex from the cancellous bone (laminotomy) either *up to* the mandibular angle (Trauner and Obwegeser 1957) or *including* the mandibular angle (Dal Pont 1961). The goal is to reposition the fragments while maintaining a sufficiently large area of bone-to-bone contact.

6.1.1 Advantages

The benefits of enlarging the area of interfragmental contact are fully realized only when the technique of functionally stable internal fixation is integrated into the treatment concept. The early mobilization and primary bone healing provided by this technique can dramatically lower the incidence of recurrence[20] and of arthrogenic dysfunction.[21] Moreover, the period of in-

[20] Two of 29 patients had a complete recurrence, four a partial recurrence. All the recurrences were retrognathias with or without an open bite.
[21] None of the patients with a preoperative joint click had similar complaints when seen at follow-up.

termaxillary fixation is reduced to 1-2 weeks in difficult cases, while in normal cases the patient is able to open the jaw immediately after surgery.[22] This results in a substantially shorter hospital stay[23] and an earlier return to work[24]. Generally there is no need for postsurgical orthodontic treatment. (Güdel 1986).

6.1.2 Disadvantages

The foregoing advantages must be weighed against the potential for intraoperative complications and late sequelae. Various disadvantages have been cited, including heavy blood loss,[25] the technical difficulty of the sagittal split,[26] and postoperative edema.[27] A relatively high incidence of postoperative nerve deficits also has been reported. Experience indicates that these problems can be minimized by following a standardized technique, although the Dal Pont operation is associated with a significant incidence of hypesthesia of the inferior alveolar nerve[28] (Güdel 1986).

6.1.3 Planning

The fragments are in their definitive position at the time the lag screws are inserted. This fact shifts the emphasis in treatment away from postoperative care toward preoperative preparation.

About half the patients will require presurgical orthodontic treatment. It is assumed that the correct use of teleradiographs and models is known.

Accurate positioning of the articular segment is of major importance when the internal fixation is performed. We achieve this by determining preoperatively the size of the bone fragment that is to be excised. For this purpose Schmoker (1975a) designed a "simulograph" device based on the principle of the diascope. Also, since projections to a flat surface poorly simulate the three-dimensional result of the osteotomy, various devices have been developed for restoring the articular segment to its presurgical

---

[22] The IMF was released at the end of the operation in 25 cases and retained for an average of 14 days in the remaining 4. These included 3 patients with a cortical fracture.

[23] The average length of hospitalization was 6.5 days.

[24] Lost job time: 2 weeks: 11%;
3 weeks: 22%;
4 weeks: 44%;
6 weeks: 22%

[25] None of the 29 patients operated upon required a blood transfusion.

[26] Three cortical plate fractures occurred in the 58 sagittal osteotomies. It should be added that the operations were performed in a teaching hospital.

[27] Recall the average 6.5-day length of hospitalization.

[28] There was one case in which intraoperative nerve injury was observed. Postoperative hypesthesia was documented in 16 of 58 sagittal splits, with symptoms still persisting in ⅓ of patients after one year.

position. These devices utilize the maxilla as a stable reference, from which the distance to the ascending ramus is determined in centric occlusion. Following the osteotomy the proximal segment is repositioned in accordance with the distance previously determined. Spiessl and Tschopp (1974) developed a forklike device with a scale that attaches to the maxillary arch splint and retains the divided ramus in its original position. Leonard et al. (1985) use a "proximal segment orienting device" (PSOD) with a paddle extension (Fig. 367), which offers a simple and reliable means of establishing the position of the proximal segment.

Seto's technique of segmental repositioning (Seto and Matsuura 1984) (Fig. 368) is even simpler, as it uses a detachable miniplate to reproduce the normal distance between the fixed reference (maxilla) and the ascending ramus. In place of the simple miniplate, Raveh et al. (1983) use a specially

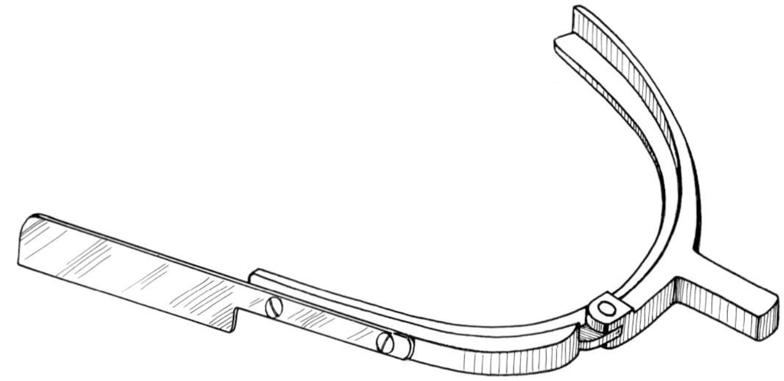

Fig. 367. Proximal segment orienting device (PSOD) of Leonard (Leonard et al. 1983)

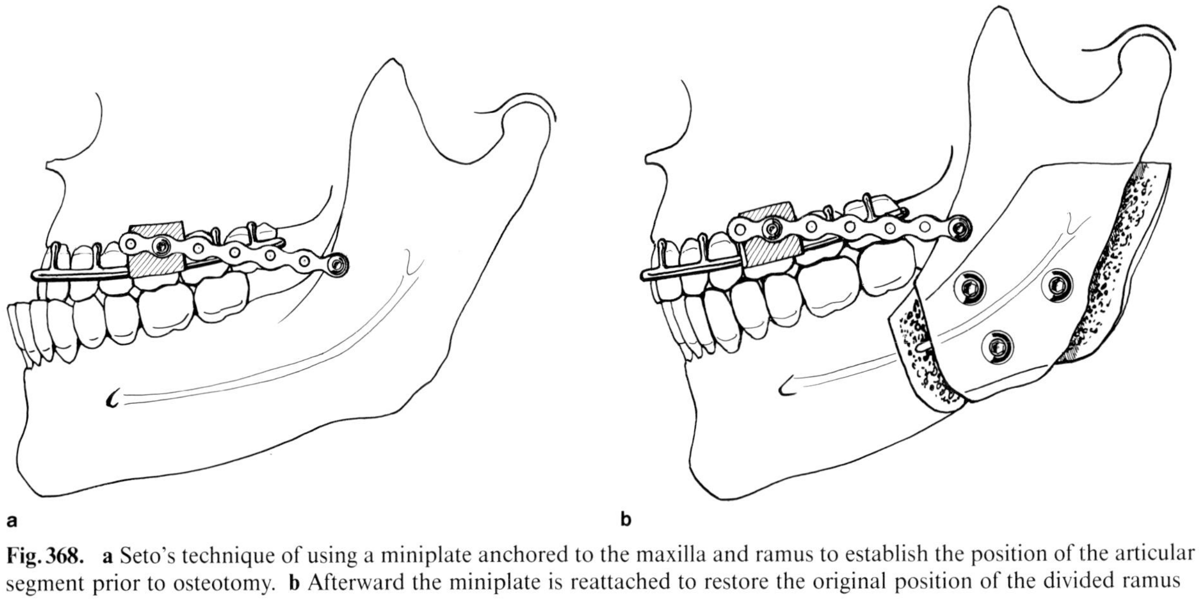

Fig. 368. **a** Seto's technique of using a miniplate anchored to the maxilla and ramus to establish the position of the articular segment prior to osteotomy. **b** Afterward the miniplate is reattached to restore the original position of the divided ramus

designed holding device with two anchoring elements and an adjustable midpiece to restore the normal distance. The stability of this device allows for even more accurate repositioning.

Initially we used the "centrostat" for this purpose, which employed a fixed reference system based on the calvarium and mandibular ramus (Spiessl 1981). A better and simpler variant of this principle utilizes the standard mandibular external fixation device (see Figs. 85-93).

Follow-up studies have shown, however, that there is virtually no difference between two- and three-dimensional positioning or between simple and more complex devices in terms of the postoperative joint function that is achieved.

Fears that screw fixation would incite arthrogenic complaints have not been confirmed either clinically in 29 patients (Güdel 1986) or by stereographic joint studies in operated patients using the TMJ system (personal communication from Gensheimer and Graber 1980).

Leonard followed 57 patients clinically over a 5-year period and made comparative pre- and postoperative CT measurements of the angle between the long axis of the condyles and the midsagittal plane (nasoauricular plane) and also the intercondylar angle (anteriorly open angle). These studies clearly show that repositioning of the divided ramus, as with the PSOD (Leonard et al. 1985), yields results that are functionally acceptable.

6.1.4 Instrumentation

Because of the parapharyngeal and extravisceral position of the ascending ramus (in the craniovertebral space), special retractors with a large offset are needed to permit atraumatic retraction of the soft tissues and provide a clear view for division of the bone. These retractors are supplied in the special ASIF set for sagittal ramus osteotomies (see Fig. 101).

The forked retractor (Fig. 369 left) is a modified Langenbeck retractor whose terminal, angulated blade carries fingerlike extensions. When the retractor is in place, the superior part of the ramus lies between the extensions, the longer "finger" providing a view into the pterygomandibular space and the shorter into the submasseter space (see Figs. 372 and 374).

The other type of retractor is a modified Hohmann elevator whose curved tip fits around the edge of the mandible and whose trough-shaped arm functions as a tissue protector. Two models are available: a medial retractor (Fig. 369 right and Fig. 373) to protect the maxillary artery and trigeminal nerve branch, and a lateral model (Fig. 369 center) designed for retraction of the masseter and the buccal soft tissues.

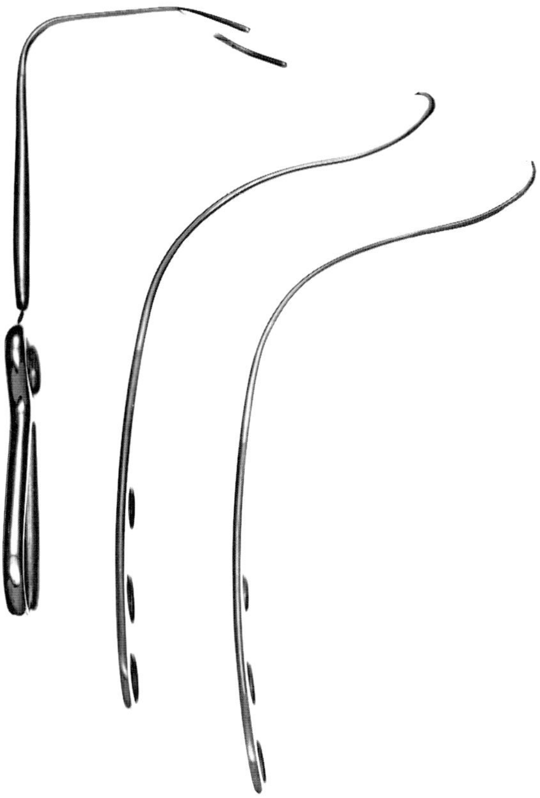

Fig. 369. *Left:* Forked retractor; *right:* medial prognathism retractor; *center:* lateral prognathism retractor

6.1.5 Anatomic Aspects of the Sagittal Split Osteotomy

Our systemic technique for the sagittal split osteotomy begins with exposure of the osteotomy sites according to strict anatomic criteria. Disregard for anatomy can have significant adverse consequences. Thus, for example, division of the buccinator muscle not only results in heavy intraoperative bleeding and subsequent anaesthesia of the buccal mucosa but also leads to troublesome scarring of the pterygomandibular fold and buccal sulcus with a prolonged restriction of jaw opening.

This muscle is preserved by releasing only its attachment on the buccinator crest (Fig. 370, 4) during division of the mucoperiosteum in the vestibule. Then the bony retromolar sulcus (fossa) posterior to the buccinator crest is exposed (Fig. 370, 3). The mucosa along the pterygomandibular fold is incised, and the underlying buccinator muscle is dissected free on the submucosal plane. The mobilized muscular wall is elevated from the anterior surface of the ramus as far as the coronoid process using a periosteal elevator that is bent on the flat and conforms to the curvature of the retromolar fossa; retraction is maintained with the swallowtail retractor. The

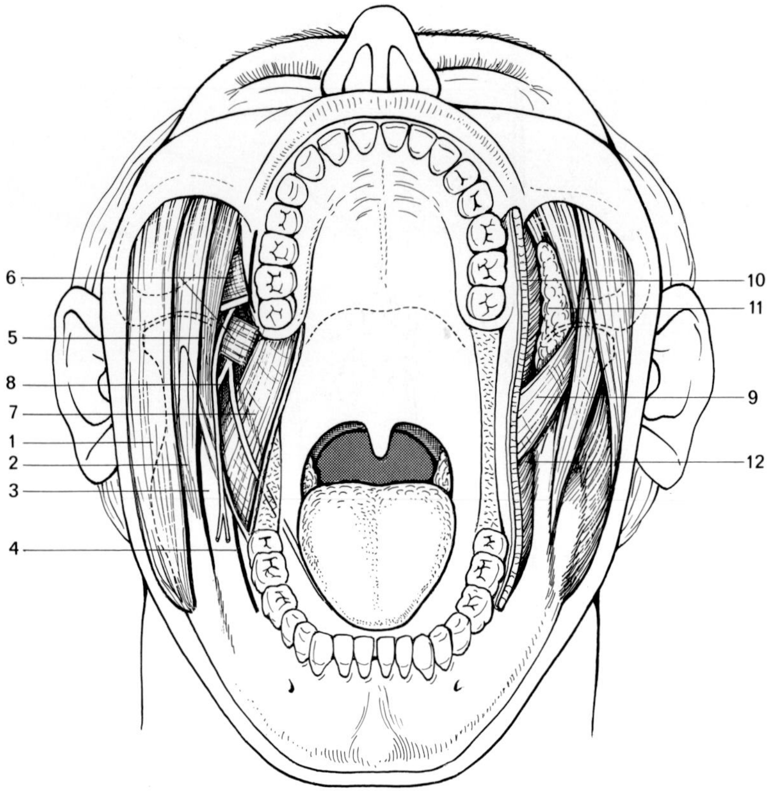

Fig. 370. *Left: 1* masseter, adherent medially to the *2* superficial limb of the temporalis muscle, *3* retromolar sulcus, *4* buccinator crest, *5* deep limb of temporalis muscle, *6* pterygoideus externus muscle with the buccal nerve between its heads, *7* pterygoideus internus muscle, *8* pterygomandibular space with the inferior alveolar and lingual nerves. *Right: 9* buccotemporal fascia (of Zenker), *10* buccinator muscle, *11* buccal space with Bichat's fat pad, *12* buccotemporal space (of Zenker)

rest of the procedure is dictated by the following anatomy, whose depiction in Fig. 370 is based on original anatomic specimens.[29]

On the left side of Fig. 370, the cheek is windowed to give a view of the four muscles of mastication. The outermost is the masseter (1), which is fused medially with the *superficial* limb of the temporalis muscle (2). The latter covers the anterior border of the ramus as far as the oblique line. Medial to the retromolar sulcus is the *deep* limb of the temporalis (5), which passes along the temporal crest and covers the mandibular foramen.

Intraoperatively the two limbs of the temporalis are split, and the adherent tendon fibers are sharply detached from the two bony margins - the crest and anterior border of the ramus. The anterior surface of the crest must be cleanly denuded to allow a strictly subperiosteal approach to the supralingular pterygomandibular space (8). The neurovascular "interpterygoid lamina" (Fig. 371) is carefully retracted medial along with the intact periosteum. To ensure preservation of this lamina and the nerves and blood vessels within it, we take down the sharp edge of the temporal crest with a pear-shaped bur (Fig. 372) so that the elevator can be inserted more easily beneath the intact periosteum.

[29] I am grateful to Prof. von Hochstetter, head of the Division of Topographic and Clinical Anatomy, Department of Surgery, University of Basel, for his assistance in the preparation of the diagram.

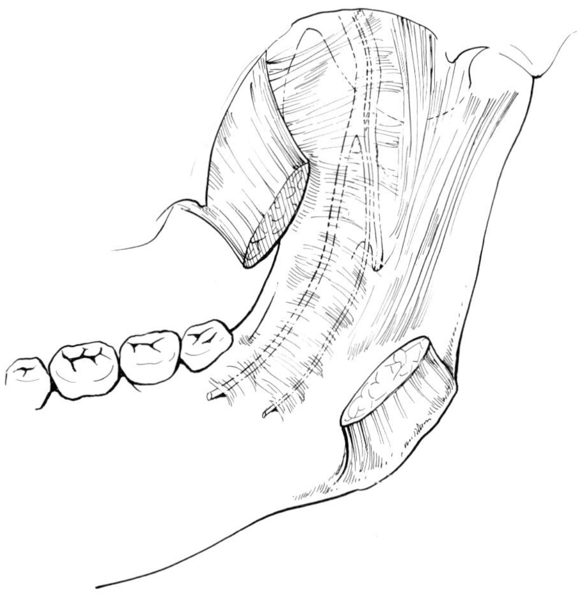

Fig. 371. The interpterygoid lamina. The mandibular periosteum and the medial muscular fascia of the pterygoideus internus muscle enclose a fibrous intermediate layer containing the inferior alveolar nerve, lingual nerve, mylohyoid nerve and bloodvessels

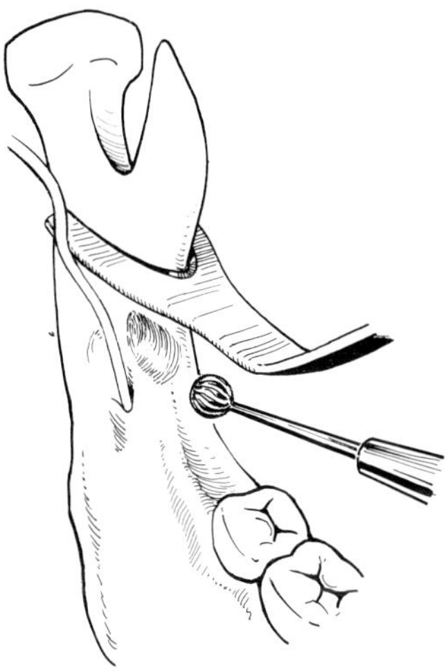

Fig. 372. Part of the temporal crest is burred away to facilitate subperiosteal elevation of the interpterygoid lamina and soft tissues and give a direct view of the posterior border of the ramus

Burring away the crest just below the base of the coronoid process affords a direct view into the pterygomandibular space as far as the posterior border of the ascending ramus. This makes it far easier to perform the osteotomy *under visual control.*

We use the alveolar part of the maxilla as a guide to determining the site for ablating the crest. An imaginary tangent to the maxillary dental arch, extended distally, will intersect the mandibular foramen when the mouth is widely open (Fig. 373). The supra*lingular* approach to the pterygomandibular space is made just above this imaginary line (see Fig. 370, 8).

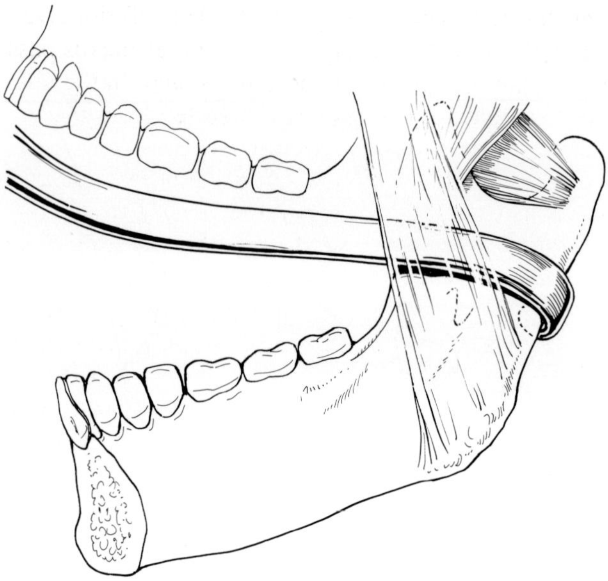

Fig. 373. Using the medial prognathism retractor to establish the supralingular approach. The dental arch of the maxilla serves as a guide for the level of the approach

Another way to determine the site is by exposing the *antilingula* deep to the masseter. The antilingula is a bony prominence on the lateral surface of the ramus (Fig. 374). Yates et al. (1976) were able to positively identify the antilingula in 44% of 70 macerated mandibles. In 41% the feature was present but indistinct.

In the anatomic specimen (see Fig. 370) the pterygoideus internus and externus muscles are shown detached from the medial surface of the ascending ramus. The buccal nerve emerges from between the heads of pterygoideus externus (6) and runs along the deep limb of the temporalis into the muscular wall of the buccinator, which is removed in the specimen. This important sensory nerve is spared by avoiding transverse division of

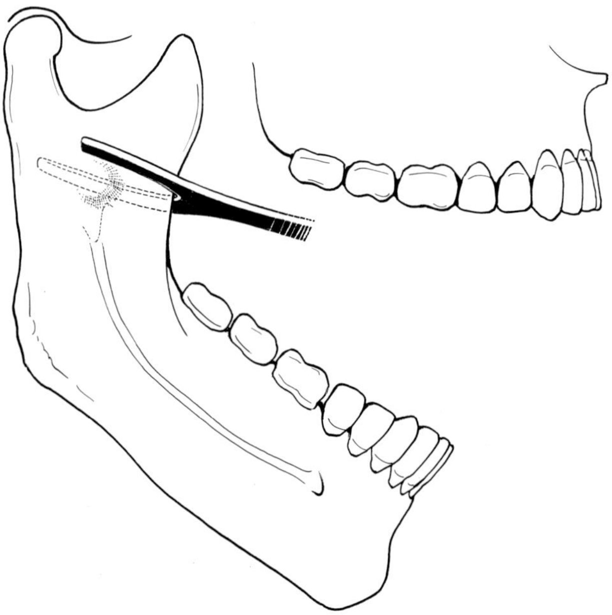

Fig. 374. The "antilingula" as an anatomic landmark for establishing the osteotomy line. Insertion of the forked retractor requires subperiosteal mobilization of the masseter muscle, at which time the antilingula can be identified

the buccinator muscle, as described above (see p. 337 ff.). The inferior alveolar and lingual nerves and the maxillary artery with its venous plexus pass between the pterygoidei to enter the pterygomandibular space. In the anatomic specimen the interpterygoid lamina has been dissected from the nerves and vessels to demonstrate this space (see also Fig. 371).

The right half of Fig. 370 shows the two limbs of the temporalis muscle in the foreground. A fascial sheet (9) (buccotemporal fascia of Zenker), often reinforced by tendon slips from the temporalis (buccal insertion of the temporalis), sweeps laterally to the buccinator muscle (10). This transverse aponeurotic fascia between the temporalis and buccinator muscles forms the boundary of the "buccal space" (11) for the Bichat fat pad and demarcates it from the "buccotemporal space" of Zenker below (12). Injury to this fascial sheet allows buccal fat to herniate into the buccotemporal space (supralingular area), making it very difficult to perform the osteotomy in that area. Besides the buccotemporal organ (of Kievitz and Zenker), the buccotemporal space contains the buccal nerve (8), the buccal artery, and a dense venous network that communicates with adjacent veins – the facial and inferior alveolar veins and the pterygoid venous plexus. Thus, it is important to elevate the strongly adherent periosteum of the supralingular area atraumatically at the inlet to the buccotemporal space, aided by ablation of the temporal crest (see Fig. 372), in order to avoid heavy bleeding and nerve injury.

6.1.6 Technique of the Sagittal Split Osteotomy (Laminotomy)

Before the cut is made on the medial aspect of the ramus, the bone along the oblique line is removed until the corticocancellous junction is identified (Fig. 375). Working from above downward, we cut a groove 5–8 mm deep using a large fissure bur. This will give the space needed to guide the osteotome precisely along the corticocancellous boundary. The groove is joined with the medial (buccotemporal) and lateral (submasseter) transverse cuts, and then the outer cortical bone is split off following the principle of *splitting by separation.*

Separation along the trajectorial boundary in the area of the intraosseous canal is accomplished manually with osteotomes (Fig. 376). The split should not be carried farther distally until the mandibular canal has been visualized. It should be noted that the pre- and postangular zones represent "safe" areas where the osteotome can be advanced along the corticocancellous junction without danger of nerve injury (Fig. 377).

We prefer the term "laminotomy" for the procedure, as it carries the connotation of detaching the cortical plate as a means of preserving the underlying nerve. The laminotomy forms the true technical principle of the Dal Pont operation. The term "sagittal split" originally implied enlarging the areas of the fragments. It does not express the point of the operation that we consider to the critical: preservation of the nerve canal, analogous to the neurosurgical procedure of laminectomy, whose aim is to expose and preserve the spinal cord.

Leonard et al. (1985) perform the cut with a power saw instead of an osteotome. They bur away an area of cortex about 5 × 5 mm in size at the

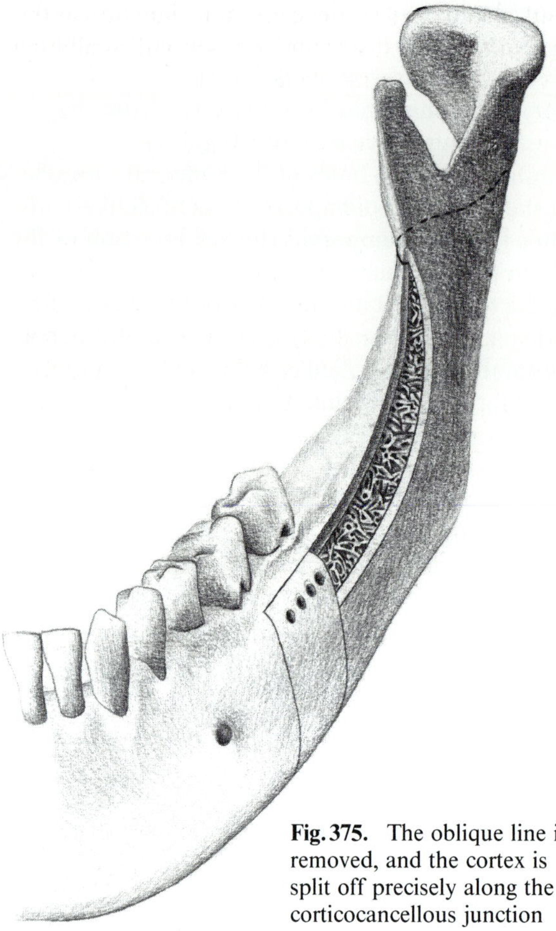

Fig. 375. The oblique line is removed, and the cortex is split off precisely along the corticocancellous junction

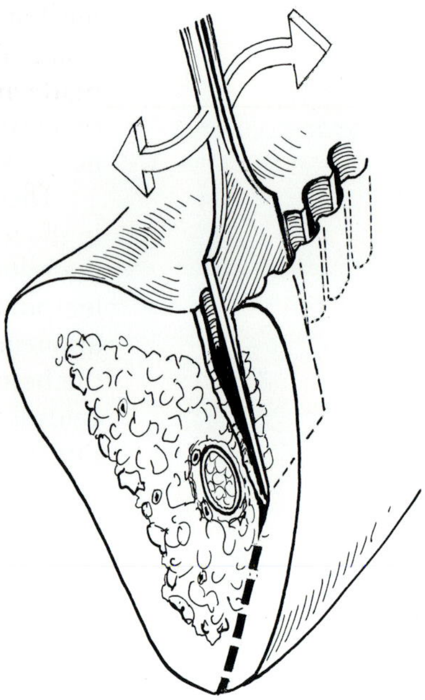

Fig. 376. *Splitting by separation:* Manual spreading in both directions with the osteotome separates the fine bony trabeculae from the outer cortical plate (lamina dura)

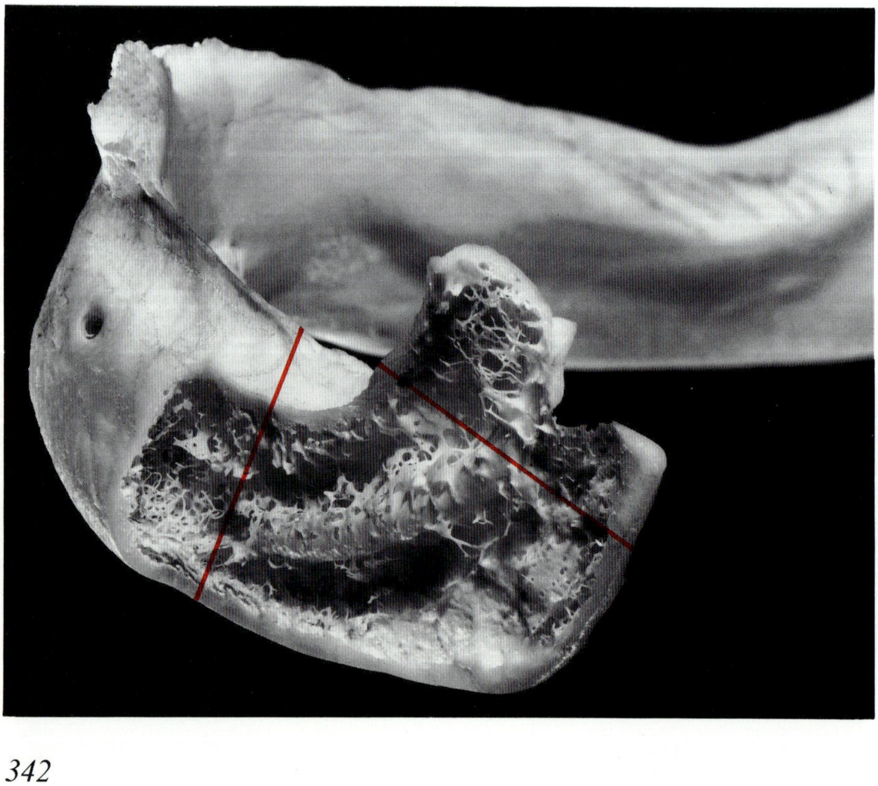

Fig. 377. Risk of nerve injury is minimal in the pre- and postangular zones

level of the second molar and identify the corticocancellous junction at that point. Then they split off the outer cortex, starting with a small oscillating blade and finishing with a long reciprocating blade.

6.1.7 Lag Screw Fixation

Rigid retention of the new occlusion (intermaxillary fixation with wire acrylic splints and wire ligatures) is an integral part of the internal fixation that follows. After the ramus fragment has been shortened according to the preoperative plan and placed in its original anatomical position (see p. 335), it is held against the body of the mandible with a special reduction forceps (see Fig. 379). A vertical stab incision is made in skin tension lines over the mandibular angle (Fig. 378), and the subcutaneous soft tissues are separated with a fine scissors in the direction of the marginal facial nerve branch until the osteotomy site is reached.

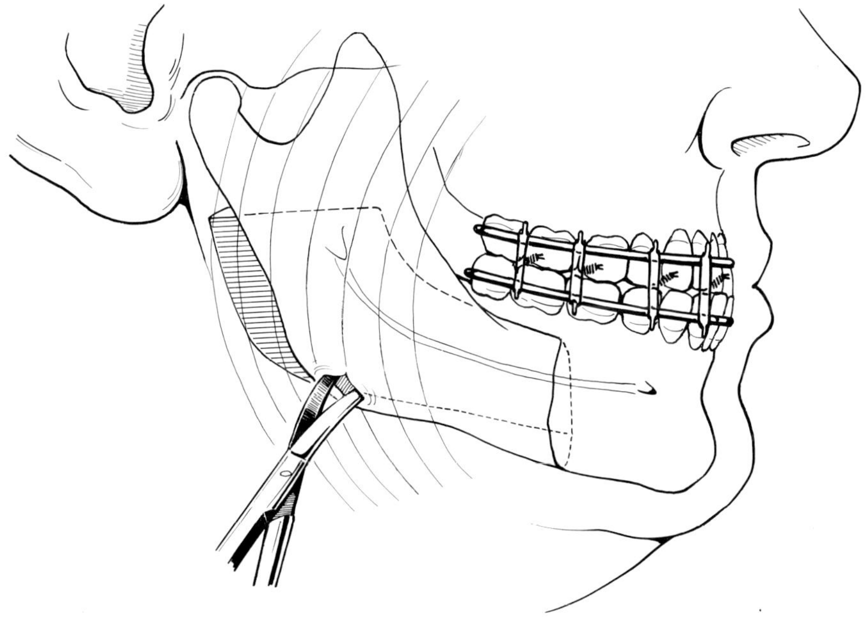

Fig. 378. A stab incision give access for insertion of the transbuccal instruments. The skin incision is 1 cm long and follows tension lines. Using the gridiron principle, the edges of the incision and the subcutaneous tissue are separated along the course of the marginal facial nerve branch down to the muscular layer. Then the fascia and periosteum are smoothly divided in the direction of the masseter fibers for the length of the skin incision. Sufficient access is developed for insertion of the trocar sleeve. It would be wrong to pierce the overlying muscle forcibly with the trocar point. Sufficient access is needed for correct placement of the three screws

A trocar with handle and metal point is introduced through the incision and is used to drill and fixate the fragments perpendicular to the bony surface. Figure 379 shows the drill sleeve inserted into the predrilled 2.7-mm gliding hole. The sleeve functions as a guide for the 2.0 mm bit used to drill the compression hole in the far cortex.

The individual steps of the percutaneous lag screw fixation are illustrated in Fig. 380:

a) The trocar with point attached is inserted through the stab incision.
b) The point is removed, and a cheek-retracting ring is attached to the trocar.
c) The drill sleeve (2.7 mm) is inserted.
d) The gliding hole is drilled in the near cortex (proximal fragment) with the 2.7-mm extra-long drill bit.
e) The 2.0-mm drill sleeve is introduced through the 2.7-mm gliding hole.
f) The compression hole is drilled in the far cortex (distal fragment) with the 2.0-mm extra-long drill bit.
g) Screw length is determined with the extra-long depth gauge.
h) The compression hole is threaded with the 2.7-mm extra-long tap.
i) The 2.7-mm cortex screw is inserted as a lag screw.

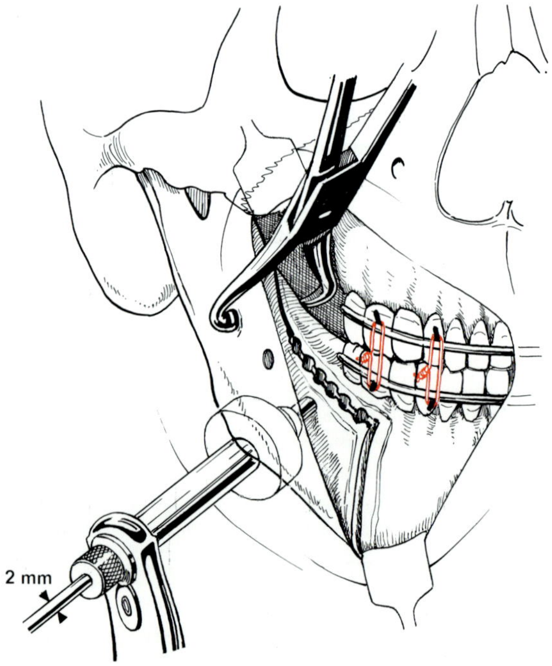

Fig. 379. Transbuccal drilling of the compression hole through the inserted 2.0-mm drill sleeve. The 0.5-mm wire ligatures provide for rigid retention of the occlusion

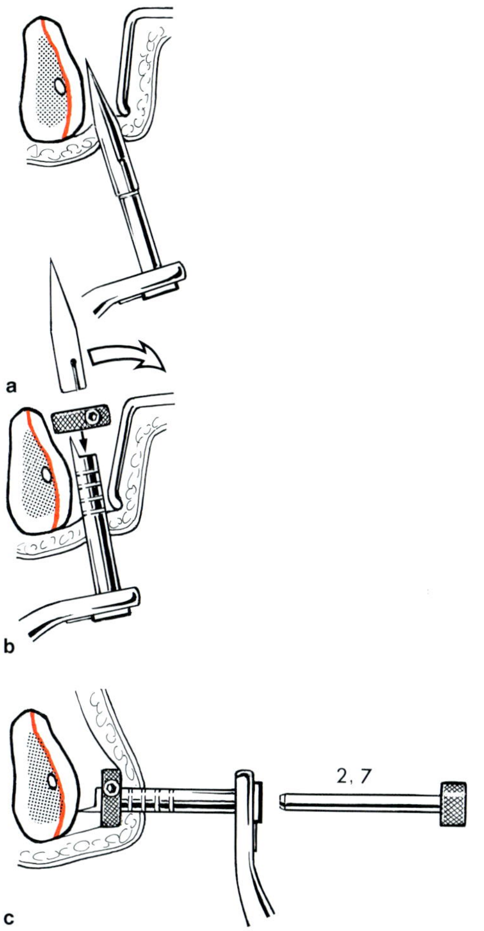

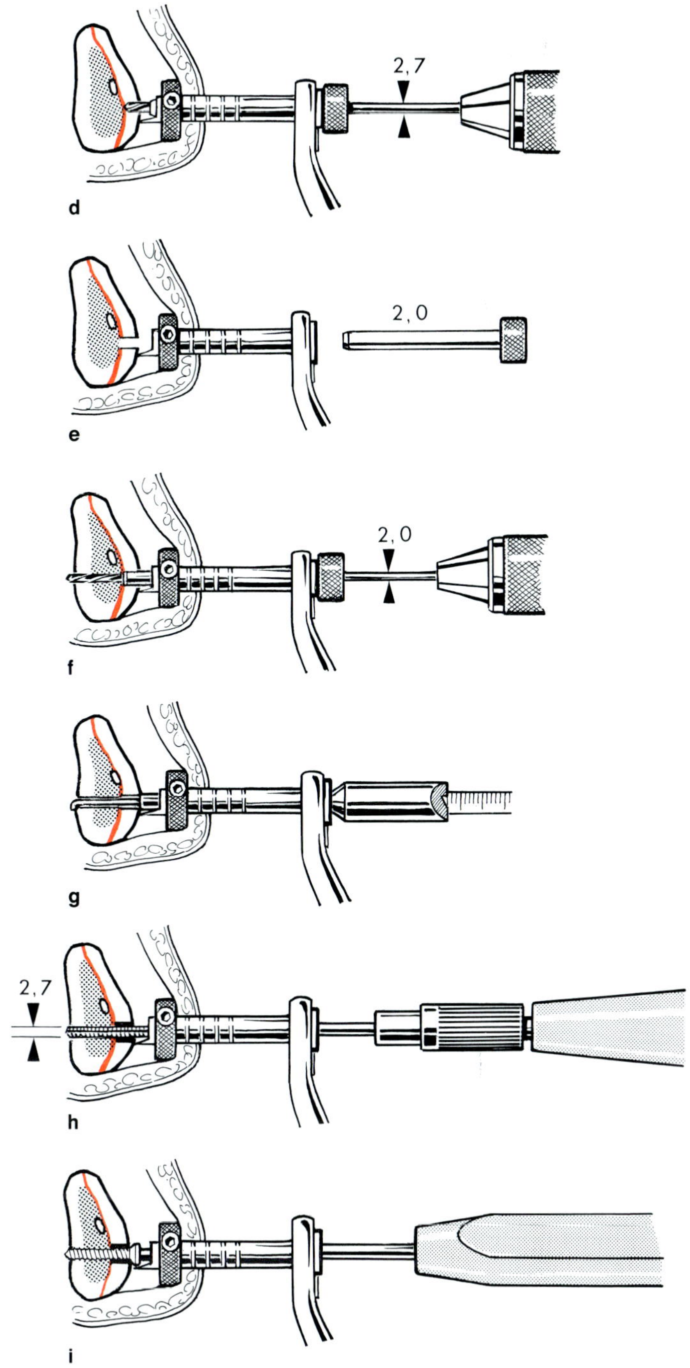

Fig. 380 a–i. Steps involved in percutaneous lag screw fixation (see text)

6.1.8 On Lag Screw Fixation as a Possible Cause of Sensory Disturbances

Surgeons at many centers have found that use of the 2.7-mm screws gives a stability that permits immediate mouth opening while providing the mechanical stability necessary for primary bony union. This is evidenced by a significantly lower rate of relapse. We caution against substituting miniscrews for the 2.7-mm screws, as this would sacrifice stability and the attendant biochemical advantages.

It has been suggested that interfragmental compression has major causal significance in postoperative sensory disturbances, but we find these claims unconvincing. Nerve deficits following sagittal split osteotomy were reported with much greater frequency before the advent of lag screw fixation than today (Spiessl 1976b). This implies that the nerve trauma is caused essentially by the sagittal spliting itself. We expect that the incidence of postsurgical neuropathies will decline substantially when the "laminotomy" technique of the sagittal split (see p. 341) becomes more widely practiced.

Occasionally it is stated that the scar left by the stab incision is a problem. This can be avoided by performing the lag screw fixation through an intraoral approach. However, this is an acceptable option only if it will afford the same quality of fixation that can be achieved extraorally. The intraoral approach should not be used if it entails a compromise of stability.

6.1.9 Removal of the Lag Screws

Güdel (1986) found only *one* loose screw in a series of 153 screw removals performed one year or more after insertion. In theory at least, screws made of titanium or sapphire (Seto and Matsuura 1984) may be left in place indefinitely (see p. 137). Clearly, this would be a major advantage in view of the significant rate of infection that is associated with implant removal – 7 of 58 exposed mandibular angles in the series of Güdel. This infection rate contrasts markedly with that after the primary operations, which was zero in the above series.

This discrepancy in infection rates apparently relates to traumatization of the muscle tissue (masseter) under the conditions of a "minimal" surgical approach and to oral infection of the hematoma. The intraoral incision is widely opened, whereas the external stab incision is made just large enough to accommodate the screwdriver. This limits the freedom of action of the screwdriver, which must be relatively long to reach the screws, distributed as they are over a relatively wide area. We recommend routine infection prophylaxis consisting of 24 h of *vacuum drainage* and a *preoperative* single dose use of a broad spectrum antibiotic.

6.1.10 Indications: Shortening and Lengthening Osteotomy

The sagittal split osteotomy may be used to shorten or lengthen the mandible as required. So far the principles of the operation have been illustrated for a *shortening osteotomy* (backward sagittal split) of the mandibular body (see p. 333 ff.). This procedure is indicated for:

- overdevelopment of the lower face; cardinal symptom: *prognathism;*
- unilateral overdevelopment of the mandible; cardinal symptom: *deviation of the midline,* prominent and laterally deviated chin, facial asymmetry;
- underdevelopment of the midface that cannot be corrected by *osteotomy* of the maxilla; cardinal symptom: *pseudoprognathism.*

The *lengthening osteotomy* (forward sagittal split) is indicated for:

- underdevelopment of the lower face; cardinal symptom: *retrognathia;*
- apparent underdevelopment of the lower face; cardinal symptom: *distal bite;*
- unilateral underdevelopment of the lower face; cardinal symptom: *cross-bite,* receding and deviated chin, facial asymmetry.

6.1.11 Details on the Forward Sagittal Split

Distal bite is corrected by simple advancement of the peripheral mandibular fragment. Simple plaster models are adequate for preoperative planning.

Retrognathia is the product of a gnathic and dentoalveolar anomaly. Besides the receding chin (Fig. 381), the shortened mandible results in a

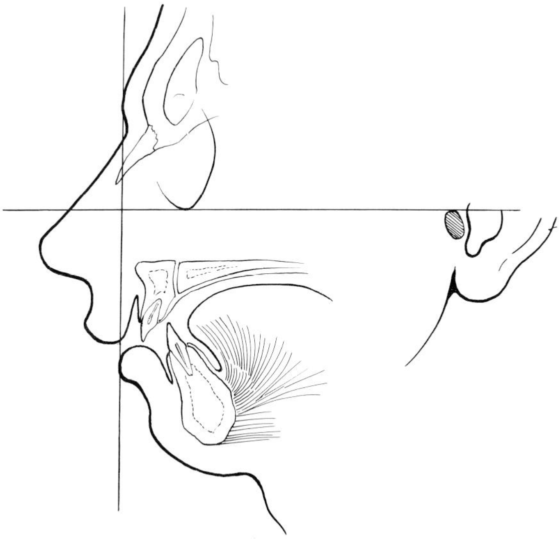

Fig. 381. Retrognathia with compensatory elevation of the anterior mandible

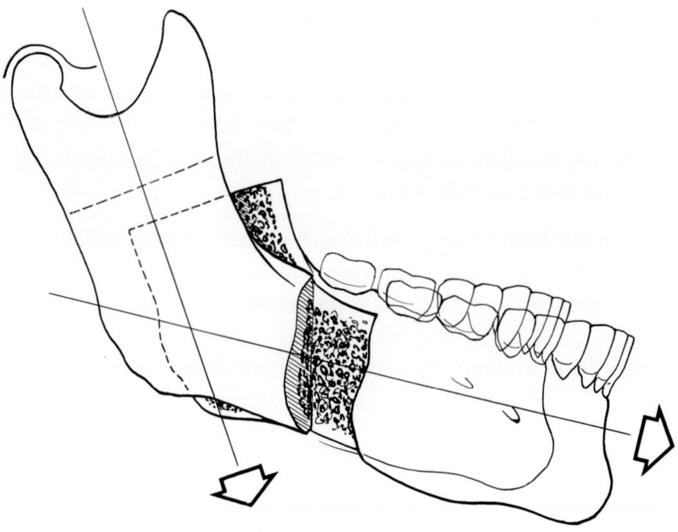

Fig. 382. The mobilized fragment is slid forward and downward for correction of the retrognathia

deep bite with compensatory elevation of the mandibular anteriors, which touch the gingiva palatal to the upper incisors. Orthognathic correction consists in biaxial elongation: forward along the horizontal ramus and downward along the ascending ramus (Fig. 382).

In addition to the sagittal split, corrective osteotomies are necessary in the area of the anterior alveolar process and the chin prominence. Also, the plane of occlusion is leveled by the use of an occlusal splint with a bite plane.

The complexity of the procedure makes it necessary, during planning, to determine

- the necessary degree of horizontal and vertical lengthening,
- the shape of the mandibular angle,
- the segmental model if anterior tooth height is excessive,
- the shape of the occlusal splint,
- the fixation technique: splinting and internal fixation,
- the method of leveling the occlusal plane,
- the need for genioplasty (may be done in a second operation).

An occlusal splint (a lingual splint with bite plane prepared from the preoperative study model) is used to ensure accurate positioning and fixation of the fragments and to even the plane of occlusion (Fig. 383). Intermaxillary fixation is not employed.

While the advancement and rotation of the mandible yields a normal anterior overbite, it leads to nonocclusion in the molar region (posterior open bite). The plane of the occlusion is leveled by adding an acrylic bite plane to the splint (Fig. 384). During postoperative care, the height of the bite plane is progressively reduced to stimulate self-correction of the open

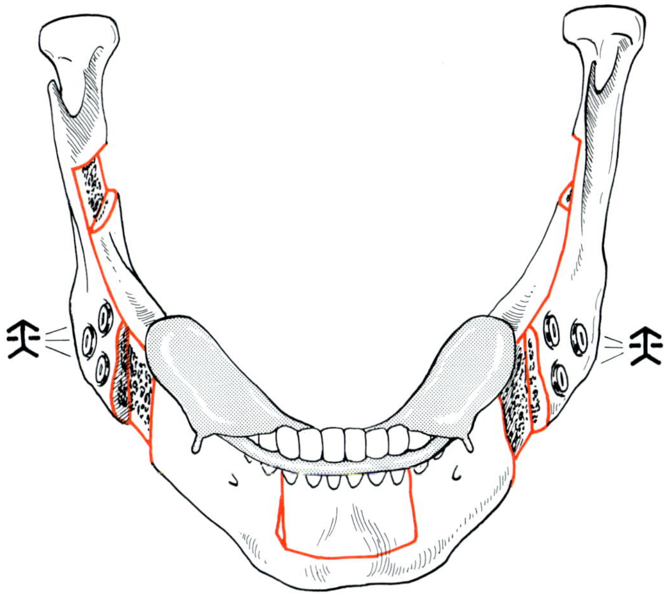

Fig. 383. The occlusal splint provides a guide for definitive positioning of the body and anterior segment. The ramus fragments are definitively fixed with three lag screws per side

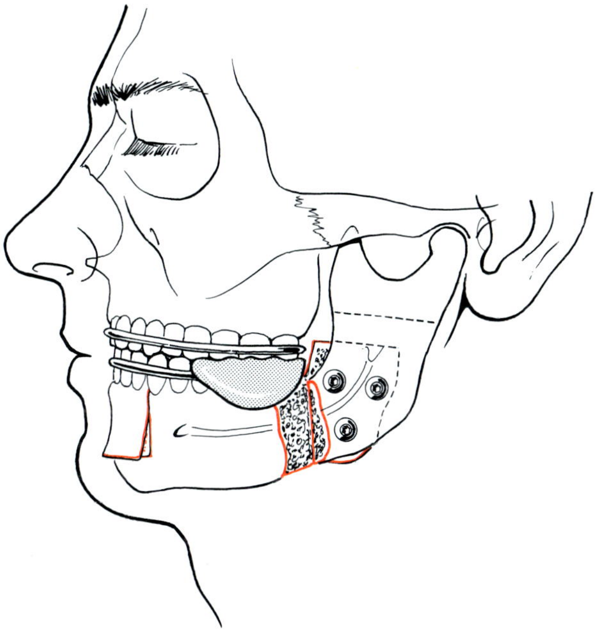

Fig. 384. An acrylic bite plane compensates for the posterior open bite caused by advancement of the lower dental arch. The appliance also supports the newly established anterior overbite during early mobilization of the jaw

bite deformity. Figure 385 illustrates the successive reduction of the bite plane over a 9-months period and the result at 1.5 years.

During internal fixation, the placement of the lag screws is determined by the new position of the nerve canal relative to the proximal fragment. Often the oblique line is the only site where two lag screws can be accommodated; the third screw is inserted basally (Fig. 386).

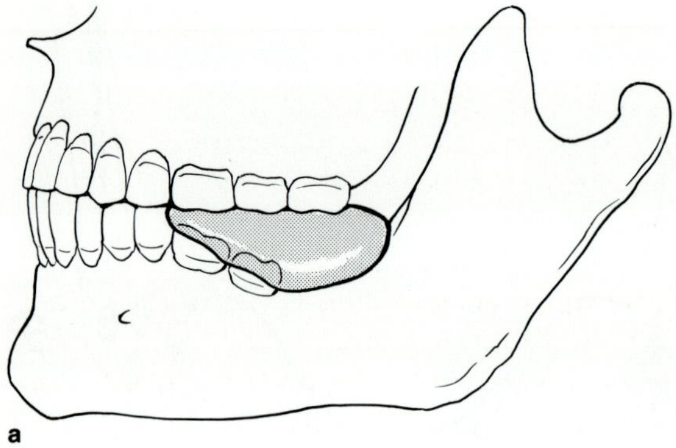

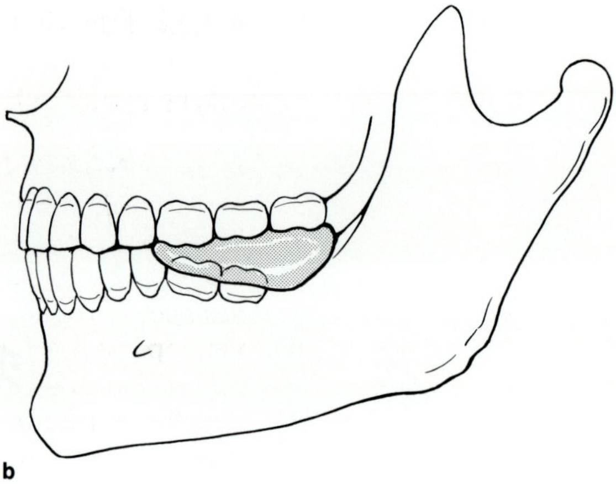

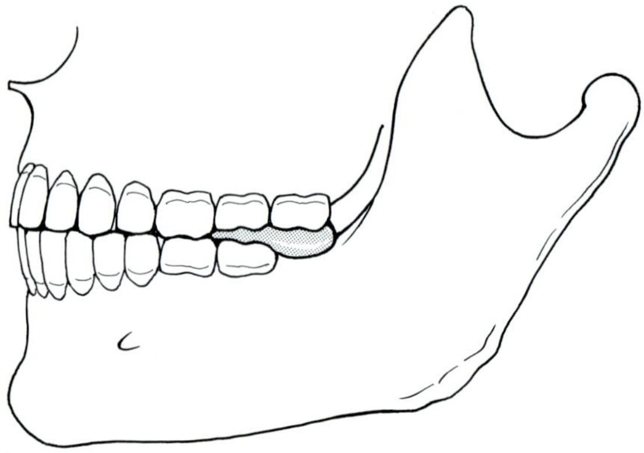

Fig. 385 a–c. Successive reduction of the acrylic bite plane corrects the posterior open bite by utilizing the self-correcting mechanism of the antagonists

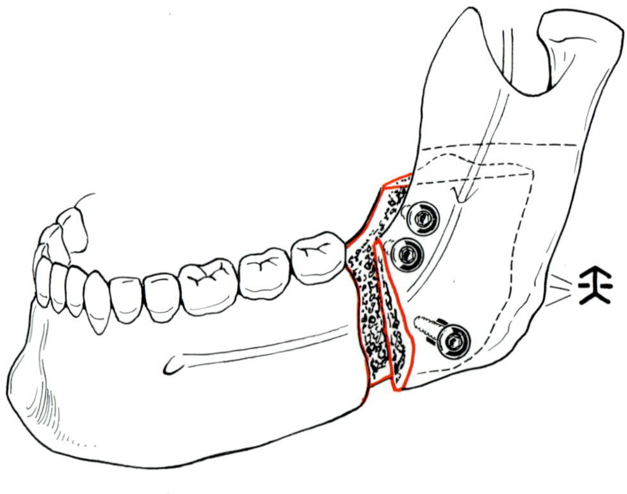

Fig. 386. Lag screw fixation of the surgically advanced mandible. Generally two screws are placed on the tension side along the oblique line

6.1.12 Functionally Stable Advancement with a Bone Graft

6.1.12.1 Method

Even today the "bird-face" deformity is occasionally seen as a sequel to mandibular osteomyelitis with involvement of the TMJ (fibrous ankylosis). The condition is marked by an extreme hypoplasia in which the body of the mandible is severely shortened while the ramus is narrowed and thinned. A sagittal split cannot be performed on the rudimentary rami in the hope of obtaining adequate advancement. A useful alternative in the case of fibrous ankylosis is the inverted L-shaped osteotomy with the interposition of an autogenous corticocancellous bone graft (Schuchardt 1958, 1960; Immenkamp 1957). In the case of bony ankylosis, see p. 326ff.

We perform the osteotomy through an extraoral approach, bypassing the antilingula (Fig. 387) and severing the tendinous lamina of the medial pterygoid muscle. Usually the tenotomy alone will permit adequate mobilization of the fragments.

The extraoral incision is carefully covered, and the peripheral fragment is advanced into the desired occlusion using a sharp hook placed behind the anterior arch. A forceful, jerking movement may be needed to overcome the resistance of the floor of the mouth muscles and integument.

Intermaxillary fixation is accomplished with 0.6-mm wire ligatures.

Following advancement of the mandibular body, the bone graft is performed through the extraoral incision under aseptic conditions. The size and shape of the discontinuity are determined with a malleable template, then the iliac bone graft is tailored to fit the gap. The long edges of the bone graft are made concave so that they will seat more firmly against the distracted ramus fragments (Fig. 388).

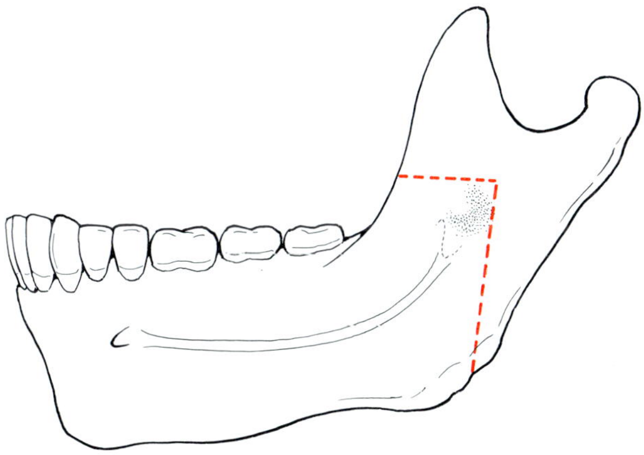

Fig. 387. L-shaped osteotomy (after Wassmund 1952). Landmark: antilingula (stippled)

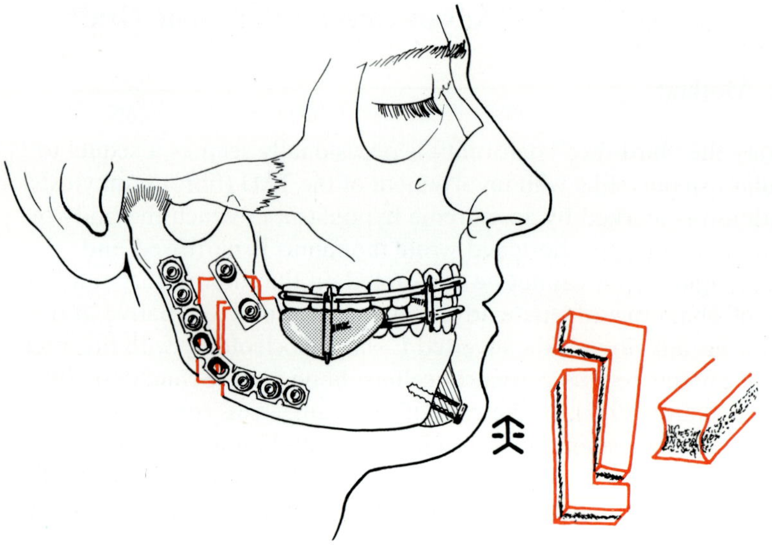

Fig. 388. Correction of "bird-face" deformity (receding chin associated with extreme retrognathia) by a functionally stable advancement procedure. A bone graft is interposed between the distracted fragments and secured in place with a tension band plate and stabilization plate. An additional graft is used to augment the chin. *Insert:* L-shaped corticocancellous grafts with concave edges

6.1.12.2 Preliminary Fixation of the Fragments

The fragments are temporarily wired together with 0.7 gauge cerclage wire in preparation for the definitive fixation. Before inserting the bone graft, we drill a hole in the upper part of the peripheral fragment and pass the wire through the hole and around the entire proximal fragment. We then interpose the bone graft and tighten the wire loop. The hollowed edges of the graft will keep the fragments from slipping.

6.1.12.3 Functionally Stable Fixation

For the definitive fixation, a small two-hole tension band plate is combined with a basal reconstruction plate to create a functionally stable assembly (Fig. 388). This functional stability is important for graft healing and especially for rehabilitation, since the "bird-face" deformity is commonly associated with a fibrous ankylosis that responds well to early functional therapy.

6.2 Lateral Ostectomy

6.2.1 Principle

Lateral ostectomy involves the bilateral excision of a segment of the mandibular body for the correction of prognathism (Hullimen, quoted in Wassmund 1935; Angle 1898/99; Pichler 1919; Dingman 1944). We rarely practice this operation today, and others use it only in selected cases. For this reason we shall mainly focus our attention on the technique for fixation of the fragments.

6.2.2 Indications

Lateral ostectomy is performed for the correction of:

- prognathism with an extremely long mandibular body and a moderately obtuse or normal gonial angle;
- prognathism with an open bite as far back as the molar region;
- prognathism with a deep bite.

6.2.3 Preoperative Planning

Preoperative simulation covers the following points:

1) performance of the ostectomy on the study model;
2) the preparation of technical aids
   - for making the incisions and tailoring the ends of the fragments: lead template,
   - for establishing the occlusion: occlusal splint,
   - for the fixation: three-part arch splint and, if necessary, prebent compression plates (DCP).

6.2.4 Operation

The ostectomy is performed by an intraoral approach or a combined intra-extraoral approach. In both approaches great care is taken to preserve the inferior alveolar nerve and to tailor the bone ends so that they will appose cleanly and give the desired occlusion. Both are more easily accomplished in the combined intra-extraoral approach.

6.2.5 Preliminary Fixation of the Fragments

The occlusion established in the study model is the guide for positioning the fragments after the ostectomy. The three fragments are secured in their new position with the occlusal splint and three-part arch splint. First the section of the arch splint are loosely approximated with 0.6-mm wire ligatures (Fig. 389 a), then the lingual occlusal splint is inserted (Fig. 389 b).

To check the tendency of the fragments to undergo torsion, we first wire the central fragment to the occlusal splint with two encircling ligatures (0.7 mm) and then fasten the lateral fragments to the splint using one ligature per side.

A perfect fit of the occlusal splint confirms that the fragments are correctly aligned on the oral side (see Fig. 389 a). On the vestibular side, the

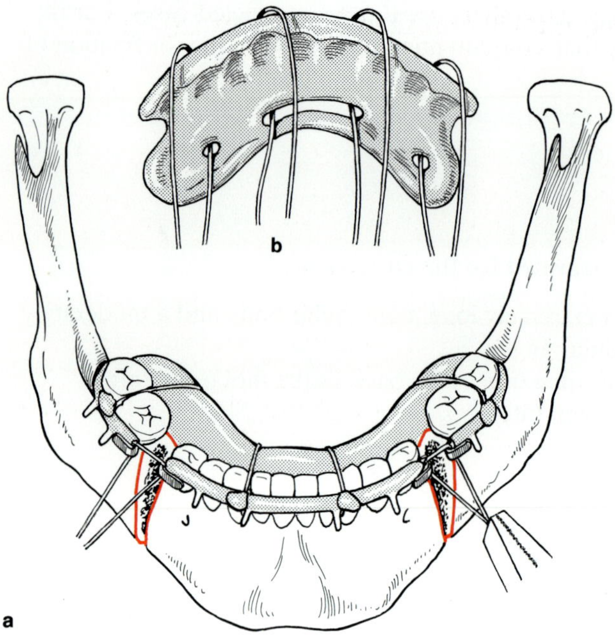

Fig. 389. **a** The three fragments are loosely approximated with simple wire ligatures between the divided arch bars. The ostectomy has resulted in partially incongruent bone ends. The lingual occlusal splint with four wire ligatures fixes the fragments in the desired position. **b** The occlusal splint is fabricated preoperatively from the study model used to simulate the osteotomy

three sections of the arch splint are rigidly interconnected by tightening the wire ligatures and applying a stabilizing acrylic veneer. At this point the occlusal splint is removed, and the occlusion is retained with wire ligatures (0.5 mm) passed between the maxillary and mandibular splints. Care is taken to remove the pharyngeal pack and suture the wound in the lingual mucosa before the intermaxillary fixation is applied.

6.2.6 Functionally Stable Internal Fixation

The disadvantage of the exclusive intraoral approach becomes apparent at the time of internal fixation, which can be difficult even when the perfacial instruments are used (see Figs. 101 and 380). Because of the lack of congruity between the bone ends and the deficient bony buttress, a six-hole DCP is employed (Fig. 390).

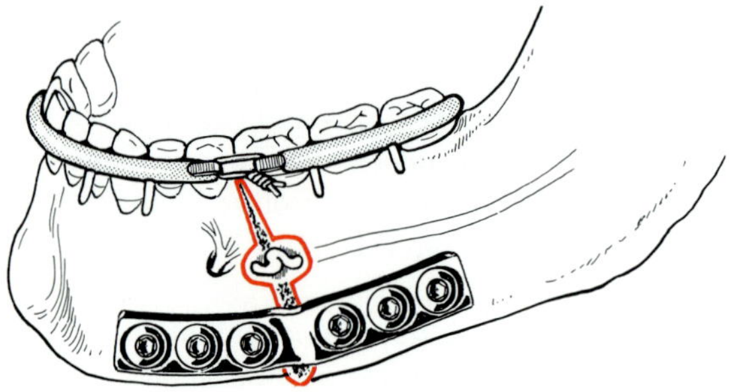

Fig. 390. Functionally stable internal fixation of Dingman's osteotomy by the plate and tension-band principle (Dingman 1944)

6.3 Anterior Ostectomy Combined with Sagittal Split

6.3.1 Principle

The mandible is narrowed and shortened by ectomy the symphyseal segment and by sagittal splitting of the ascending rami.

6.3.2 Indication

The procedure is indicated for extreme prognathism with a bilateral crossbite (overdeveloped mandible and deficient maxilla, Fig. 391).

6.3.3 Preoperative Planning

Simulation on the study model shows that occlusion cannot be achieved by either a lateral ostectomy or a sagittal split osteotomy alone. Both osteotomies, possibly combined with shortening of the chin prominence, are needed to obtain a satisfactory result. Often a simultaneous Le Fort Osteotomy is indicated.

6.3.4 Operation

The sequence of steps is as follows:

1) median ostectomy by the intraoral approach and temporary fixation of the apposed fragments with two 2-mm Kirschner wires,
2) sagittal split osteotomy (laminotomy),
3) rigid intermaxillary fixation,
4) lag screw fixation,
5) compression plating.

6.4.3.1 Technique of Ostectomy

With the aid of the metal template applied basally, we outline the area to be excised with drill holes placed through both cortices. The drill holes in the outer cortex are then interconnected with an oscillating saw, at which point the outer cortical fragment with attached cancellous bone is easily broken off with an osteotome. Next the inner cortex is removed with a rongeur, sparing the periosteum. Periosteum is removed only from the inferior border of the mandible; it is left on the mental spine and the symphysis, which are fused to the aponeurosis. A little rest of the inner cortex and the posterior mental spine are preserved along with the aponeurosis of the genioglossus and geniohyoid muscles (Fig. 392).

The cut ends of the bone are beveled at a divergent angle so that they will appose over a maximum area and the two halves of the tension-band splint will fit the bite rim. Then the chin fragments are held together with a Kirschner wire (2.0 mm).

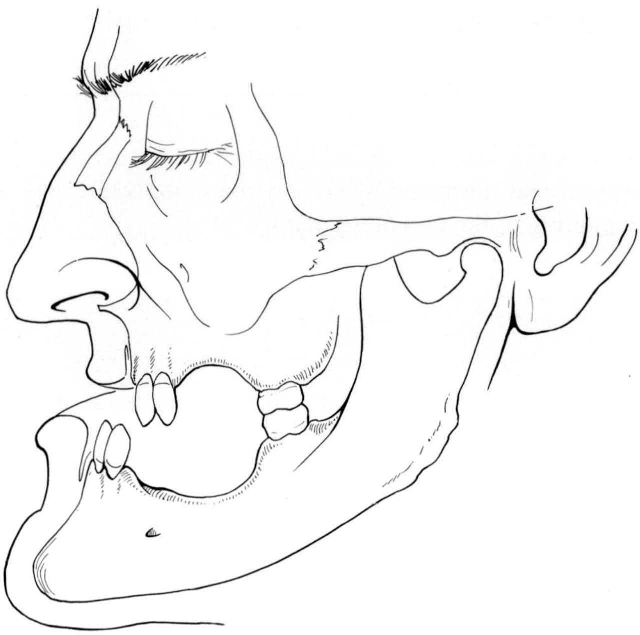

a

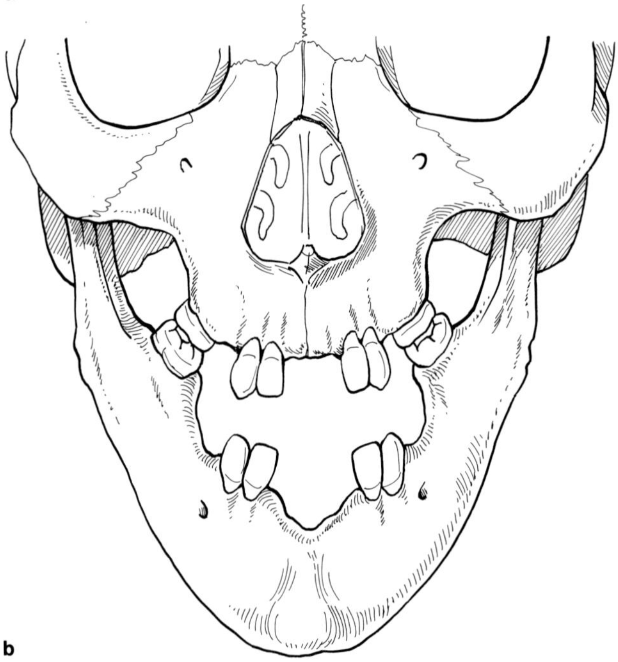

b

Fig. 391 a, b. Status prior to operation (see text)

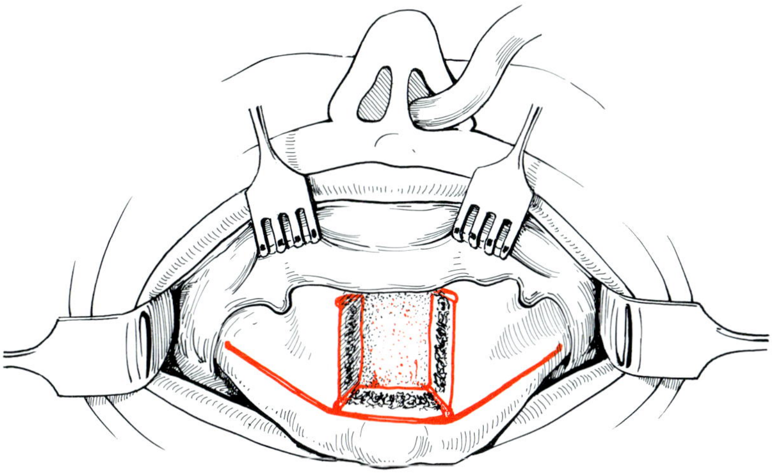

Fig. 392. Box-shaped osteotomy preserving the aponeurosis of the genioglossus and geniohyoid muscles

6.3.4.2 Internal Fixation

This tentative fixation facilitates the sagittal split and lag screw fixation (see p. 345). The chin is definitively fixed with a four-hole DCP (Fig. 393).

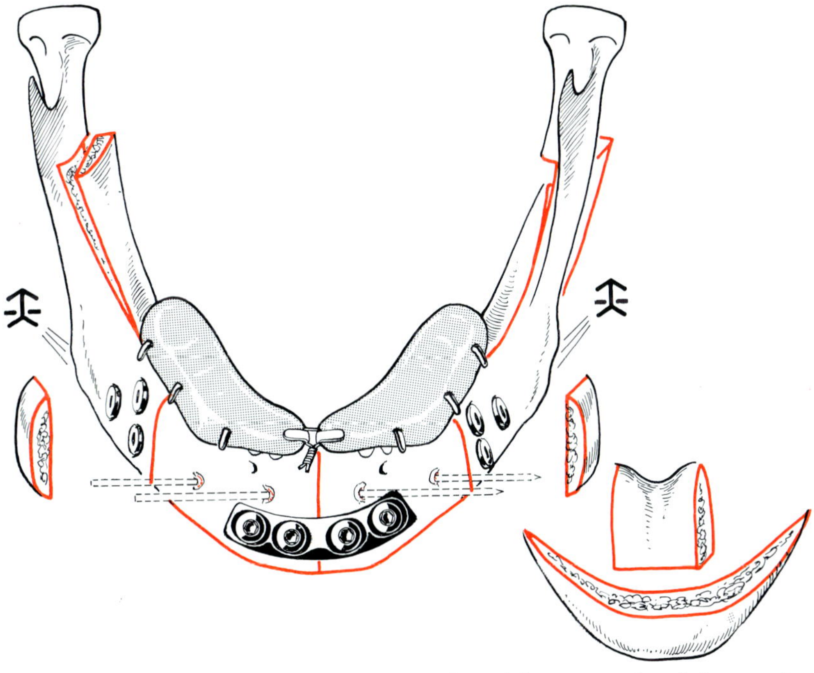

Fig. 393. Combination of plate and lag screw fixation of the narrowed and shortened mandible: 1) preliminary fixation of the narrowed mandible with a "key splint" and Kirschner wires, 2) occusal fixation of the fragments after the sagittal split, 3) plate fixation (after removal of the Kirschner wires if the position of the fragments needs to be adjusted on the midline), 4) lag screw fixation

6.4 Triple Basoalveolar Ostectomy

6.4.1 Principle

The body of the mandible is shortened and narrowed by step ostectomies in its basal and alveolar portions.

6.4.2 Indication

Prognathism with bilateral crossbite and an intact anterior dental arch.

6.4.3 Preoperative Planning

This complex anomaly of dentoalveolar and gnathic origin requires orthodontic consultation during planning so that necessary presurgical orthodontic treatment can be provided. The result of this preliminary treatment can be simulated on a wax model. Similarly, models of the body and rami can be prepared from the teleradiograph and directly measured values of the mandibular index. The dentoalveolar and gnathic model fabricated from wax and acrylic teeth reflects the true size and shape of the jaw. The location and extent of the triple ostectomy can be determined so accurately on the model that an anatomically and functionally optimum result can be achieved (see Hockenjos and Komposch 1974).

6.4.4 Operation

We shorten the dental arch by excising one premolar segment per side, for example, and osteotomize the frontal alveolar process from the body of the mandible. We additionally shorten the jaw base by removing a central section from the mental trigone whose width equals the total width of the two excised premolar segments (Fig. 394).

6.4.5 Internal Fixation

With the aid of a previously fabricated occlusal splint, the three fragments are placed in the desired occlusal position and fixed with a divided wire acrylic splint. The basal ostectomy site is compression plated (see Fig. 394).

Unlike the median resection (Fig. 392), the step ostectomy is performed entirely through an intraoral approach.

The principle of the step osteotomy is also applied in cases that require expansion of the mandibular arch. This procedure creates distraction spaces into which autogenous bone grafts are interposed: a corticocancellous graft basally and cancellous bone chips in the alveolar process. The operation is performed by an intraoral approach.

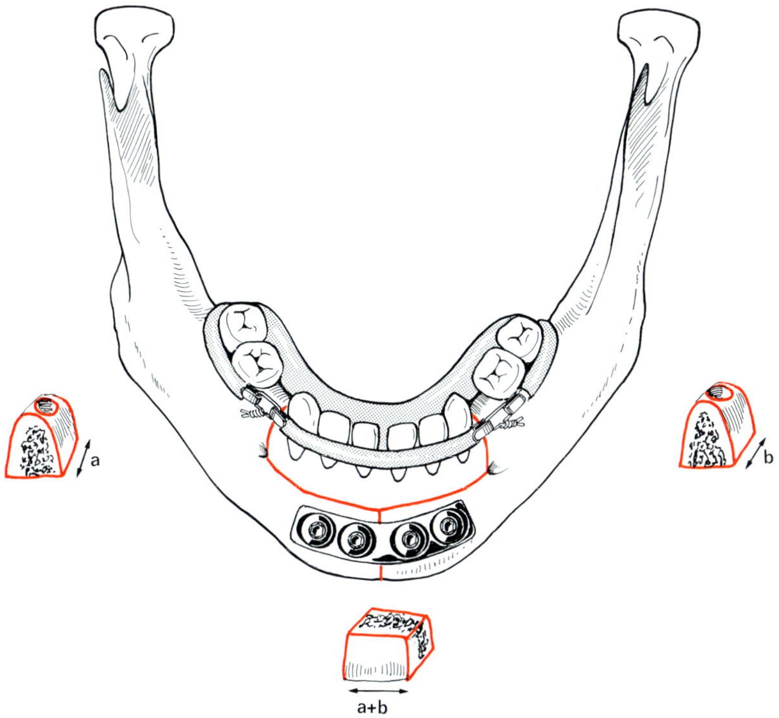

Fig. 394. Internal fixation of a triple osteotomy performed to narrow and shorten the mandible

6.5 Genioplasty

The chin is as important as the nose in its impact on the profile. It is a uniquely human feature which has evolved since the time of Homo heidelbergensis, who showed no evidence of a chin whatsoever. As a general rule, excessive prominence of the chin is perceived to be less objectionable aesthetically than a recessive chin.

Evaluating the appearance of the chin is a highly subjective matter, but an objective assessment can be made on the basis of the chin projection angle. The basic types of anomaly are the *receding, prominent,* and *deviated* chin. Corrective procedures include *sliding osteotomy* and *ostectomy* on the one hand and *grafting* and *implantation* on the other. The procedures may be performed alone or in conjunction with other orthopedic interventions. These operations, such as grafting and implantation, are beyond this scope of this text, and we shall limit our remarks to aspects of internal fixation.

6.5.1 Lag Screw Fixation

The steplike position of the fragments is maintained with lag screws. This mode of fixation requires a 5-mm-thick corticocancellous layer for drilling a compression hole that can accommodate an emergency screw (see p. 115). Paramedian screws are usually adequate for approximation of the fragments (Figs. 395 and 396). Three screws may be appropriate for fixation of the advanced mandibular border (Fig. 397).

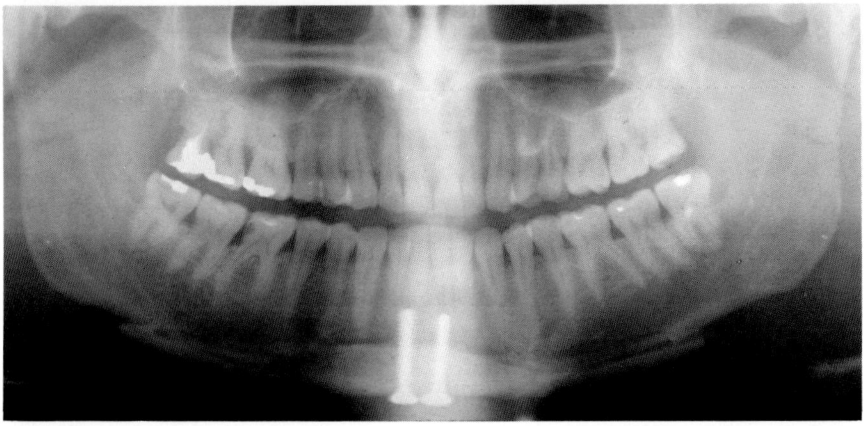

Fig. 395. Paramedian lag screw fixation following setback of the mental trigone

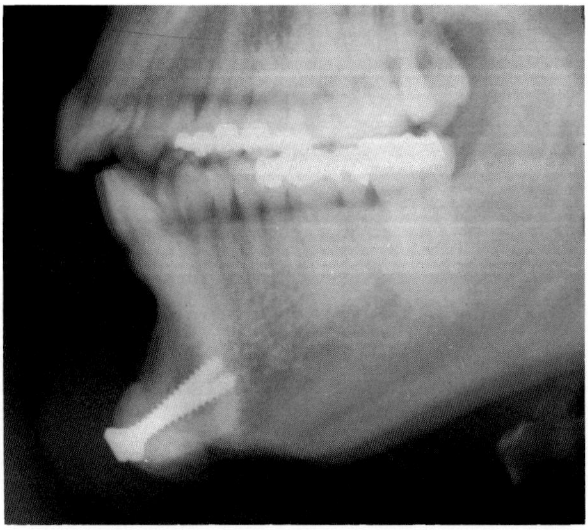

Fig. 396. Lag screw fixation following upward advancement of the chin prominence

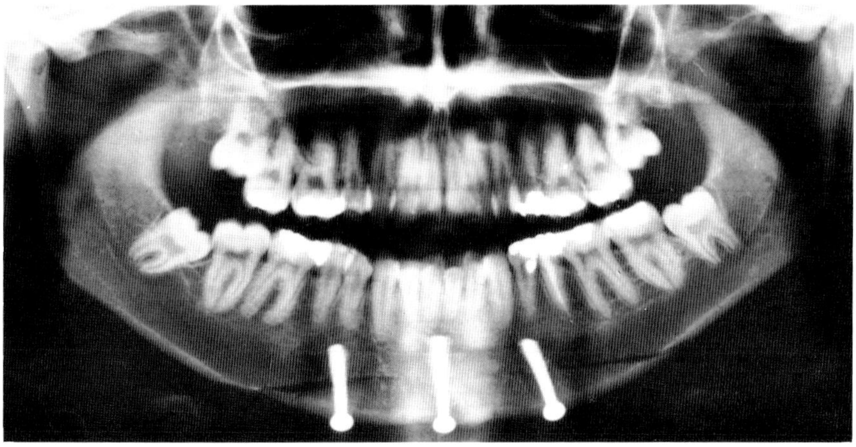

Fig. 397. Lag screw fixation after forward advancement of the mandibular border

6.6 Concluding Remarks

Our discussion of functionally stable internal fixation in orthognathic surgery has intentially been limited to a few illustrative cases. Our main intent was to suggest the many potential applications of ASIF principles in this field and especially to make it clear that osteotomy and stable fixation form a therapeutic unit.

Bibliography

Aebi F (1985) Vergleich verschiedener Zuggurtungsschienen und intermaxillären Fixationen bei der Osteosynthese der Mandibula. Med. Dissertation, Universität Basel

Aebi M, Regazzoni P, Rahn BA, Harder F (1984) Experimental model for bone allografts with and without immunosuppression and microsurgical revascularisation. Helv Chir Acta 51:641

Allgöwer M (1971) Weichteilprobleme und Infektionsrisiko der Osteosynthese. Langenbecks Arch Chir 329:1130

Allgöwer M, Border JR (1983) Advances in the care of multiple trauma patient - introduction. World J Surg 7:1

Allgöwer M, Perren SM, Rüedi T (1971) Biophysikalische Aspekte der normalen und der heilenden Knochencorticalis. Langenbecks Arch Chir 328:109

Andrä A, Grabowski R (1978) Zur Wahl der Operationsmethode bei sagittaler Über- und Unterentwicklung des Unterkiefers. Zahn Mund Kieferheilkd 66:3

Angle EH (1898/99) Double resection for treatment in mandibular protrusion. Dent Cosmos Nr. 8; ibid (1903) 45:268

Ansell RH, Scales JJ (1968) A study of some factors which affect the strength of screws and their insertion and holding power in bone. J Biomech 1:279

Arnold M (1985) Postoperative Okklusions- und Dysfunktionsstudie als Qualitätskontrolle der funktionsstabilen Osteosynthese am Unterkiefer. Med. Dissertation, Universität Basel

Ariyan S (1979) Further experiences with the Pectoral major myocutaneous flap for immediate repair of defects from excisions of head and neck tumours. Plast Reconstr Surg 64:605

Bakamjian VY (1965) A two-stage method for pharyngooesophageal reconstruction with a primary pectoral skin flap. Plast Reconstr Surg 36:173

Bandi W (1972) Chondromalacia patellae und femoro-patellare Arthrose. Schwabe, Basel

Bandi W (1980) Probleme der Indikationsstellung zur Osteosynthese von Oberarmschaftbrüchen. Z Unfallheilkd 3:141

Baumann R (1973) Die dreidimensionale extraorale Kieferschiene. Med Dissertation, Universität Bern

Benninghoff A (1927) Über die Anpassung der Knochenkompakta an geänderte Beanspruchung. Anat Anz 63:289

Benninghoff A (1931) Über die Entstehung funktioneller Strukturen. Verh Anat Ges 39:62

Birke WP (1972) Unsere Erfahrungen mit der modifizierten perkutanen Osteosynthese nach Becker. Dtsch Stomat 22:31

Border JR (1984) Advances in the care of the patient with blunt multiple trauma. Am Coll Surg 69/10

Bornand F (1984) Die funktionsstabile Osteosynthese am Unterkiefer. (Ergebnisse der Nachuntersuchung von 130 Fällen 1977 - Juni 1981). Med Dissertation, Universität Basel

Brack AA (1980) Sekundär-Tumoren. Die Absiedelung von Fernmetastasen in die Kieferknochen - Symptome, Diagnose, Therapie. Med Dissertation, Universität Basel

Brinker WO, Hohn RB, Prieur WD (1984) Manual of internal fixation in small animals. Springer, Berlin Heidelberg New York Tokyo

Brunner C, Weber BG (1981) Besondere Osteosynthesetechniken. Springer, Berlin Heidelberg New York

Brussatis (1985) Defektüberbrückung durch kortikospongiöse Transplantate. Vortrag am Symposium „Defektüberbrückung an Knochen und Weichteilen", Berlin 31.10./1.11.

Burke JF (1963) Preoperative antibiotics. Surg Clin North Am 43:665
Claudi B, Schläpfer F, Cordey J, Perren SM, Allgöwer M (1979) Die schräge Plattenzugschraube, in vivo-Messungen der Stabilität an queren Osteotomien des Tibiaschaftes. Helv Chir Acta 46:177
Contzen H, Straumann F, Paschke E (1967) Grundlagen der Alloplastik mit Metallen und Kunststoffen. Thieme, Stuttgart
Converse JM, Warnitz FW (1942) External skeletal fixation of the mandibular angle. J Bone Joint Surg 24:154
Coutelier L (1969) Recherches sur la guerison des fractures. Arscia, Bruxelles
Dal Pont G (1961) Retromolar osteotomy for the correction of prognathism. J oral Surg 19:42
Danis R (1949) Théorie et pratique de l'osteosynthèse. Masson, Paris
Decker S, Rehn J, Düring M von, Decker B (1976) Morphologisch experimenteller Beitrag zur Kenntnis der Vorgänge bei der Verpflanzung von autologer Beckenkammspongiosa bei Hunden. Arch Orthop Unfallchir 85:303
Dingman RO (1944) Surgical correction of mandibular prognathism, an improved method. Am J Orthod 683
Dittel KK, Weller S (1981) Zur Problematik des polytraumatisierten Patienten. Akt Traumatol 11:35
Dumbleton JH, Black J (1975) An introduction to orthopaedic materials. Thomas, Springfield
Elmiger V (1979) Stabilitätsabhängiges Heilungsbild bei experimentellen Kieferfrakturen. Med Dissertation, Universität Bern
Eschmann A (1974) Die funktionsstabile Osteosynthese am Unterkiefer. (Nachuntersuchungsergebnisse bei 81 kontrollierten Fällen von 1966 bis 1973). Med Dissertation, Universität Basel
Euw A von (1982) Die funktionsstabile Osteosynthese. Ergebnisse der Nachuntersuchungen von 85 Fällen (1974–1976). Med Dissertation, Universität Tübingen
Flynn MB (1979) Morbidity and mortality of mandibular resection for malignant disease. In: McCoy et al. (eds) Yearbook of plastic and reconstructive surgery. Chicago
Frenkel G (1961) Die perkutane Osteosynthese nach Becker und ihre Indikation nach 6jähriger Erfahrung in der Unterkieferbruchbehandlung. Dtsch Zahnärztl Z 16:706
Fromm U (1980) Die Kompressionswirkung von Rundlochplatten und dynamischen Kompressionsplatten am intakten und osteotomierten Knochen in vitro. AO-Bulletin
Ganz R, Perren SM, Rüter A (1975) Mechanische Induktion der Knochenresorption. Fortschr Kiefer Gesichtschir 19:45
Gautier E et al. (1984) Porosity and remodelling of plated bone after internal fixation: Result of stress shielding or vascular damage? In: Ducheyne P et al. (eds) Biomaterials and Biomechanics (1983). Elsevier, Amsterdam
Gerber H, Perren SM (1980) Evaluation of tissue compatibility of in vitro cultures of embryonic bone. In: Winter GD et al. (eds) Advances in biomaterials. Wiley, New York
Grätz K (1986) Eine neue Klassifikation zur Einteilung von Unterkieferfrakturen. Med. Dissertation, Universität Basel
Gruber UF (1983) Ist eine Antibiotikaprophylaxe in der Chirurgie sinnvoll? JAMA 2:328
Güdel M (1986) Nachuntersuchung bei 29 Progenie-Patienten. Med Dissertation, Universität Basel
Gunst MA (1980) Interference with bone blood supply through plating of intact bone. In: Uhthoff HK (ed). Current concepts of internal fixation of fractures. Springer, Berlin Heidelberg New York
Gunst MA, Rahn BA, Rüedi T, Perren SM (1982) Blutversorgung der Knochenkortikalis nach Osteotomie. Helv Chir Acta 49:229
Habel G, Rahn BA, Perren SM, Krüger E (1980) Tierexperimentelle Untersuchungen zur Unterkieferersatzplastik in Abhängigkeit von Verplattungssystem und Beschaffenheit des Transplantatlagers. In: Hierholzer G, Zilch H (Hrsg) Transplantatlager und Implantatlager bei verschiedenen Operationsverfahren. Springer, Berlin Heidelberg New York (16. Jahrestagung der Deutschen Gesellschaft für Plastische und Wiederherstellungschirurgie)
Hanslik L (1969) Die operative Behandlung gelenknaher Frakturen osteoporotischer Knochen. Mschr Unfallheilkd 72:514
Harnisch H, Gabka J (1962) Beitrag zur Indikation der extraoralen Verschraubung. Dtsch Zahnärztl Z 17:315

Hierholzer G, Allgöwer M, Rüedi T (1985) Fixateur externe-Osteosynthese. Springer, Berlin Heidelberg New York Tokyo
Hockenjos C (1974) Fernröntgenologischer und klinischer Befund bei erschwerter Nasenatmung. Med. Dissertation, Universität Freiburg i. B.
Hockenjos C, Komposch G (1974) Die Simulation bei der Planung und Vorbereitung von kieferorthopädisch-chirurgischen Behandlungen. Fortschr Kieferorthop 35: 113
Hörster G (1985) Die infizierte Corticalisnekrose - theoretische Aspekte und klinische Relevanz. Vortrag beim Symposium Defektüberbrückung an Knochen und Weichteilen. Berlin, 31.10./1.11.85
Immenkamp A (1957) Chirurgische Kieferorthopädie. In: Häupl K et al. (Hrsg) Die Zahn-, Mund-, und Kieferheilkunde. Bd 3/1. Urban & Schwarzenberg, München
Janecka JP (1984) External stabilisation of the mandible with the mini-H-fixator. Plast Reconstr Surg 73/5:840
Jaques WA (1976) Preventive antibiotics in elective maxillofacial surgery. In: Spiessl B (ed) New concepts in maxillofacial bone surgery. Springer, Berlin Heidelberg New York
Johnson KD, Ladambi A, Seibert GB (1985) Incidence of adult respiratory distress syndrome in patients with multiple musculoskeletal injuries: Effect of early operative stabilization of fractures. J Trauma 25:375
Junier N (1980) Support mécanique permettant la charge fonctionelle du maxillaire inférieure. Med Dissertation, Universität Basel
Karnofsky DA (1948) The use of nitrogen mustards in the palliative treatment of carcinoma. Cancer 634
Knothe H, Dette GA (1984) Antibiotika in der Klinik. Äsopus, S 6
Köle H (1968) Ästhetische Operationen im Mund- und Kieferbereich. In: Gohrbrandt E et al. (Hrsg) Handbuch der plastischen Chirurgie. Bd 2, Lfg 11. De Gruyter, Berlin
Krompecher S (1937) Die Knochenbildung. Fischer, Jena
Kroon F (in preparation) Effects of three dimensional loading on stability of internal fixation of mandibular fractures
Küppers K (1971) Analyse der funktionellen Struktur des menschlichen Unterkiefers. Springer, Berlin Heidelberg New York (Ergebnisse der Anatomie und Entwicklungsgeschichte, Bd 44, Heft 6)
Lambotte A (1913) Chirurgie opératoire des fractures. Masson, Paris
Leonard MS, Ziman P, Bevis R et al. (1985) The sagittal split osteotomy of the mandible. Oral Surg 60:459
Lewin WWC (1913) Die innere Struktur der Mandibula der Anthropinen und Anthropoiden in mechanischer Beleuchtung. Ludwig, Bonn
Liebermann ZH, Byrd DL, Davidson TJ (1981) Immobilization of mandible in oral cancer therapy. In: McCoy FJ et al. (eds) Year book of plastic and reconstructive surgery. Chicago, p95
Litwan M (1984) Die operative Versorgung von Kieferwinkelfrakturen. Eine Nachuntersuchung. Med Dissertation, Universität Basel
Litwan M, Spiessl B (im Druck) Die extraorale Versorgung der Kieferwinkelfrakturen
Lorenz O (1953) Nagelung bei Kieferfrakturen nach Roger Anderson. Med Klin 48: 1350
Mathis H (1956) Dic Behandlung der Frakturen der zahnlosen Kiefer. Fortschr Kiefer Gesichtschir 2:92
Matter P (1980) Der posttraumatische und postoperative Knocheninfekt. Osteosynthese und Endoprothese. Jahrbuch Schweiz Naturforsch Ges 2:60
Matter P (1986) AO/ASIF Dialogue 1:1
Matter P, Brennwald J, Perren SM (1974) Biologische Reaktion des Knochens auf Osteosyntheseplatten. Helv Chir Acta [Suppl 12] 1:36
Matti H (1929) Über modellierende Osteotomie und Spongiosatransplantation. Schweiz med Wochenschr 49:1254
Matti H (1932) Über freie Transplantationen von Knochenspongiosa. Langenbecks Arch Chir 168:235
McGregor IA (1980) Fundamental techniques of plastic surgery. Livingstone, Edinburgh London New York
Merrit K, Brown SA (1980) Tissue reaction and metal sensitivity. An animal study. Acta Orthop Scand 51:403
Morscher E, Gerber B, Fasel J (1984) Surgical treatment of spondylolisthesis by bone

grafting and direct stabilization of spondylosis by means of a hook screw. Arch Orthop Trauma Surg 103:175
Müller KH, Rahn BA (1983) Knochenheilung nach stabiler externer Osteosynthese. Unfallheilkunde 86:341
Müller ME, Ganz R (1973) Hämatogene Osteomyelitis. Pädiatr Fortbild Prax 36:173
Müller ME, Perren SM (1972) Callus und primäre Knochenheilung. Med Unfallheilk 75:442
Müller ME, Allgöwer M, Schneider R, Willenegger H (1969/1977) Manual der Osteosynthese. 1. u. 2. Aufl. Springer, Berlin Heidelberg New York
Müller ME, Allgöwer M, Schneider R, Willenegger H (1970/1979) Manual of internal fixation. 1st and 2nd edn. Springer Berlin Heidelberg New York
Müller R (1968) Die schicksalsmäßige Entwicklung der nicht chirurgisch behandelten Coxarthrose. Med Dissertation, Universität Zürich
Niederdellmann H (1980) Rigid internal Fixation by means of lag screws. In: Krüger E, Schilli W (eds) Oral and maxillofacial Traumatology. Bd 1. Urban & Schwarzenberg, München
Niederdellmann H, Schilli W (1980) Zugschraubenosteosynthese zur Behandlung der Kieferwinkelfraktur. Akt Traumatol 10:105
Öst O (1968) Palliativoperationen bei Knochenmetastasen. Melsunger Med Mitteilungen [Suppl 2] 42:1
Ohnsorge J (1970) Die Fixation von Metallendoprothesen am Knochen mittels Knochenzement ohne thermische Schädigung des Kontaktgewebes. Langenbecks Arch Chir 327:855
Pauwels F (1935) Der Schenkelhalsbruch, ein mechanisches Problem. Enke, Stuttgart
Pauwels F (1948) Bedeutung und kausale Erklärung der Spongiosaarchitektur in neuer Auffassung. Ärztl Wochenschr 3:379
Pauwels F (1965) Gesammelte Abhandlungen zur funktionellen Anatomie des Bewegungsapparates. Springer, Berlin Heidelberg New York
Perren SM (1971) Biomécanique de la compression interfragmentaire. In: Boitzy A (ed) Osteogenese et compression. Huber, Bern
Perren SG, Cordey J (1977) Die Gewebsdifferenzierung in der Frakturheilung. Unfallheilkunde 80:161
Perren SM, Huggler SM, Russenberger A et al. (1969a) The reaction of cortical bone to compression. Acta Orthop Scand [Suppl] 125:3
Perren SM, Russenberger M, Steinemann S, Müller ME, Allgöwer M (1969b) A dynamic compression plate. Acta Orthop Scand [Suppl] 125:29
Perren SM, Ganz R, Rüter A (1972) Mechanical induction of bone resorption. 4th International osteological Symposion, Prague, September 1972
Perren SM, Hayes WC, Eliasson E (1974) Biomechanik der Plattenosteosynthese. Med Orthop Tech 94:56
Perren SM, Rahn B, Cordey J (1975) Mechanik und Biologie der Frakturheilung. Fortschr Kiefer Gesichtschir 19:33
Perren SM, Ganz R, Rüter A (1975) Oberflächliche Knochenresorption um Implantate. Med Orthop Tech 95:6
Petzel JR (1980) Die chirurgische Behandlung des frakturierten Collum mandibulae durch funktionsstabile Osteosynthese. Fortschr Kiefer Gesichtschir 25:84
Pfister U, Rahn BA, Perren SM, Weiler S (1979) Vaskularität und Knochenumbau nach Marknagelung langer Röhrenknochen. Akt Traumatol 9:191
Philps R (1987) Die geschlossene und offene Unterkieferfraktur. (Eine retrospektive Studie zum Krankengut von 1976–1982). Med Dissertation, Universität Basel
Pichler H (1919) Doppelte Unterkieferresektion in einem Fall von Progenie. Vjschr Zahnheilkd 35:1
Pohler OEM (1983) Degradation of metallic orthopedic implants. In: Rubin LR (ed) Biomaterials in reconstructive surgery. Mosby, St. Louis
Pohler OEM, Straumann F (1975) Charakteristik der AO-Implantate aus rostfreiem Stahl. AO-Bulletin
Prein J, Remagen W, Spiessl B, Ühlinger E (1985) Atlas der Tumoren des Gesichtsschädels. Zentrales Referenzregister des DOESAK. Springer, Berlin Heidelberg New York Tokyo
Prein J, Remagen W, Spiessl B, Ühlinger E (1986) Atlas of the tumours of the facial skeleton. Central Registry of DOESAK. Springer, Berlin Heidelberg New York Tokyo

Puranen J (1966) Reorganization of fresh and preserved bone transplants. Acta Orthop Scand, Supp. 82
Rahmanzadeh R (1972) Zur Operationstechnik der Femurkopfprothese. Mschr Unfallheilk 75, H. 5:213
Rahn BA, Cordey J, Prein J, Russenberger M (1975) Zur Biomechanik der Osteosynthese der Mandibula. In: Fortschr Kiefer Gesichtschir 19:37
Rahn BA (1982) Bone healing: Histologic and physiologic concepts. In: Sumner-Smith G (ed) Bone in clinical orthopaedics. Saunders, Philadelphia
Rahn BA (1985) Osteosynthese und Knochenreaktion. In: Staubesand J (Hrsg) Benninhoff Anatomie. Urban & Schwarzenberg, München
Raveh J, Redli M, Markwalder TM (1984) Operative management of 194 cases of combined maxillofacial-frontobasal fractures. J oral maxillofac Surg 42:555
Raveh J, Roux M, Sutter F (1983) Resultate nach sagittaler Spaltung am Unterkiefer und gleichzeitiger Oberkieferosteotomie unter Anwendung eigener Methoden. Schweiz Mschr Zahnheilk 93:734
Raveh J, Stich H, Sutter F (1985) Titanplasma-beschichtetes Hohlschrauben- und Rekonstruktionsplatten-System (THRP) zur Überbrückung von Kieferdefekten. Chirurg 56:337
Raveh J, Sutter F (1984) Defektüberbrückung unter lingualem Zugang und Knochentransplantatfixation am Unterkiefer mit dem THRP-System. Schweiz Mschr Zahnheilk 94:134
Regazzoni P (1982) Osteosynthesen an Röhrenknochen: Technische und biologische Untersuchungen zur Stabilität und Heilung. Med. Habilitationsschrift, Universität Basel
Riegger J (1980) Die Zugschraube zur Behandlung der Kieferwinkelfraktur. Med Dissertation, Universität Freiburg i. B.
Ritter G, Grünert A (1973) Experimentelle Untersuchungen zu den mechanischen Eigenschaften des Knochens im Hinblick auf die Druckosteosynthesen. Arch orthop Unfall-Chirurgie 75:302
Rittmann WW, Perren SM (1974) Cortical bone healing after internal fixation and infection. Springer, Berlin Heidelberg New York
Rowe NL, Killey HC (1955) Fractures of the Facial Skeleton. Livingstone, Edinburgh London
Schenk RK (1986) Histophysiology of bone remodelling and bone repair. Perspectives on biomaterials. OCC Lin and EYS Chao (Eds). Elsevier, Amsterdam
Schenk RK, Müller J, Willenegger H (1968) Experimentell-histologischer Beitrag zur Entstehung und Behandlung von Pseudarthrosen. Hefte Unfallheilk 94
Schenk RK, Willenegger H (1963) Zum histologischen Bild der sogenannten Primärheilung der Knochenkompakta nach experimentellen Osteotomien am Hund. Experientia 19:593
Schenk RK, Willenegger H (1964) Zur Histologie der primären Knochenheilung. Langenbecks Arch Chir 308:440
Schewior TH, Schewior H (1984) Mechanische und methodische Aspekte des Fixateur externe aus Ringen und Kirschnerdrähten (nach Wittmoser und Ilisarov). Alternativprinzip zur Plattenosteosynthese. Akt Traumatol 6:237
Schmoker R (1975a) Zur Operationsplanung bei Progenie- und Retrogeniefällen. Schweiz Mschr Zahnheilk 85/6:598
Schmoker R (1975b) Experimentelle Untersuchung zur Stabilität und intraoperativen Kompression bei der Osteosynthese von Unterkieferfrakturen. AO-Bulletin
Schmoker R (1976) The eccentric dynamic compression plate. An experimental study as to its contribution to the functionally stable internal fixation of fractures of the lower jaw. AO-Bulletin
Schmoker R (1983a) Der Craniofixateur externe zur funktionsstabilen Fixation des Mittelgesichts – Erfahrungsbericht nach Anwendung in über 50 Fällen. Dtsch Z Mund Kiefer Gesichtschir 7:241
Schmoker R (1983b) Mandibular reconstruction using a special plate. J maxillofac Surg 11/3:99
Schmoker R (1986) Die funktionelle Unterkieferrekonstruktion. Springer, Berlin Heidelberg New York Tokyo
Schmoker R, Spiessl B (1973) Exzentrisch-dynamische Kompressionsplatte. Schweiz Mschr Zahnheilkd 83:1496
Schmoker R, Spiessl B (1976) Infektion nach Osteosynthese von Unterkieferfrakturen. Kasuistik, Ursache, Verhütung, Behandlung. Akt Traumatol 6:297

Schmoker R, Spiessl B (1978) Fehlermöglichkeiten bei der Osteosynthese von Unterkieferfrakturen. Dtsch Z Mund-Kiefer-Gesichtschir 2:129
Schmoker R, Spiessl B, Gensheimer T (1976) Funktionsstabile Osteosynthese und Simulographie bei der sagittalen Osteotomie des aufsteigenden Astes. Eine vergleichende klinische Untersuchung. Schweiz Mschr Zahnheilkd 86:582
Schmoker R, Eulenberger J, Spiessl B, Mathys R (1977) Entwicklung und tierexperimentelle Untersuchung einer Kieferköpfchenprothese. Dtsch Z Mund Kiefer Gesichtschir 1:86
Schmoker R, Spiessl B, Trzeciak W (1979) Verriegelungsplastik am Kiefergelenk zur Behandlung der Hypermobilität. Schweiz Mschr Zahnheilkd 89:213
Schmoker R, Allmen G von, Tschopp HM (1982) Application of functionally stable fixation in maxillofacial surgery according to the ASIF principles. J Oral Maxillofac Surg 40:457
Schuchardt K (1958) Erfahrungen bei der Behandlung der Mikrogenie. Langenbecks Arch Chir 289:651
Schuchardt K (1960) Experiences with the surgical treatment of some deformities of the jaws: Prognathia, micrognathia and open bite. In: Wallace AB (ed) Transactions of the international society of plastic surgeons. Livingstone, Edinburgh
Schüle H (1957) Schienung von Unterkieferfrakturen mittels extraoraler Verschraubung. Dtsch Zahnärztl Z 12:933
Schweiberer L (1970) Experimentelle Untersuchungen von Knochentransplantaten mit unveränderter und mit denaturierter Knochengrundsubstanz. Hefte Unfallheilk (Beiheft) 103
Schweiberer L, Klapp F, Chevalier H (1975) Platten- und Schraubenosteosynthese bei Frakturen und Pseudarthrosen des Ober- und Unterschenkels. Chirurg 46:155
Séquin F, Texhammar R (1980) Das AO-Instrumentarium. Anwendung und Wartung. Springer, Berlin Heidelberg New York
Seto K, Matsuura M (1984) A new concept of mandibular osteotomy. Odontologia (Japan) 19/3:315
Seto K, Oguchi H (1985) Progress in the jaw bone reduction and fixation method. Dental J 22:163
Slotman GJ, Cummings FJ, Glicksman AR et al. (1986) Preoperative simultaneously administered cis-platinum plus radiation therapy for advanced squamous cell carcinoma of the head and neck. Head Neck Surg 8:159 Jan/Feb, 159
Somlo T (1982) Über die Operationsplanung bei Progenie- und Retrogeniefällen (Simulographie). Dtsch Z Mund Kiefer Gesichtschir 6:259
Spiessl B (1972a) Probleme der Wiederherstellung nach Tumoroperationen im Kiefer-Gesichts-Bereich. Therapiewoche 22, 23:1917
Spiessl B (1972b) Rigid internal fixation of fractures of the lower jaw. In: Chapchal G (ed) Reconstruction surgery and traumatology. Karger, Basel München Paris London New York Sydney
Spiessl B (1975) Funktionsstabile Osteosynthese bei Unterkieferfrakturen – Problematik und Technik. Forschr Kiefer Gesichtschir 19:68
Spiessl B (1976a) Erste Erfahrungen mit einer Kiefergelenkprothese. Fortschr Kiefer Gesichtschir 21:119
Spiessl B (ed) (1976b) New concepts in maxillofacial bone surgery. Springer, Berlin Heidelberg New York
Spiessl B (1978) Die Unterkiefer-Resektionsplatten der AO. Ihre Anwendung bei Unterkieferdefekten in der Tumorchirurgie. Unfallheilk 81:302
Spiessl B (1980a) Das Problem der Nonunion bei Frakturen des atrophierten Unterkiefers. Schweiz Mschr Zahnheilk 90:627
Spiessl B (1980b) A new method of anatomical reconstruction of extensive defects of the mandible with autogenous cancellous bone. J maxillofac Surg 8:78
Spiessl B (1980c) Die Osteosynthese zur frühfunktionellen Behandlung komplizierter Unterkieferfrakturen. Jahrbuch Schweiz Naturforsch Ges 2:70
Spiessl B (1981) Verfeinerte Technik der Progenie-Operation. Fortschr Kiefer Gesichtschir 26:96
Spiessl B (1982) The sagittal splitting osteotomy for correction of mandibular prognathism. Clin Plast Surg 9:491
Spiessl B (1983) Maxillofacial injuries in polytrauma. World J Surg 7:96
Spiessl B, Hochstetter A von (1982) Unspezifische pyogene Infektionen im Kiefer-Gesichts-Bereich. In: Allgöwer M (Hrsg) Allgemeine und spezielle Chirurgie, 4. Aufl. Springer, Berlin Heidelberg New York

Spiessl B, Schroll K (1972) Gesichtsschädel. In: Nigst H (Hrsg) Spezielle Frakturen- und Luxationslehre, Bd 1/1. Thieme, Stuttgart

Spiessl B, Tschopp H (1974) Chirurgie der Kiefer. In: Naumann HH (Hrsg) Kopf- und Hals-Chirurgie. Bd 2: Gesicht und Gesichtsschädel. Thieme, Stuttgart

Steinemann S (1968) Résistance à la corrosion par piqûres de l'acier inoxydable au chrome-nickel-molybdène- élaboré normalement à haute fréquence et refondue sous laitier electroconducteur (ESR). Rev Métallurg 65:651

Texhammar R, Schmoker R (1984) Funktionsstabile maxillofaziale Osteosynthesen. Springer, Berlin Heidelberg New York Tokyo

Trauner R, Obwegeser H (1957) The surgical correction of mandibular prognathism and retrognathia with consideration of genioplasty. Oral Surg 10:677, 787, 899

Trentz O, Tscherne H (1978) Kriterien für die Operabilität von Polytraumatisierten. Unfallheilkunde 81:451

Tscherne H (1969) Operative Frakturbehandlung. Langenbecks Arch Chir 324:348

UICC (1979) TNM Klassifikation der malignen Tumoren. 3. Aufl. Springer, Berlin Heidelberg New York

UICC (1985) TNM-Atlas. Illustrierter Leitfaden zur TNM/pTNM-Klassifikation maligner Tumoren. Springer, Berlin Heidelberg New York Tokyo

Ullik R (1953) Die Indikation für die Nagelung von Kieferbrüchen nach Roger Anderson. Zentralbl Chir 78:1012

Urist MR, Urist JM, Dubuc FL (1970) Quantitation of new bone formation in intramuscular implants of bone matrix in rabbits. Clin Orthop 68:279

Urist MR, Mikulski A, Boyd SD (1975) A chemosterilized antigen-extracted autodigested allo-implant for bone banks. Arch Surg 110:416

Vogel R (1984) Interfragmentäre Druckwerte bei der Anwendung verschiedener dynamischer Kompressionsplatten (Eine experimentelle Studie am Unterkiefer). Med Dissertation, Universität Basel

Walkhoff O (1900/1901) Der menschliche Unterkiefer im Lichte der Entwicklungsmechanik. Dtsch Mschr Zahnheilk 19:529, 222

Wassmund M (1935) Lehrbuch der plastischen Chirurgie des Mundes und der Kiefer. Heusser, Leipzig

Weber BG (1979) Frakturbehandlung bei Kindern. Springer, Berlin Heidelberg New York

Weber BG, Cech O (1973/1976) Pseudarthrosen. Pathophysiologie, Biomechanik, Therapie, Ergebnisse. Huber, Bern Stuttgart Wien

Willenegger H (1973) Präliminäre Überbrückungsosteosynthese bei der Resektion von Knochentumoren. Helv Chir Acta 40:185

Willenegger H (1975) Verplattung und Marknagelung bei Femur- und Tibiaschaftfrakturen: Pathophysiologische Grundlagen. Chirurg 46:145

Winter S (1987) Entwicklung eines neuen Fixateur externe für den Unterkiefer. Med Dissertation, Universität Hamburg

Wolff G, Dittmann M, Ruedi T, Buchmann B, Allgoewer M (1978) Koordination von Chirurgie und Intensivmedizin zur Vermeidung posttraumatischer respiratorischer Insuffizienz. Unfallheilkunde 81:524

Wolter D, Hutzschenreuter P, Burri C (1974) Einbaustudien autologer Spongiosa am Kompaktknochen in Abhängigkeit von der übertragenen Menge und des anliegenden Gewebes. Langenbecks Arch Chir [Suppl Chir Forum] 225

Wolter D, Hutzschenreuter P, Burri C, Steinhardt B (1975) Einbau autologer Spongiosa am Kompaktaknochen in Abhängigkeit von der Vitalität der transplantierten Zellen. Langenbecks Arch Chir [Suppl Chir Forum] 383

Yates C, Olson D, Guralnick W (1976) The antilingula as an anatomic landmark in oral surgery. Oral Surg 41/6:705

Zuber P (1982) Interfragmentäre Druckwerte bei Anwendung von Zuggurtungsschiene und dynamischer Kompressionsplatte. Med Dissertation, Universität Basel

Further literature in Müller ME, Allgöwer M, Schneider R, Willenegger H (1970/1979) *Manual of Internal Fixation*, 1st and 2nd edn, Berlin Heidelberg New York Tokyo

Subject Index